P9-CLB-930

Community
Mental Health
Social Action and Reaction

Please remember that this is a library book,
and that it belongs only temporarily to each
person who uses it. Be considerate. Do
not write in this, or any, library book.

WITHDRAWN

Community Mental Health
Social Action and Reaction

Edited by
Bruce Denner
Community Mental Health Program
at the Illinois Mental Health Institutes

Richard H. Price
Indiana University

WITHDRAWN

HOLT, RINEHART AND WINSTON, INC.
New York   Chicago   San Francisco   Atlanta
Dallas   Montreal   Toronto   London   Sydney

Copyright © 1973 by Holt, Rinehart and Winston, Inc.
All rights reserved
Library of Congress Catalog Card Number: 72–88162
ISBN: 0–03–085651–5
Printed in the United States of America
4 5 6   090   9 8 7 6 5 4 3 2

362.22
D399c

WITHDRAWN

PREFACE

The boundaries of the community mental health movement are as amorphous and ill-defined as the boundaries of the communities we live in. We all have an intuitive sense of what the words "community" and "mental health" mean, but we have not yet generated a language which can describe all the forms of mental illness both from the point of view of the individual and from that of his community. At the present time we struggle along with an uncertain mixture of sociological, psychological, and medical concepts many of which are derived from quite disparate ideological and theoretical points of view. And this situation is likely to remain unchanged for years to come. Perhaps the best we can do now is to articulate the critical ideological, theoretical, and practical problems associated with community mental health thought and practice.

The text is organized around three central issues: a) the impact of the community movement on the definition of mental illness, b) the changing concept of the practitioner role, and c) the political consequences of community involvement.

The papers in Part 1 argue that we must give up individualistic concepts of mental illness and view community disorders in terms of social problems and social conflicts. The papers in Part 2 explore the consequences for the role of the mental health worker. Two trends are described, namely, the emergence of the paraprofessional and the community advocate. The heart of this text, Part 3, contains a number of case histories which describe the cycle of social action and community reaction which is set off when this new breed of mental health practi-

v

29094

tioner attempts to apply community concepts by organizing neighborhoods through the development of community mental health centers.
Although this process seems to flow fairly smoothly in homogenous, stable
small towns and rural areas, in urban sections of the larger cities the reactions of the local people have been anything but passive and accepting. Although the mental health establishment likes to see itself as organizing the community, once the action begins it is often difficult to distinguish between actor and reactor. What seems to emerge is a series of
social-political events in which mental health people and neighborhood
people are swept along by the forces of social change.

It is our hope that the reader will come away with an attitude of
patience and pluralism towards both the profession and the communities
this profession hopes to transform. For it must be kept in mind that the
practice of community mental health cannot be understood as the mere
technical application of a set of abstract principles. The community mental health movement has not only unleashed political forces, but is itself a political force in communities across the country. For better or
for worse psychological intervention has become a political act.

We would like to acknowledge the help of a number of people in
the preparation of this book. Dennis and Pat Bouffard helped greatly in
assembling the manuscript and in the necessary clerical work; Mary
Price and Loretta Denner provided invaluable editorial assistance; and
finally, Janet Peckinpaugh, Darlene Stucky, and Donna Littrell patiently
typed the several drafts of the manuscript.

B. D.

R. H. P.

CONTENTS

Community
Mental Health
Social Action and Reaction

INTRODUCTION

In recent years we have seen drastic social change shake the complacency of the human service professions. Radical spokesmen have disrupted professional meetings, university students have demanded that the professions become more relevant to societal needs, and many of those within and outside the professions have begun to question seriously whether the human service disciplines are (or should be) apolitical and value-free.

In effect the critics have been saying that the human service professions—psychiatry, psychology, social work, the ministry—have been more concerned with their own development than with the needs of the people. The professions have put most of their time and effort into working with low-risk clients—the stable, slightly neurotic middle class. The "others" have been considered either incurable or not educated enough to benefit from therapeutic services. In some instances this line of argument is very convincing. Certainly one might expect the poorly educated, nonverbal, or nonintrospective person to reject the traditional psychoanalytic regime that involves free association, plenty of time, and ambiguous goals. Yet society invests too much of its resources in training and maintaining the human professions to have only the chosen few profit from these services.

Traditionally the human professions have responded to the countless "others" by placing them in large institutions, out of the public eye, where everyone could assume that something positive was happening. Occasionally, when an exposé appears, people are shocked to hear that not only is there little therapy but it is also common for the inmates' condition to deteriorate over time. The traditional professional response, however, has been to place the blame on society. The professional argues very persuasively that there are insufficient funds to support the numbers of therapists, social workers, and nurses that would be required to cure these very sick people. Of course, the same explanation can account for the legions of untreated poor and socially isolated people living outside the asylum's walls. They cannot afford to purchase professional service either.

Although the public at large may have remained ignorant of con-

1

ditions within the mental hospitals, since the turn of the century one pressure group in particular, the mental hygiene movement, has been calling for reform. But these concerned individuals did not really have significant effect until the federal government became involved in the nation's mental health with the enactment of the Community Mental Health Centers Act of 1963. This act allocated large sums of money for the creation of community-based facilities that would offer a variety of mental health services to the community as well as provide consultation to all agencies that touch on mental health problems. With the creation of this new community institution there emerged new therapeutic techniques and methods. But more important than the development of new techniques was the working notion that therapists cannot sit back and passively wait for the sick to request treatment. The new therapists have embraced a public health model. In short, mental illness is viewed as a health hazard, a danger to the community, and something that the community must eradicate for the sake of its own well-being.

Definitions of Community Mental Health

The notion that mental illness can be wiped out through concerted community effort is not new. It seems as if society goes through certain periods when it believes that environment is the major determinant of human problems. During such times professionals and nonprofessionals work together to improve what they feel are the detrimental aspects of a community.

Levine and Levine's (1970) study of the settlement-house movement at the turn of the century suggests that the community mental health centers of today are the settlement houses of yesterday. Unlike the settlement houses, however, which were mostly financed by church groups, private gifts, and charity drives, the mental health center is the creation of government at the federal, state, and local levels. The political structure of a center varies, but it is commonly understood that a community-based center has the following aims: (1) determining the prevalence of the various types of mental illness, (2) launching preventive programs that lower the incidence of these diseases, and (3) mobilizing the entire community's resources to combat mental disease. To accomplish these ends the therapeutic team cannot wait for the individual to declare himself ill and in need of treatment. He must go out into the community and work with illness in its natural setting. The assumption is that the worker must bring his service to the people. The therapist working only with patients who come to his office voluntarily is equating mental illness with "patienthood"; that is, anyone who wishes to go into psychotherapy has a mental problem. But the community mental health professional must find his answer in terms of norms or standards of behavior so that certain types of deviation can be labeled "mental illness."

As any student of abnormal psychology knows, there is little agreement among mental health professionals as to the exact meaning of the term "mental illness." In fact, some theorists (Szasz, 1961) have argued that the notion is a myth used to oppress those whom society finds undesirable (more about this later). Nevertheless, modern psychiatry and psychology presume that mental illness does exist and have described numerous disease entities. Those who believe in the utility of the term mental illness try to distinguish "mental illness" from other socially prohibited behaviors. The clearest distinction is made between mental illness and abnormal behavior, and "criminal" behavior. Murder, theft, and rape are prohibited by law. Those who engage in these behaviors are deviant but not *necessarily* sick. Of course, it is maintained by some that criminals are sick—at least certain kinds of lawbreakers are—and the courts do recognize an "insanity" defense.

Besides criminality, there are other forms of behavior that society does not approve, but neither are they considered to be signs of mental illness. Included here are the many types of personal deviance and eccentricity that neither offend, disturb, nor perhaps even interest most people. Other forms of deviance are breaches of approved etiquette. You can eat with your hands, blow your nose in the street, and fail to tip a waitress without being called "sick." Polite society may see you as immature, disgusting, or a fool, but few would recommend psychiatric treatment.

The question of why people go to a psychiatrist cannot be answered simply. Apparently many factors are at work besides the presence of symptoms, especially social class and friendship patterns (Kadushin, 1969). However, it is safe to say that most people think of mental illness as a way of explaining others' behavior when it seems bizarre, irrational, and impulsive (Mechanic, 1962). "Mental illness" is invoked as an explanation when no other explanation fits. The case of the "insane" criminal is particularly illustrative. If a man robs a bank and in the process kills a guard, he's likely to be convicted of robbery and murder. He is likely to spend the rest of his life behind prison walls. His criminal behavior is perfectly intelligible: Money is stolen because it is an asset. However, if this same man were to enter a bank, kill everyone within, but make no attempt to steal the money or rob the customers, he would most likely be judged insane and sent to a mental hospital. We would think him to be mentally ill not because he murdered, but because he murdered with no apparent purpose. If a clever district attorney could convince us that this seemingly senseless slaughter was part of an overall (logical) plan to disrupt the banking business, then we might consider this man to be a cold-blooded genius. Similarly, individuals who assassinate famous statesmen are often considered to be mentally ill until it can be shown that they are in the pay of a foreign enemy.

Usually an observer will begin to consider a person to be "mentally ill" when he cannot see any plausible motives for the person's behavior. Once the observer entertains the notion that a person is mentally ill, he is apt to look for two kinds of supporting evidence: evidence that the individual in question is suffering from intense interpersonal stress or some organic pathology. The press often reports a doctor's belief that a mass murderer suffers from brain damage (as in the Whitcomb case) or from chronic stress (as in the My Lai incident). Presumably most people find comfort in thinking that mass murder is an act not *willed* by a rational mind but an impulsive response brought on by stress and physical abnormality, although the basis of this distinction is questionable.

Clearly, the community mental health practitioner faces no easy task in defining community mental health. Should he stay with the traditional psychiatric classification scheme, current community tolerance for deviance and eccentricity, or just use individual, subjective evaluations of personal distress? Whether he chooses one or other method, or some combination of both, he must come up with a set of criteria that allow him to select clients from the total population of potential clients. There are various ways in which workers in this field have responded to the question of who is the client.

Working with clients in the community. Many types of therapeutic activity are considered to be a form of community mental health intervention because they are community based. Included are the traditional casework activities such as finding employment, housing, and companionship for patients living at home or preparing to leave a mental hospital. In these cases the mental health worker may still maintain an intrapsychic interpretation of the patient's problems. That is, the worker may talk about his client's problems as if they existed within the client himself. But the treatment focuses on the interpersonal consequences of the psychopathology, seeking to improve the patient's social reality. Also included here are group-centered therapeutic endeavors in which the mental health worker does not relate to any individual but to a community group. Gang workers and street workers are the clearest example of this sort of effort. Interestingly, many gang workers may persist in thinking about the problems of the gang in intrapsychic terms even though no individuals, as such, are ever under treatment. Thus, numerous mental health workers feel a part of the community movement because they work with patients in the community rather than in the clinic or psychiatrist's office.

Community agencies as clients. Another traditional activity of the therapist is consultation. The guiding assumption is that someone with much experience can train a number of inexperienced people together. Thus, the experienced therapist multiplies his influence by the number of people with whom he consults. Consulting can take place with other therapists in private practice or with workers in various types of institutions such as schools, police departments, the courts, employment agencies, business organizations, and rehabilitation services. Typically, the consultant tries not to "take over" a case, but rather to foster independent decision making by the consultee. Some consultants have offered the notion that the individual consultees are not the true client. Instead, they claim the whole agency is the client. The implications of this assertion are not always clear. What is probably meant is that the consultant must not act in the interest of any one worker but in the interest of the total organization. For example, a consultant may be called in to assist a school teacher in her evaluation of her students. The consultant, however, cannot merely think in terms of the students, but must consider the entire classroom relationship (teacher–students, student–student, and so on) and perhaps even the relationship of this classroom to other classrooms and to the entire schooling process.

The total community as client. Once the leap is made to consulting with whole agencies, there is little reason to stop there. Why not consult with entire communities? This sort of therapeutic intervention can take two forms. One might look at a community as a system of services. These services may be performed by public or private organizations, but, one way or another, these services must satisfy the needs of the people for housing, transportation, medical aid, sanitation, education, law enforcement, recreation, and so forth. [A good example is Key's (1966) involvement in urban renewal.] Clearly there is a psychological aspect to each of these needs. It does not take much imagination to think of ways in which the delivery of community services can cause or prevent mental disturbances. Housing must be planned so as to avoid overcrowding. Traffic should move through the city with a minimum of noise and congestion. Hospitals must treat patients as people, not objects. Police should not harass residents in the name of "law and order." Recreational sites should encourage free play. If one adopts the point of view that the psychological health of the community is the responsibility of the planners and governing officials, it follows that consultants should be called in on the policy-making level.

A more restricted form of community intervention, and one that avoids a too-deep entanglement with government officials, is the troubleshooter who uses a crisis-oriented model (Caplan, 1964). In this case, the mental health worker does not attempt to delineate how the community services are to operate but instead attempts to solve the social problems created by improperly functioning care-delivery systems. Thus, the consultant may become involved with poverty programs and deal with the issues of work attitudes among the poor and the psychological impact of living on welfare. Or the consultant might speculate about the causes of crime. In the last decade "juvenile delinquency" represented the greatest concern, but now drug abuse is stealing the spotlight. In each case the task of the troubleshooter is to formulate the problem in terms that city, state, and federal officials can understand, and then to propose ways of alleviating the difficulty. Sometimes all that is called for are renewed efforts by already established agencies, though new programs are frequently called for that demand reorganization of traditional services.

Thus, what community mental health means in any particular setting is largely determined by how the particular mental health workers cope with the basic problem of determining who is the client. As long as the professional views the individual person as the client, traditional therapeutic efforts can be employed and supplemented with some efforts in the community, such as helping the patient obtain employment. But once the professional views entire agencies or towns as "the client," it is questionable whether he can continue to do therapy in any conventional sense. Has not this type of community worker abandoned therapy for politics?

The social and political implications of the community movement are perhaps best seen from three vantage points: Who goes into treatment, who performs the treatment, and what constitutes the therapeutic treatment?

The making of the client. If mental illness is conceptualized as a form of deviant behavior and thought, with negative social and personal consequences, mental illness is very widespread indeed. Furthermore, if one endorses a preventive approach, that is, if one conceives of mental illness as a progressive disease that is best treated in its early stages, then all people from all walks of life are potential clients. Since everyone shows some behavioral and thought disturbance at one time or another, and most of us begin to decompensate under severe stress, the mental health clinic must be prepared to serve the total population. It should be obvious that the public would never subsidize such an operation. There is already a manpower shortage in the mental health field. There would obviously be difficulties in finding enough therapists if everyone were a patient. Hence, the issue of who should be served becomes critical.

A humanitarian response to this problem would be to insist that the most needy deserve first attention. There would certainly be disagreement over who should be considered the "sickest." As we have implied, the criteria are vague. But in the end a good case could be made for the severely regressed, hospitalized, psychotic individual who is wasting away in the back wards of our overcrowded institutions. But one could just imagine society's response if all efforts were focused on these individuals. Many would argue that "it is like throwing good money after bad," since it is widely believed that these unfortunates are incurable. In any case, even great changes would not be very visible. Would the public be impressed if, after an enormous investment of time and money, a psychotic patient began to dress himself but remained incapacitated in every other respect?

The problem of who should receive treatment can be dealt with pragmatically: Treat those who would benefit most from being under treatment. There is, of course, the empirical question relating to the kind of therapy that would work best with a particular client. Researchers are not even close to answering this question. Nevertheless, certain attitudes prevail.

It is generally accepted that children, especially preadolescent school children, are most amenable to change. Most school systems employ psychological consultants. If the community really took seriously the notion of treating the entire school population to improve the mental health of all children, their behavior could be monitored and evaluated in accordance with developmental scales of psychopathology. Treatment plans could be devised and instituted in the classroom. Parents could be included in the treatment or merely informed about it. The children need not even know what is happening to them. The therapeutic program could be blended into the educational curriculum with minimum difficulty and little publicity. Such a plan is not a mere pipe dream. There are reports in the literature of "redtagging" (Cowen et al., 1967) problem children in order to measure their psychological adjustment through the school years. Diagnosis is but one step away from therapy, although diagnostic information alone is an insufficient basis for launching a program of therapy.

A pervasive program of this kind [Rae-Grant & Stringer's (1969), for example] does, at least on the surface, seem very appealing. If all children are in therapy, then none are singled out as "sick," and the stigma associated with being mentally ill might then be removed. There is less resistance to therapy done under the guise of education because people are less resistant to a teacher's instruction than they are to a therapist's interpretations.

Fine, but do we really want the school system to place all school-age children in therapy? It may be in society's interest to bring all children up to certain levels of healthy functioning, but is it necessarily in the child's or his parents' interest? What are the consequences of delegating this task to a bureaucracy (though it might have the best intentions)? Would not the school system abuse its power by labeling "mentally ill" all those who disrupt the orderly process or undermine the governing power? Being truant or publishing an underground newspaper could possibly be considered psychopathological. What recourse would the parents have if they disagreed with the school's interpretation of their child's behavior, assuming that the school would even confide in them? And what of the children—do they have the right to resist the externally imposed change? If so, the child must have a way, which is recognized to be legitimate, of challenging the authorities without being dismissed as merely "defensive" or "belligerent."

Another possible pragmatic answer to the question of who should be under treatment begins with the recognition that there are many people in the United States today who by conventional standards are doomed to live unrewarding, debasing, backward, self-destructive lives. The causes are many, but there is a psychological component as well. One may conveniently assume that mental illness contributes to racism, the "culture of poverty," alcoholism, drug addiction, and all forms of rebellious antisocial behavior. And if one considers these deviants to be presocial, like children, then one cannot seriously expect them to participate in their own cure except insofar as they follow the doctor's orders. In fact, it has sometimes been argued that it may be against the public interest to create resistance by emphasizing the therapeutic aspect of any community endeavor.

One might maintain that the underprivileged have been ignored by the private practitioner and that such people have a right to treatment. Any number of therapeutic programs could be devised. Currently there is much interest in launching an attack on the problem of drug addiction. An examination of such programs reveals that their advocates see drug abuse as but one symptom of a defective life-style. The programs' real aims involve turning these young adults away from an offensive life-style (the hippie syndrome) and persuading them that the middle-class way is ultimately more rewarding. The same sort of thinking is implicit in many of the poverty programs, for example, Head Start and the Job Corps. Efforts to change certain aspects of a person's life-style all too easily tend toward efforts to change the entire person. And this tendency increases as the efforts fail or the people appear to resist the change.

To balance the picture it should be emphasized that many community mental health programs take the side of the client, for example, the Woodlawn Project in Chicago (Sabshin, 1969) and the Lincoln Hospital involvement in the South Bronx Model Cities program (Peck & Kaplan, 1969). In these programs the therapist becomes the client's advocate, and, in a sense, society becomes the patient. This process is clearly seen in community programs based in minority group neighborhoods where mental health workers fight discrimination, police harrassment, City Hall's indifference to problems, and related forms of oppression.

The question posed earlier in this section was: Who should receive the treatment? It was not our intention to formulate an answer. The regressed psychotic, the disturbed school child, and the forgotten American all deserve prompt attention. Our point is that the question goes beyond the bounds of behavioral science. Surely the social and biological sciences have unearthed facts that are pertinent. But the facts alone do not settle the issues. Who should receive help is a political and social problem and should be debated in the social–political arena. Expert opinion is one thing, but control by a professional body of experts is something else. Our inclination is to build in safeguards so that no person is ever forced into becoming a client and every man has an opportunity to become one.

It should be recognized that the community mental health movement is not merely reaching out to clients who have passed their days on waiting lists. The movement has the potential of artificially creating whole new caseloads by transforming the status of large numbers of people. If some community mental health therapists had their way, people who seem self-destructive (drug addicts, hippies), people who resist social change (tenants who respond poorly to urban renewal), people who present a threat to the state (Black Panthers, KKK) would all be analyzed, forced into therapy, and transformed according to the socially approved modes and norms of behavior.

The making of a therapist. The traditional therapist was a man of grace and wisdom. Troubled people sought his aid, so that he might ease their pain while setting them on a path of personal growth. Very few among us have the personality required for such a frustrating and thankless task. And since the community movement has drastically increased the number of clients, it is not surprising that methods have been devised to increase the number of mental health workers. What is surprising is the unusual array of people who are seen as performing therapeutic services. In the past, the mentally ill were treated in specially designated places by specifically trained professionals. Hospital aides and other ancillary helpers were not considered to be directly therapeutic. Today, not only are such respectable people as ministers, nurses, school teachers, and probation officers being trained in the art of therapy, but it has also already been proposed that bartenders, bus drivers, and barbers be trained. These new workers have been called urban agents (Kelly, 1969), and their "new career" can be seen as therapeutic for them as well (Pearl & Riessman, 1965).

Of course all of these programs are being carried out under the watchful eye of the medical and psychological professions. The people they train are called "paraprofessionals," which suggests a subordinate status. But, just as the psychologist was once content to work under the psychiatrist, but is no longer, so should one expect the paraprofessionals to voice their demands for independence. This rebellion is more likely, given the fact that nonprofessionals are often as effective as the professional (Rioch et al., 1963).

There is another issue associated with the presence of paraprofessionals in the community. The paraprofessional's services are typically free or nearly so. This creates the danger of a dual system of therapeutic services, namely, professionals for those who can afford them and paraprofessionals for the poor. Of course, it may turn out that some free paraprofessionals are more effective than costly professionals.

Encouraging people to perform therapeutic services in their spare time or as an adjunct to their daily work can create other serious difficulties. Denner has worked with a volunteer group that responded to the lack of psychiatric care for adolescents in a small town by setting up a service that provided surrogate parents and friends. Some workers were natural therapists, and the group's motivation was high. The workers received some training and supervision but retained their independence from the professionals. When a problem arose, it usually stemmed from the fact that these people were part-time mental health workers. The other aspects of their lives—their business, social, and political interests—easily contaminated the relationship with their client. Moreover, most of the policy decisions were based not on any body of facts but on a sense of what was good for the community. But unlike highly visible, elected public officials, who must be responsive to community opinion or be voted out of office at the next election, this group was able to operate out of public view and community control. They affiliated themselves with the juvenile court and used the judge as a protective shield whenever parents became unhappy with the way their child was being treated. Obviously a system of controls is needed to protect the public against these vigilantelike community groups.

There was a time when only the selected few could legitimately practice the art of psychotherapy. The professionals who once were so reluctant to share their techniques with the public are now only too anxious to train people from all walks of life. But can the public really trust this new breed of therapist? We expect professionals to be better than the average person. They should have higher personal standards, be more ethical, be more trustworthy than the neighbor next door. We can allow ourselves to believe in a man who dedicated himself to years of study, passed numerous examinations, and successfully completed the arduous process of obtaining his credentials. But what trust can be placed in a person who finished a four-month training program? As more and more people become therapists by new and shortcut routes, the public may begin to wonder whether they wish to relate to these new therapists as they did with their sage and learned predecessors.

The therapeutic act. If new types of diseases are being treated and a new breed of therapist is being created, it only makes sense that new forms of therapy are being practiced. The classical therapist used words sparingly. He reflected, questioned, doubted, and sometimes criticized his patient. In time, after many sessions, he would deliver an elaborate interpretation that proved that even through those long periods of silence he had been listening. The therapist would only reluctantly interfere in his client's life. Involvement was taboo because it was said to limit objectivity.

Today, by contrast, this sort of detachment is no longer considered a virtue. Indeed, it may be seen as nontherapeutic and, in any case, unrealistic. We cannot ask the school teacher to dissociate himself from his pupil's life. The housewife working in the storefront clinic cannot just *listen* and *sympathize* with people's complaints. Many of the new paraprofessionals perform therapy as negotiator, broker, reformer, and social activist. Calling a rent strike could be the therapy decided upon.

The community-oriented therapist has become a man of action, and such therapy is action-oriented. More than ever, the cry is heard for changing the patient's social behaviors. Whereas in the past therapy might end in symptom removal, today symptoms may be ignored entirely if the patient's employment record improves. Therapy may consist of teaching people how to win friends and influence people, how to be successful at a job interview, how to meet a member of the opposite sex, and how to avoid being cheated by door-to-door salesmen. Therapy has gradually blended with social action. Across the country, in cities of all sizes, there are telephone crisis lines, referral centers, walk-in storefront clinics, and the like, which attempt everything from suicide prevention (presumably a medical specialty) to befriending a lonely soul. The more action-oriented programs involve ombudsmen who will hear grievances and even fight City Hall. And who can debate the fact that improving a person's life is therapeutic? Of course there are still those who would distinguish between therapy as a special healing process and the many human acts that have a therapeutic effect. There are therapies, for example, psychoanalysis, that have been worked out in such sufficient detail that the therapist works within the limits of specific, prescribed methods. However, most psychotherapies currently practiced are so very vague that almost anything that helps the patient can be considered part of the therapeutic system. Therefore, a clinician could claim that he is still within his area of expertise when he leads his "patients" in an effort to oust a racist police captain. He is not claiming merely that political acts are therapeutic to the parties involved but that political acts are therapy.

The community enthusiasts have drastically increased the scope of the therapist's activity. He is no longer confined to his office and restricted to those behaviors and experiences that the patient wishes to introduce. The community therapist, especially one with a notion of preventive medicine, can become involved in the total life of the client. No aspect of the client's life is irrelevant; no problem is extraneous. However, this orientation can bring the therapist into direct conflict with other professionals—lawyers, for example. According to a recent report (Langsley & Kaplan, 1968) on the use of a family-crisis method for keeping potential patients out of a state hospital, the conflicts between community therapists and lawyers clearly arise. The therapists were shocked at the suspicious and protective behavior of the lawyers. The therapists took the point of view that they had no vested interests and wanted to help everyone. The lawyers, on the other hand, tended to see themselves aligned with one person or another. Somehow the lawyers could not accept the notion that one person (in this case, the family therapist) could be the agent of both the wife and the husband when they were in open conflict. We share these lawyers' concerns and doubts. We wonder if community workers can really work for entire families, agencies, and towns simultaneously, and we wonder if the neutral-sounding term *therapy* is being used to camouflage well-known forms of legal and political action.

Community Mental Health: A Social–Political Movement

In his recent book, *The Manufacture of Madness* (1970), Szasz worries about the direction of the community movement. He sees clear parallels between present and past in cases where the state has promised to create a golden age by curing all sickness and purging all evil; however noble the program and its planners, in the end the deviants are sacrificed in the name of the public good. Those who would dismiss Szasz's dark vision argue that scientific institutions can never become as blind as religious and military ones. Perhaps, but there is much more to community mental health than scientific theory and empirical data. And that is our point. The changing definitions of client, therapist, and therapy, the new (and not so new) forms of community intervention, and the social-action approaches to mental health are not really scientific acts. Scientists may be making the decisions based on empirical knowledge, but the acts are social–political in nature. The problems of community mental health are not solely technological problems, and hence they cannot be solved in social science laboratories. In this introductory essay we have tried to demonstrate that the problems associated with launching community programs are human problems; and the most critical decisions are based not on scientific theory but social philosophy.

This is not to suggest that there is an agreed-upon social philosophy that underlies and pervades all the various community projects. Yet one does recognize a certain commitment to a public health ideology in many of the programs. This ideology casts the physician or some surrogate in the role of public protector of the community's mental health, and most often without consulting the community. The emphasis is often on the prevention of new cases, and thus the community specialist feels a strong obligation to the whole population, the currently sick as well as the potentially ill. It is comforting to know that physicians are at work preventing the outbreak of contagious diseases by setting up sanitary standards, draining marshes, and inspecting supermarkets. On the other hand, it is unsettling to think that public officials would concern themselves with our mental well-being. There is something private and sacred about our minds, and it gives us an uneasy feeling when others in power claim that they wish to protect us against ourselves.

Yet we would not reject the community movement (as Szasz seems inclined to do) even though it is more social philosophy than science. The alternative of having private practitioners see one voluntary client at a time is even more dismal and even less responsible. In any event, there is no turning back. The professionals cannot stop this movement, for the truth is that they did not even start it. First Congress and then the President suggested an all-out community effort and the creation of a new community institution, the base-center unit. Naturally, mental health workers who had been community-oriented saw their opportunity, and soon others did too. As might be expected, the professions have assumed (and in some cases insisted upon) leadership. All this activity may very well be in the public interest, but the public's response is yet to be heard.

We have no quarrel with community modes of intervention except insofar as they are imposed upon an unknowing public. But more is required than informing the public. Somehow, in ways yet to be developed adequately, the public must be involved in the planning and management of community programs. Some programs have attempted this, with rather disastrous results. Certainly, in the short run, it is far more efficient not to ask the poorly educated, the man-in-the-street, to join the inner circle of social scientists and physicians who have taken the responsibility for the community's health.

But should scientists and physicians solely assume such responsibility? The answer to this question may vary with the type of program. Diagnostic, evaluative surveys that collect data and nothing more may be of little interest to the public at large. On the other hand, parents might be more concerned over therapeutic programs that influence the school's curriculum. This is all obvious. Public acceptance of programs should never be taken for granted. Nor should the mental health planners invite the public in only when they think it appropriate. The public should be present at the program's inception and not be expected only to play watchdog. Casting the layman in the role of critic will only serve to increase the natural bitterness between professional and nonprofessional. Similarly, giving the nonprofessional odd jobs or making him an ancillary member of the therapeutic team is making way for future reaction. The time is past when the people are going to accept mental health and social programs delivered from above. As Silberman (1964) points out, "welfare colonialism" and related forms of social manipulation are self-destructive. How long can we placate the public by putting them on powerless advisory boards and mystifying them with pseudoscientific jargon? Of course, these conflicts would be avoided if the professional retreated from the arena in which public policy is formed. But it is not possible to engage in community mental health practice without forming and reforming public policy. In fact, as time goes on, it becomes increasingly clear that methods of community intervention that do not derive from the model of public policy formation are blind technological forms that are likely to destroy the community in the name of mental health.

REFERENCES

Caplan, G. *Principles of preventive psychiatry.* New York: Basic Books, 1964.

Cowen, E. L., Gardner, E. A. and Zax, M. *Emergent approaches to mental health problems.* New York: Appleton, 1967.

Kadushin, C. *Why people go to psychiatrists.* New York: Atherton Press, 1969.

Kelly, J. The mental health agent in the urban community. In A. Bindman and A. Spiegel (Eds.), *Perspectives in community mental health.* Chicago: Aldine, 1969.

Key, W. Controlled intervention—The helping professions and directed social change. *American Journal of Orthopsychiatry,* 1966, *36,* 400–406.

Langsley, D. G., and Kaplan, D. M. *The treatment of families in crisis.* New York: Grune & Stratton, 1968.

Levine, M., and Levine, A. *A social history of helping services.* New York: Appleton, 1970.

Mechanic, D. Progress in community mental health: Sociological issues. Mimeographed paper, 1962.

Pearl, A., and Riessman, F. *New careers for the poor.* New York: Free Press, 1965.

Peck, H., and Kaplan, S. A mental health program for an urban multiservice center. In M. Shore and F. Mannino (Eds.), *Mental health and the community.* New York: Behavioral Publications, 1969.

Rae-Grant, Q., and Stringer, L. Mental health programs in the schools. In M. Shore and F. Mannino (Eds.), *Mental health and the community.* New York: Behavioral Publications, 1969.

Reiff, R., and Reissman, F. The indigenous nonprofessional: A strategy of change in community action and community mental health. *Community Mental Health Journal Monographs, No. 1.* New York: Behavioral Publications, 1965.

Rioch, M., Elkes, C., Flint, A., Usdansky, B., Newman, R., and Selber, E. National Institute of Mental Health pilot study in training mental health counselors. *American Journal of Orthopsychiatry,* 1963, *33,* 678–689.

Sabshin, M. Theoretical models in community and social psychiatry. In L. Roberts, S. Halleck, and M. Loeb (Eds.), *Community psychiatry.* Garden City, N.Y.: Anchor Books, 1969.

Scheff, T. The role of the mentally ill and the dynamics of mental disorder. *Sociometry,* 1963, *26,* 436–453.

Silberman, C. *Crisis in black and white.* New York: Random House, 1964.

Szasz, T. *The myth of mental illness.* New York: Hoeber, 1961.

Szasz, T. *The manufacture of madness.* New York: Hoeber, 1970.

PART

1

The Politics of Defining Deviance

The papers included in Part 1 give the reader a feeling for what has been called the "third revolution" in mental health, namely, the community movement. Psychiatry emerged as a scientific discipline in the late nineteenth century; it was followed by the psychoanalytic movement, and now community mental health promises to transform both theory and practice.

In order to understand a "revolution" one must first come to grips with its ideology and conceptual framework. Both Ryan and Reiff explore the traditional psychiatric ideologies and possible innovative revisions stemming from a community point of view. Ryan's basic argument is that the community approach is not really consistent with a medical analysis of deviant behavior. In this paper, Ryan asks us to reject the "exceptionalist" viewpoint of the medical profession and view mental health in the context of universal social problems that are a function of social arrangements, social power, and the like. He also asks us to stop "Blaming the Victim," that is, to stop analyzing social problems in such a way that the victims are blamed for having the problems. He points out that concepts like "cultural deprivation" that are used to explain the failure of ghetto school children place the burden of reform upon the victimized slum inhabitants.

Reiff also is calling for a new perspective on mental health. He points out that the traditional psychiatric point of view that considers mental health and illness to be on a continuum and the traditional preoccupation with "self-actualization" will never make sense to large segments of the population. He asks us to consider that the average person mightily resists seeing his problems in emotional terms and that many people, especially low-income people who are supposed to be reached by these new community programs, are much more concerned

17

with the hostile environment than they are interested in their intra-psychic life.

Warren obviously embraces Reiff and Ryan's community ideology. He advocates a broad mental health planning perspective in which mental health centers work within the context of large-scale social programs such as Model Cities. Warren points out that mental health administrators, in contrast to administrators of social programs, are more inclined to focus on approaches that emphasize individual change. Working in the context of a Model Cities program would surely counteract this tendency.

The Brower, Taber, and Visher and Harris papers elaborate further possibilities. Brower, after examining the economic, political, and social climate of the ghetto, concludes that powerlessness is the critical issue. His analysis suggests that mental health programs should focus on the forms of community organization and development that maximize local control.

Taber also is impressed by the sense of powerlessness of the ghetto inhabitant. However, he views the situation from an ecological perspective in which abnormal behavior is considered to be an interaction between the individual ghetto dweller and his surrounding network of social systems. Consequently, he works with natural groups that exist in the community and attempts to foster positive mental health without making people into patients. Taber describes two projects—one with an adult social group and another with a teen-age gang, but in both cases the message is the same. Taber is saying that community workers must consider individual symptoms in the context of the person's life, his family system, and the larger community systems.

Obviously, Visher and Harris are also persuaded that the most effective way of dealing with individuals who are not usually seen in traditional mental health settings is to work with their reality-based problems, such as chronic unemployment. Their paper describes a program of mental health consultation for personnel at youth and adult opportunity centers located in the poverty areas of a major city. It is well known that staff in these agencies are demoralized by the lack of resources both within the community and among the clients. Thus, Visher and Harris elected to support these critical people in the hope that a change in their attitudes would result in their being more effective and would consequently uplift the mental health of the clients.

Kiesler, although operating in an entirely different setting, is also imbued with the notion of working through others to provide psychiatric help. Kiesler's concept of programming for prevention is illustrated in a rural Minnesota community mental health center that could never hope to provide enough therapists for one-to-one counseling for the majority of the people even if they wanted such service. Rather than welcome referrals, the staff tried to act as consultants to the "firing line professionals," for example, physicians, probate judges, sheriffs, clergymen, and so on. They found that many referrals had less to do with the conditions of the person and more to do with the attitudes of the professional on the firing line. The strategy of working with the caretakers rather than the patients seems to be as effective in a rural setting as it is in an inner-city ghetto.

In summary, the papers included here formulate a number of models for community mental health theory and practice. The traditional models for mental health delivery systems based on the traditional medical approach are contrasted with the social reform and social action approaches to community well-being. What is glaringly obvious in all of these papers is that the shift from an individual, medical analysis of deviance to a social, humanistic concern with discrimination and oppression has been inspired more by a shift in social–political thought rather than by the scientific analysis of hard experimental data. That is, the redefinition of mental illness in social terms is a social–political act and as such must have social and political consequences. The authors of the articles in this section have gone to great pains to show the liberating influence of these redefinitions. But, as we will see in subsequent articles, redefining deviance is a political act that has sewn the seeds of social–political strife.

EMOTIONAL DISORDER AS A SOCIAL PROBLEM: IMPLICATIONS FOR MENTAL HEALTH PROGRAMS

1

William Ryan

The overriding problems in the mental health field are manifold and well documented: the manpower shortages, the maldistribution of care, the deprivation of care suffered by the poor and the black, the fragmentation of services and lack of coordination in programming, and the continuing uncertainty as to how well, in fact, the services we provide meet the needs of those who are in distress.

The community mental health center, to the extent that it is a new kind of institution, is a social invention designed to solve these problems, and, to a substantial and encouraging extent, it is beginning to do so. There is some reason, then, to be optimistic. But there are reasons to be pessimistic that are, at least to me, more compelling and persuasive. For every new center program that is creative and innovative there are, I fear, a half dozen that are being assimilated to past practices, that are in fact merely providing more of the same. For every community mental health professional who is approaching these problems in an imaginative and inventive way there are several who are too bound by their professional identities and ideologies to do much more than spruce up and put a fresh coat of paint on their old-model methods.

In the following pages, I would like to make several points that bear on this issue. First, I would suggest that we are handicapped and blocked in dealing with the basic problems of the mental health field by *ideological* barriers, by distortions and deficiencies in our viewpoint, our way of thinking, our assumptions about the phenomena with which we are supposedly dealing. Second, I will propose that it is more fruitful and effective to think about mental health under the category of social problems than under the category of medical diseases. And, finally, I would like to summarize an ideological analysis of the problem of the mental health of the poor in some detail, as an example of how our

This is a revised version of a paper presented at the 1970 annual meeting of the American Orthopsychiatric Association, San Francisco. Reprinted from *American Journal of Orthopsychiatry*, 1971, *41*, 638–645. Copyright © 1971, the American Orthopsychiatric Association, Inc. Reproduced by permission. William Ryan is Professor and Chairman, Psychology Department, Boston College.

thinking about issues is deficient and hampers us in the development of appropriate programs.

Defining a social problem is not so simple as it may seem, as John Seeley (6) has pointed out. To ask "What is a social problem?" may seem to be posing an ingenuous question, until one turns to confront its opposite: "What human problem is *not* a social problem?" Since any problem in which people are involved is social, why do we reserve the label for some problems and withhold it from others? The phenomena we look at are bounded by the act of definition. They become a social problem only by being so considered. In Seeley's words, "*naming* it as a problem, after naming it as a *problem*."

In addition to the issue of what is a social problem, there are additional issues of what *causes* social problems, and, then, perhaps most important, what do we do about them. C. Wright Mills (2) has analyzed the ideology of those who write about social problems and demonstrated its relationship to class interest and the preservation of the existent social order. By sifting the material in thirty-one widely used textbooks in social problems, Mills was able to demonstrate a pervasive, coherent ideology with a number of common characteristics. First, the textbooks present material about these problems in simple, descriptive terms, each problem unrelated to the others, and none related in any meaningful way to other aspects of the social environment. Second, the problems are selected and described largely in relation to predetermined norms. The norms themselves are taken as givens and no effort is made to examine them. Nor is there any thought given to the manner in which norms might themselves contribute to the development of the problems. Within such a framework, then, deviation from norms and standards comes to be defined as failed or incomplete socialization—persons haven't learned the standards and rules or haven't learned how to keep them. A final, variant theme is that of adjustment or adaptation. Those with social problems are viewed as unable or unwilling to adjust to society's standards.

By definining social problems in this way, the social pathologists are, of course, ignoring a whole set of factors that might ordinarily be considered as relevant, such as unequal distribution of income, social stratification, political struggle, ethnic and racial group conflict, and inequality of power. This ideology concentrates almost exclusively on the failure of the deviant. To the extent that society plays any part in social problems, it is said somehow to have failed to socialize the individual, to teach him how to adjust to circumstances, which, though far from perfect, are gradually changing for the better.

This ideology, identified by Mills as the predominant tool used in *analyzing* social problems, also saturates the majority of programs that have been developed to *solve* social problems in America. These programs are based on the assumption that *individuals* "have" social problems as a result of some kind of unusual circumstances—accident, illness, personal defect or handicap, character flaw or maladjustment—that exclude them from the ordinary mechanisms for maintaining and advancing themselves.

Health care in America, for example, has been predominantly a matter of particular remedial attention provided individually to the more or less random group of persons who have become ill, whose bodily functioning has become deviant and abnormal. In the field of mental health, the same approach has been, and continues to be, dominant. The social problem of mental disease has been viewed as a collection of individual cases of deviance, persons who—through unusual hereditary taint or exceptional distortion of character—have become unfitted for the normal activities of ordinary life.

This has been the dominant style in American social welfare and health activities, then: to treat what we call social problems, such as poverty, disease, and mental illness, in terms of the individual deviance of the special, unusual groups of persons who had those problems. There has also been a competing style, however, much less common, not at all congruent with the prevalent ideology, subordinate, but continually developing parallel to the dominant style. Adherents of this approach tended to search for causes in the community and the environment rather than individual defect, to emphasize predictability and usualness rather than random deviance, to think about preventing rather than merely repairing or treating, to see social problems, in a word, as social.

In the field of disease, we have the public health approach, whose practitioners sought the cause of disease in environmental factors such as the water supply, the sewage system, and the quality of housing conditions. In the field of income maintenance, this secondary style of solving social problems focused on poverty as a predictable event, on the regularities of income deficiency, and on the development of usual, generalized programs affecting total groups.

These two approaches to the solution of social problems have existed side by side, the former always dominant, but the latter gradually expanding, slowly becoming more and more prevalent.

Elsewhere (3, 4, 5) I have proposed the dimension of *exceptionalism–universalism* as the ideological underpinning for these two contrasting approaches to the analysis and solution of social problems. The *exceptionalist* viewpoint is reflected in arrangements that are private, voluntary, remedial, special, local, and exclusive. Such arrangements imply that problems occur to specially defined categories of persons in an unpredictable manner. The problems are unusual, even unique; they are exceptions to the rule; they occur as a result of individual defect, accident, or unfortunate circumstance; and they must be remedied by means that are particular and, as it were, tailored to the individual case.

The *universalistic* viewpoint, on the other hand, is reflected in arrangements that are public, legislated, promotive or preventive, general, national, and inclusive. Inherent in such a viewpoint is the idea that social problems are a function of the social arrangements of the community or the society and that, since these social arrangements are quite imperfect and inequitable, such problems are both predictable, and, more important, preventable, through public action. They are not unique to the individual, and their encompassing of individual persons does not imply that those persons are themselves defective or abnormal.

Generally speaking, mental health services have, in the past, been organized and arranged in an exceptionalistic fashion. This would be perfectly appropriate if we considered mental illness an illness—a genuine disease—and decided that it was a disease of mysterious and unpredictable proportions. Given the tremendous quantities of evidence amassed in recent years that suggest the conclusion that emotional disorder is, rather, a social problem, with a relatively predictable pattern of incidence, one would argue that mental health services should be organized in a universalistic fashion. What would that mean?

First, it would mean less and less reliance on the private, voluntary sector and much heavier emphasis on public programs based on clear legislative sanctions. Second, it would require an expansion of scope so that mental health programs would concern themselves not merely with remedial treatment activities directed toward a special, unusual, deviant population, but rather with preventive efforts directed toward an entire population. It would also mean that the group taking responsibility for planning and decision making with respect to the organization of services would be expanded in a parallel fashion so that the community as a whole, through some type of representative mechanism, would have the responsibility and the power to decide the form and structure and priorities of mental health programs.

We find the greatest degree of readiness to view emotional disorder as a social problem among those who have concerned themselves with the mental health of the poor.

In observing the growing interest in the relationship between poverty and mental health, my own mood has ranged from exhilarated gratification through puzzlement to a growing sense of concern and dismay. I see signs that the mental health approach to the problems of the poor is being gradually fitted into the same mold that contains and cripples most other approaches to the poor. The central event in this constraining and crippling process is conceptual or, rather, ideological, what I have called elsewhere "Blaming the Victim" (5).

Briefly, "Blaming the Victim" is an intellectual process whereby a social problem is analyzed in such a way that the causation is found to be in the qualities and characteristics of the victim rather than in any deficiencies or structural defects in his environment. In addition, it is usually found that these characteristics are not inherent or genetic but are, rather, socially determined. They are stigmas of social origin and are therefore no fault of the victim himself. He is to be pitied, not censured, but nevertheless his problems are to be defined as rooted basically in his own characteristics. Some of the common stigmas of social origin that are used to blame the victim are the concept of cultural deprivation as an explanation for the failures of ghetto schools to educate poor and black children and the concept of the crumbling Negro family as a basic explanation of the persistence of inequality between blacks and whites in America today. "Blaming the Victim" is differentiated from old-fashioned conservative ideological formulations, such as Social Darwinism, racial inferiority, and quasi-Calvinist notions of the prospering elect. It is a liberal ideology.

The theoretical—or, more properly, ideological—formulations that are beginning to attain dominance in considerations of the mental health of the poor show unmistakable family resemblances to the Culture of Poverty cult and the other victim-blaming ideologies.

An important element in this ideology is the assumption that it is the early experiences of the poor, the failures of mothering, the inconsistent patterns of discipline, the exposure to deviant values and behavior patterns that account for their apparent excessive vulnerability to emotional disorder.

These assumptions, this ideology, boil down to a process of relating mental disorder to social class by relating psychosexual development to presumed cultural features of a subgroup of the population. It derives from the extreme and continuing influence of W. Lloyd Warner in American thinking about social class, in which social class is defined largely in terms of prestige, life style, social honor.

There are other views about social stratification that have been far less influential but that might in the long run prove more fruitful for understanding the complexities of relationship between class and distress. Max Weber's (7) conception of stratification, for example, which is followed rather closely by C. Wright Mills and others, maintains that there is not one but three dimensions of social ordering. These are *class*, the extent to which one controls property and financial resources and maintains a favorable position in the marketplace; *status*, the manner in which one consumes resources and the extent to which one is accorded social honor (this is the predominant element in Warner's view of social class); and *power*, the extent to which one (or, more commonly, a group of persons, a "party") is able to control and influence the community's decisions.

Now, if one limits one's thinking about relationships between social stratification and emotional disorder to *status* questions (largely disregarding *class* and *power* issues), one starts seeking explanations in terms of status elements, such as child-rearing practices, values, life style, and so on. One is inclined to conclude that the poor are more subject to emotional disorder than the affluent because their patterns of parenting are deficient, their values are different, their time orientation is different and they cannot defer need-gratification, their life styles emphasize violence and sexual promiscuity, they have ego deficiencies as a result of their childhood experiences in the culture of poverty, and so forth.

One hears and sees these kinds of formulations more and more frequently in mental health settings. I fear that an ideology is developing in which the mental health problems of the poor (which one might reasonably have expected would be related to poverty) are being analyzed through status-oriented formulations of class differences, with the result that these problems are being conceptually transformed into one more category of intrapsychic disorder. The consequences of such transformations are predictable. The evidence that appears to relate disorder to environmental circumstances is being rapidly assimilated to preexisting patterns of intrapsychic theorizing, and the *status quo* is being maintained—which, after all, is the purpose of ideology.

When one focuses on status and life-style as explanatory variables, one omits at the same time the other elements that determine social stratification—power and money. Lack of money as a cause of emotional disorder can be conceptualized through the mediating concept of stress. Stresses relating to lack of money—poor and crowded housing, nutritional deficiencies, medical neglect, unemployment, and so on—have been found as correlates of disorder rather regularly. Moreover, there is evidence that certain kinds of stressful events, such as illness, which can be merely inconvenient for the well-to-do, are often disastrous for the poor. Some of Dohrenwend's (1) recent work contains some intriguing ideas on the possible relationship between poverty, stress, and emotional disorder. He sets forth the hypothesis that reaction to stress is ordinarily cyclical and time-limited and that most emotional symptomatology evidenced in such reactions is temporary. A prevalence study at a given point in time, then, would tend to include substantial numbers of such temporary stress reactions. If one assumes that stresses in the lives of the poor are both more prevalent and more severe than those in the lives of the more prosperous, one would expect that, at a given point in time, the poor as a group would exhibit more stress reactions and would therefore demonstrate a higher prevalence of emotional disorder. This is one example of the way in which the class-oriented, which is to say the money-oriented, method of dealing with stratification can be introduced into the process of theorizing about the relationship between poverty and mental health.

The third leg of the stratification stool—power—can be dealt with principally through the mediating concept of self-esteem. There is an overwhelming array of theoretical and empirical literature suggesting that self-esteem is a vital element in mental health and, further, that self-esteem is based on a sense of competence, an ability to influence one's environment, a sense of mastery and control over events and circumstances that affect one's life. These are psychological terms that are readily translatable into the sociological concept of power as used by Weber. To the extent that a person is powerful, then, he is more likely to be what we call mentally healthy; to the extent that he is powerless, he is likely to be lacking in this characteristic.

The functional relationship between the exercise of power, feelings of self-esteem, and mental health has been empirically observed in a number of settings—civil rights demonstrations, block organization projects, and even, according to some, in ghetto disorders.

There are, then, relationships to be found between mental health phenomena and issues of money and power that are direct, more direct than the secondary kinds of relationships hypothesized between mental health and social status and life-style. The major difference, however, is in program implications. If one makes the assumption that the relevant variable is status, one tends to work on changing the characteristics of the individual—his life-style, his values, his child-rearing practices, or the effects of the child-rearing practices of his parents. If, on the other hand, one makes the assumption that the relevant variables are money and power, one tends to work toward changing the environment, toward developing programs of social change rather than individual change.

I am dismayed and concerned that we in the mental health field are moving more and more toward a narrow view of status issues, which will permit us to conduct business as usual—focusing on changing the person—and avoid the broader view of class and power issues that would oblige us to alter our methods and start putting our resources into the business of social change.

If we did make such a shift, such a change in our ideology and our assumptions about what is wrong, what alterations would there be in our style of doing business? How might we translate the problems we confront into different kinds of needs? And what kinds of services would we develop to meet those needs?

We would, first of all, turn our attention to the patterns of social inequity and injustice that play such a major role in producing the casualties and victims who come to us for attention. Just as, in years gone by, the pioneers of public health spoke up and cried out for change in housing and sanitation and factory conditions, so would we be required to cry out about our society's basic inequalities in the distribution of money and power. In the councils of professional activity, in the councils of social welfare, and in the councils of government, ours would be a voice agitating for equality as a fundamental prerequisite for mental health.

Second, as we encounter and evaluate—or, as we used to say in the good old days, "diagnose"—our clients, we would necessarily find ourselves including in our thoughts and our repertoire of labels and categories redevelopment as well as repression, superhighways as well as superegos, police training as well as toilet training, discrimination as well as displacement, and racism as well as autism.

It would also follow that in our interactions with clients drawn from low-income and black neighborhoods, our services would have to be at least partially geared toward the fundamental issues of money and power. We would have to act to increase our clients' resources—through training and referral services to help them get a job, or a better job, through encouragement of the development of unions in unorganized settings to help them get more money, through advocating more public funds for such matters as income maintenance and public assistance, public housing, subsidized medical care, better education, increased day care facilities, and so on.

And we would have to act to increase our clients' power in the community—primarily through community organization efforts in the low-income neighborhoods of our specific catchment areas, but also through out own political, lobbying, and public educational activities.

An indispensable element in, and touchstone of, our commitment to increase the power of our constituency is the way we deal with the issue of decision making in our own centers. Power sharing—like charity—begins at home, which means citizen involvement and participation in shaping the programs and priorities of the mental health center. In a word, community control. If powerlessness gives rise to pathology, and the only cure for powerlessness is power, and we have the occasion to relinquish power to the citizens we profess to serve, the consequences are obvious. We must put our money where our mouth is.

An unexpected by-product of such a shift in orientation, that is, a reconceptualization of the great majority of mental health problems as *social* problems, flowing from structural and environmental distortions on the axis of money and the axis of power, would be the possibility of some easing of the acute shortage of manpower in the psychiatric professions. On the one hand, the mental health center would become one agency among several in an alliance of equals that could attack these problems jointly. (I say alliance of equals deliberately, to distinguish this hypothetical situation from the present case in which a psychiatric facility is seen as a dominant agency collaborating condescendingly with a group of ancillary or paramedical agencies.) And the appropriate manpower to engage in such a preventive, social, universalistic program would not have to include any substantial number of trained mental health professionals.

The latter, the psychiatrists and clinical psychologists and nurses and social workers, could then turn their attention more vigorously to the minority of mental health problems that may be considered more accurately as *medical* or *quasi-medical* in nature: the psychosomatic disorders, the metabolic disorders, the major and minor brain dysfunctions, and the most acute and refractory of the disorders that are characterized by disorientation, thought and mood disruption for which there is some evidence for genetic or other physical causation.

In summary, I am suggesting that the mental health center can fulfill its promise only if those of us in the field consciously undertake to revamp and expand our ideological framework to include the disorder of the community as well as the dysfunction of the individual. We must learn that the emotionally disturbed individual is not an unusual, abnormal, unexpectable "case," but is rather a usual, highly predictable index of the distortion and injustice that pervades our society. Only after such ideological transformation can the community mental health center become what it must become—a committed instrument for social change and social justice.

REFERENCES

1. Dohrenwend, B. 1967. Social status, stress and psychological symptoms. *Amer. J. Pub. Hlth.*, 57(4):625–632.
2. Mills, C. W. 1943. The professional ideology of social pathologists. *Amer. J. Sociol.*, 49(2):165–180.
3. Ryan, W. 1969. Community care in historical perspective: Implications for mental health services and professionals. *Canada's Mental Health* supplement #60 (March–April).
4. Ryan, W. 1969. Distress in the City. Case Western Reserve Press, Cleveland.
5. Ryan, W. 1971. Blaming the Victim. Pantheon, New York.

6. Seeley, J. 1965. The problem of social problems. *Indian Sociol. Bull.*, 2(3). *Also in* The Americanization of the Unconscious, J. Seeley. 1967. Science House, New York (pp. 142–148).
7. Weber, M. Class, status and party. *In* Max Weber: Essays in Sociology, H. Gerth and C. W. Mills, translators.

THE IDEOLOGICAL AND TECHNOLOGICAL IMPLICATIONS OF CLINICAL PSYCHOLOGY

2

Robert Reiff

For the past seven years, under a grant from the National Institute of Mental Health, I have been engaged in a program to develop mental health education, research, and services for labor and low-income groups. This rich experience has had a profound influence on my views on mental health, mental illness, the role of the psychologist, in fact, on all the pertinent questions that pose themselves when one looks at psychiatry and psychology as a social process.

The development of psychiatry and clinical psychology has been one of increasing acceptance on the part of the middle and upper classes in this country. There has also been an ever-increasing expansion of its influence on child-rearing practices, education, marriage, and so on. In fact, there is hardly an area of social living over which the umbrella of psychiatry has not been extended. On the other hand, there has been a long history of persistent alienation from psychiatry of the lower socioeconomic groups in this country. This alienation represents a critical failure on the part of psychiatry and clinical psychology. It is not merely the failure of each individual clinical psychologist, although there is the element of the individual's social responsibility involved here. Neither is it primarily a matter of the tools and skills of the clinical psychologist, although, again, this element is also involved. Basically, the problem is an ideological one. Clinical psychologists have not responded to the challenge of this alienation but have for the most part embraced the ideology of psychiatry. By ideology, I mean the body of knowledge, the set of integrated assertions, theories, and aims, primarily psychoanalytical, which constitute the individualistically oriented program for restoring to society the mentally sick and socially deviant. It is the thesis of this paper that the roots of this alienation from the low-income populations lie primarily in the middle-class ideology of contemporary psychiatry and only secondarily in its technology.

Invited address presented at the Boston Conference on the Education of Psychologists for Community Mental Health, Swampscott, Massachusetts, May 5, 1965. Reprinted from *Community Psychology*, Boston, 1966, 51–64. Robert Reiff is at the Albert Einstein College of Medicine, New York, New York.

There is a basic dichotomy between the popular point of view about mental illness and mental health and the mental health professional's point of view. Studies by Shirley Star (1957), Reiff (1960), and others have found that the popular point of view starts with normal behavior as its reference point. It seeks to explain normal behavior as the distinctive and essentially human qualities of rationality and the ability to exercise self-control. Given this premise, normal behavior is viewed as a rational response to the immediate circumstances in which the individual finds himself, which is at the same time fully within the conscious control of the person. Mental illness is defined as the extreme opposite of normality. It is behavior in which rationality is so impaired that the individual has lost control and can no longer be responsible for his acts. It is, therefore, quite logically, only the extreme form of psychosis that is considered mental illness by most workers. It follows from this that mental illness is a very threatening thing. It represents a loss of the distinctly human qualities, the ultimate catastrophe that can befall a human. Thus, in their view, mental health and mental illness are not related to each other as on a continuum, but they are discontinuous phenomena.

The psychiatric point of view starts with abnormal behavior as its reference point and extrapolates to the normal. It views mental health and mental illness as on a continuum, and it holds that personality characteristics and behavior are universal, differing only in degree. It contends that there is really no such thing as a completely normal person and that the same phenomena we see in mental illness are present in all people. In fact, mental health professionals can hardly use the word "normal" without prefacing it with the words "so-called" normal. Further, the psychiatric point of view holds that characteristic emotional patterns are not entirely within the rational control of an individual. The modifications of behavior patterns do not depend entirely on rationality, self-help, will-power, reasoning, or even purely environmental manipulations. It assumes that a large part of our motivations are unconscious or unknown to us and that until they become conscious they are unmodifiable. Finally, the professionals' point of view makes the implicit conclusion that mental illness is not necessarily an overwhelming threat, nor must it inevitably arouse fear or alarm.

While it may be reassuring to a middle-class patient to hear that the emotional mechanisms of sick people aren't so different from anyone else's, it is anything but acceptable to a healthy worker that his emotional mechanisms aren't so different from the mentally ill, especially if he holds the point of view that mental illness is about as far from normal as you can get. I am not suggesting that the validity of a scientific concept depends upon its popular acceptance, but merely that a practical concept of normality is necessary to find a basis of understanding with low-income groups essential to successful treatment as well as primary and secondary prevention. They key to developing such a practical concept of normality is the recognition that, though personality characteristics and behavior may be universal, their meaning and significance must be assessed within their social–cultural context. The failure to control violent acts of aggression has different implications for normality and illness in a civil rights demonstration, a quarrel in a working-class bar, a middle-class family quarrel, or a meeting of clinical psychologists.

Furthermore, while the worker acknowledges there is such a thing as mental illness that he equates with severely psychotic behavior, from his point of view he has difficulty accepting the concept of a neurotic emotional disturbance as an illness. The term itself is confusing to him. If he sees a raving psychotic screaming or a psychotic depressive crying and wailing, he can see how they can be called emotionally upset. In that sense it is simply a synonym for excessive emotional behavior out of control. However, if he is told that a man with a lame back or a particularly passive person who lets everybody walk all over him is emotionally disturbed, this idea of sickness is incomprehensible to him. To him there is physical illness and mental illness. In mental illness one sometimes sees severe emotional upsets. Sometimes people get upset over physical illness, death, stressful situations; but to him this is not mental illness. It is either a normal reaction to a stressful problem of living or a sign of physical or moral weakness. It follows then that the psychiatric point of view that the failure to meet the problems of living is an emotional disturbance, a milder form of mental illness to be treated by the same kind of doctor that treats the more seriously mentally ill, only alienates him. To the worker, emotional disability or impairment is either related to a physical illness and should be treated as such by the doctor; or is the result of undue stresses and strains in the environment; or it is related to a moral weakness and should be treated by a minister or priest or conquered by oneself or accepted and lived with. If one attempts to treat what is considered to be a moral weakness, the worker, with his present view, considers it a tremendous invasion of his privacy. Also, the general practitioner reinforces his tendency to identify emotional disturbance with physical illness, by making it so easy for him to find a physician to treat it as physical illness. Can present psychiatric ideology ever make an impact on the "moral weakness" problem? It can, of course, work through ministers and priests. That may help the small minority who seek help from them; but, for the most part, there is little hope of getting workers or low-income groups to accept failure to meet the problems of living as an illness; and I am not so sure that it is even desirable to do so.

Present psychiatric ideology and technology will continue to fail with low-income patients unless they shift their focus to the coping styles of low-income patients and respond to their need for more successful coping techniques. The focus should shift from how they are reacting to how they are acting, from changing their reactions to teaching them more successful actions. These changes also have implications for changing the aims and goals of treatment. The fundamental justification and aim of psychotherapy are self-actualization. Everyone should realize his full potential, and if he is not able to do so, then he should be in therapy so that he may fully actualize himself. This, of course, meets a responsive chord in the feelings of most middle- and upper-class persons about themselves and their lives. They see themselves in many possible roles, and their hope is to select those roles that enable them to actualize themselves. The view that one can realize one's full potential presupposes a view of society in which there are many possibilities and opportunities and that one need only remove the internal difficulties to make a rich, full life possible. For the most part, disturbed middle-class patients see themselves as *victims of their own selves.* Low-income people, on the other hand, are not future-oriented. They are task-oriented, concrete, and concerned primarily with the here and now. They live in a world of limited or no opportunities. There is little or no role flexibility. They see themselves as *victims of circumstance.* Self-actualization under these conditions is meaningless to them. Before they can become interested in self-actualization, they have got to believe that they can play a role in determining what happens to them. Thus, *self-determination* rather than self-actualization is a more realistic and more meaningful goal for them.

Another ideological dilemma is the domination of the relationship in therapy practice by the values and mores of a "fee-for-service" ethic. Even where the service is rendered by an agency this is true. Goffman (1961) eloquently described this relationship that he says involves a set of interdependent assumptions that fit together to form a model.

. . . When services are performed whose worth to the client at the time is very great, the server (that is, the professional mental health worker) is ideally supposed to restrict himself to a fee determined by tradition—presumably what the server needs to keep himself in decent circumstances while he devotes his life to his calling . . . . When he performs major services for very poor clients, the server may feel that charging no fee is more dignified (or perhaps safer) than a reduced fee. The server thus avoids dancing to the client's tune, or even bargaining, and is able to show that he is motivated by a disinterested involvement in his work.

The server's attachment to his conception of himself as a disinterested expert, and his readiness to relate to persons on the basis of it, is a kind of secular vow of chastity and is at the root of the wonderful use that clients make of him. In him they find someone who does not have the usual personal, ideological, or contractual reasons for helping them; yet he is someone who will take an intense temporary interest in them . . . .

. . . It therefore pays the client to trust in those for whom he does not have the usual guarantees of trust.

This trustworthiness available on request would of itself provide a unique basis of relationship in our society . . .

These implicit characteristics of the service or therapeutic relationship are understandable and acceptable to most middle-class people who themselves are often engaged in trading their expertness to other individuals. But the worker finds it difficult to trust the person who expects a fee for helping him with what he believes to be a moral problem. Children, too, have difficulty understanding; and they are confused when they discover that the therapist is paid for "being his friend." Thus the therapy relationship itself is confusing and untrustworthy in the eyes of the low-income people. The state hospitals that do not charge a fee are still based on a fee-for-service basis because in many state hospitals they require some form of pauper's oath. A person must certify that he is not able to pay. The fact remains that, for any person in a low-income group, having a mental illness means being a medical indigent.

These are but a few of the ideological differences that relate directly to psychiatric theory. There are, in addition, the ideological differences in values, goals, and styles of life of low-income groups and the professional himself. Reiff (1963, 1964) and Riessman (1964) have dealt in detail with these differences and have detailed what modifications in techniques may result in more effective work with low-income groups. But this paper focuses on the ideological failure of psychiatry because we are about to embark on new community mental health programs, and we are faced with the task of how to train clinical psychologists for these programs. It is therefore necessary to call attention to the implications of those aspects of the new community mental health programs that may not have been considered but that may vitally affect what may happen to clinical psychologists in this new setting.

Reaching the lower socioeconomic groups, and particularly the poor, has been a growing and vital concern of the professional in human services and the more enlightened public-service–minded government agencies. The increasing recognition that there is a vast multitude of people with unmet needs has resulted in two national programs—the community mental health and the antipoverty programs. Both of these programs have as their aim to tend to the problems of those in society whose needs are greatest. Both are concerned with developing programs in the community.

It is to the credit of professional and political leaders that both these programs have come into existence as a result of their sense of social responsibility, their vision, and their initiative, without the stimulus of a vocal and organized demand from the suffering people themselves. But the absence of such a demand from below poses a question of very crucial importance. What strategies can be developed to convert the very great existing need into effective demand for services? A great deal of productive thinking is going into this problem. Many new strategies relating to program, technology, and other aspects are being devised and demonstrated.

The comprehensive community mental health program enacted into legislation promises to change the whole nature and direction of treatment for mental illness in this country. The idea that the mentally ill can be treated in the community is relatively new and has become possible because of advances in drug therapy during the last ten or fifteen years. The new drugs, although they do not cure mental illness, change the behavior of the patient so as to make it possible for him to live in the community with certain kinds of support from its resources. This has led to a shift in emphasis, a change in goals, in the treatment and care of the mentally ill. Once, custodial care was the only alternative to the failure to qualify for treatment. Now, with an emphasis on a return to functioning rather than cure, rehabilitation and habilitation have become the organizing goals of the treatment process, and the alternative of institutionalization is less necessary.

Clinical psychiatry, responding to the social pressures that this situation engendered, developed its branch of social and community psychiatry so that now that legislation makes possible the development of community mental health facilities, psychiatry has a conceptual and a professional organizational structure that can take responsibility for the community mental health centers. It is significant that no comparable organizational structure has grown within the profession of clinical psychology. Instead, clinical psychologists today, for the most part, are struggling for their place in community mental health programs just as they did years ago in the clinics and hospitals of this country with a theoretical framework, an ideology and a technology, which have been basically borrowed from clinical psychiatry.

We meet here today to ask ourselves the question, "How can we train psychologists for community mental health?" The question is both belated and premature, belated because as scientists we should have been aware of and devoted ourselves to the study of the question of the failure of modern psychiatry to help those in the lower economic classes. It is premature because, without an analysis of the reasons for this failure, we run the risk of providing training and new skills that are dictated by the technological needs of the settings in which we are going to work rather than by the social and psychological needs of the poor who are mentally ill. The profession of psychology will be responding to technological challenges and not to the theoretical and ideological ones that the whole problem of mental health and mental illness in this country presents. This tendency is already seen in the fact that conferences for the training of clinical psychologists seem to be addressing themselves to the training of clinical psychologists in new settings rather than to meeting theoretical and ideological challenges.

It has been proclaimed that the community mental health development signals a revolution in mental health. Such a view is a gross exaggeration. A more sober look will reveal that the new community mental health programs are extensions of the present ideology of psychiatry, through modified goals, strategies, and techniques, over that part of society from which it has been hitherto alienated. It is in fact a process of consolidation rather than revolution, a consolidation made necessary by the realization of its failure to perform adequately its social function of restoration of those whose needs are greatest. Such a consolidation is, of course a step forward. But we must keep in mind that it solves none of the ideological problems but rather perpetuates them. It does more: It legitimates a two-class system of mental health treatment in this country—self-actualization for the rich, rehabilitation for the poor. Although the consolidation is a necessary step forward, its very necessity points to the real crisis in mental health today, and that crisis is a crisis of theory and ideology, not a crisis of technology. It is the failure to come up with a conceptual framework that integrates society and the individual, enables us to understand the individual within his social–cultural matrix so that we may intervene effectively with the individual and the social–cultural matrix to treat and to prevent mental illness.

Gerald Caplan has pointed out that primary prevention should be an integral part of community mental health programs. He sees no basic contradiction in the requirements of the clinician's role of secondary prevention, which is primarily consultation and treatment, and the requirements of social action innovation. He acknowledges that there may be difficulties but feels they are basically compatible. This view, which may be theoretically and personally attractive to clinicians, may lead to a kind of psychiatric imperialism unless it is accompanied by a rethink-

ing of some of the basic concepts of psychiatry. Philip Rieff calls attention to the fact that Goethe feared that the whole world would become
a hospital and all of us sick nurses tending to each other. This prophetic
fear is becoming realized in the view that the whole community can be
a hospital and all of us sick nurses to one degree or another. Actually,
the prospect of any really effective primary prevention programs in community mental health—at least in the ones that are being planned now
—is minimal; first, because with a few outstanding exceptions, the implementation of the community mental health program as it is taking
place now is not taking this direction and, secondly, because few clinicians, even those in community mental health, have the know-how. And
finally, even more importantly, the social criticism, reorganization, and
change needed require the concepts and technology of social scientists;
and the functions of social scientists and clinicians are, at this stage of
our knowledge, not easily integrated. This point needs stressing because
for years we have been taking the position that we want to train
scientist–clinicians, that we want to integrate the role of the scientist
and the role of the clinician; and we've had twenty years of failure. We
have started from the premise that integration is possible and desirable.
I propose that reciprocity is all that can be achieved with our present
state of knowledge, that the social function of a clinician and the social
function of a scientist are different, and that society will permit reciprocity but not integration between these two roles.

At the present time there is no theory or set of concepts that integrates the social process and the individual. Until such a time the therapist, who is the repairman, and the social scientist, who is the engineer,
perform different social funtions. These two functions have different concepts, values, motivations, interests, and aims as well as different roles.
Every social function for which there is a need tends to become institutionalized, and the process of institutionalization tends to rigidify and
restrict the role necessary to accomplish the function. The result of this
institutionalization process is to rigidly define the professional role and
to prescribe sanctions for those who may be tempted to contaminate
their function through role flexibility. Regardless of what any conference
may decide, in the absence of an integrative theory, the social forces at
work on professional roles will prevent the integration of the social scientist and the clinician.

It is necessary to recognize how the nature of society is affecting
and frequently limiting the development of our profession. We act as
though all we have to do is to decide what professional skills are necessary and that will solve the social problems. We act as though there are
no social forces other than those we set in motion operating on the profession. Yet we have already had close to twenty years of failure trying

to integrate the scientist and the clinician precisely because we failed to understand the social forces operating on these two roles that made their fusion or integration impossible. We are about to make the same mistake in community mental health as we did with clinical psychology.

The clinical psychologist is not recognized particularly by the other mental health professionals for his therapeutic skills and technology. He has never achieved recognized independent status in this area, but he is respected and recognized where clinical psychology has made a theoretical or technological impact on mental health from work that is indigenous to psychology. Modern psychoanalytic thinking, for example, has incorporated a great deal of academic developmental psychology. This is one of the heritages of psychology. Psychoanalysis draws heavily on developmental psychology. It is often called ego psychology. (The tragedy is that the new students coming out of the schools of clinical psychology today know very little about developmental psychology.) In this area, the clinical psychologist's views are often sought and listened to. In psychological testing, again an area indigenous to psychology, modern psychiatry finds the contributions of clinical psychology useful and acceptable as an independent function. But as far as treatment is concerned, the clinical psychologist is still regarded as ancillary. This point is forcefully made by Rosenbaum and Zwerling (1964) who write,

> The social scientist in his (the social psychiatrist's) milieu is not the familiar psychiatric social worker or clinical psychologist but rather the sociologist, the anthropologist, and the social psychologist. Whereas the traditional social worker and psychologist operate from within the framework of psychoanalytic theory, the social scientist operates from social system theory, and the psychoanalyst in a unit in social psychiatry is forced to work on a more truly interdisciplinary team basis.

Clinical psychologists are not seen as extradisciplinary and therefore requiring interdisciplinary team relationships, but because clinical psychologists operate within the framework of psychoanalytic theory, they are seen as an intradisciplinary substrate of psychiatry; and therefore the relationship assumes hierarchal rather than team forms. The issue is stated clearly by Klein (1963), "Will the training of clinical psychologists be geared to the nature and requirements of social or community psychiatry just as clinical psychology developed with the needs of clinical psychiatry as a critical determinant?" That in my opinion would be a serious mistake. We must accept the challenge of conceptualization, of theory building, of developing a body of systematic knowledge, a set of integrated assertions, theories, and aims based on psychological tradition and that constitute a socially oriented program for improving the psychological effectiveness of all individuals in our society to deal with the problems of living. Unless we do this, we will continue to put ourselves in the position of having to argue over our rights to employ the technological skills that are rooted in psychiatric ideology. The issue will always be posed as one of skill; and as long as we continue to justify our existence on the basis of technological skills, we condemn ourselves to an interminable power struggle in the form of a jurisdictional dispute with the other sections of the mental health skilled trades.

I am not against power struggles, but if I am going to conduct a power struggle, I want to conduct it on the basis of ideology, not on the basis of technology. A power struggle on the basis of technology results in merely a power struggle and nothing else. A power struggle on the basis of ideology, however, educates everybody; and that is why it seems to me important.

I want to spend a few minutes on an aspect of community mental health that is not talked about very much, namely, the risks in community mental health. I think it is necessary to mention these risks because we have to devise concepts and techniques to ensure against them. This seems to me one of the important functions that a psychologist can play in community mental health. For example, if we're going to send the mentally ill back into the community, what about psychic contagion? What happens to the community? What happens to the people in the community when we turn the psychotics back into the community? What happens to the children? What happens to the family? These, I think, are things we have to examine. I'm not opposed to treating the mentally ill in the community. But we have to be aware of what the risks are and to devise ways of ensuring against them.

Another risk: The community mental health program is going to spend a lot of money building new community mental health centers, and I fear we're going to have old wine in new bottles. Let me give you an example of that, because it's already happening. One of the fundamental components of the community mental health program today is the walk-in clinic. Originally, the walk-in clinic was supposed to be an effective way of dealing with the problem of waiting lists, referrals, and immediacy of service. The doors were supposed to be open twenty-four hours a day. Now I know that in many of the new community mental health clinics the walk-in clinics are becoming brief psychotherapy clinics. They are no longer walk-in clinics. They are becoming brief psychotherapy clinics because the people who man them only know psychotherapy. There is the problem of what we are going to do about the skills of the people who are going to man the new community mental health centers. They've spent a lot of years getting training. They have a great deal at stake in practicing these skills, and they're going to practice what they know. Somebody mentioned in our earlier discussions, meeting with a group of architects to design community mental health centers. Psychiatrists are telling them what their needs are, from which the architects are going to design buildings. I hope that these new buildings are only going to have one door. I'll tell you why. If a center has an emergency clinic, a walk-in clinic, and an outpatient center, there is a danger that if you walk into the emergency clinic, you will get hospitalized. If you walk into the walk-in clinic, you will get brief psychotherapy. If you walk into the outpatient clinic, you will get long-term psychotherapy. This is what is going to happen if we are not careful. The type of treatment people will get is going to depend on what door they walk into.

Another difficulty: the question of treatment techniques and how we approach the treatment of low-income people. This has often been conceptualized as crisis-oriented therapy. Now, if you examine everything that's been written on crisis-oriented therapy, you will find something interesting. The crisis is always in the individual. Nobody ever stops to think about whether there might be a crisis in the environment, in society, in the community. This is related to another problem. When I talk to social psychiatrists about social process, I find myself not talking the same language because what they mean by social process is interpersonal. Social to them is equivalent with the word interpersonal; and if they talk about social process, they're talking about something interpersonal. The fact that there's a society out there in which these interpersonal interactions take place gets little or no consideration.

There is another important development today, which is outside of the institutionalized community mental health movement, which has great potential as a competitor. The poverty program has a lot of shortcomings. I don't think it's going to wipe out poverty, and I think that a lot of the things it is doing are meaningless; but the community action program of the poverty movement, it seems to me, is going to play a crucial role in community mental health on the primary prevention level. And, it is in a much better position to succeed because it isn't bogged down by the ideology of psychiatry. Let me give you some of the principles upon which it is operating now, and you will see how it fits in much more closely with the ideology of low-income groups. The poverty movement addresses itself to the normal. It doesn't talk about sick people. The goal of the poverty movement, and particularly the community action program, is self-determination—not self-actualization. It focuses on coping techniques, not on psychodynamics. In brief, it is free of many of the characteristics of the mental health professional's ideology that make for alienation. Clinical training can be an impediment in working with the poor. A typical clinical judgment, which is more of a value judgment, is that the poor are apathetic. The poor are not apathetic at all. There is a very small section of the poor that might be termed apathetic, but the poor are busily engaged in a severe struggle for existence on a personal activist level. There are different sections of the poor that have different coping styles. That is true. There are those who are able to cope with the problem on a social level by joining social organizations such as the indigenous ethnic groups, or trade unions, or other forms of social organizations. There is a small group among the poor who struggle that way. Then there is a large group who conduct a personal activist struggle. They go down to the Welfare Department and they fight for what they think they should have. There are many mothers on ADC who conduct a successful struggle to raise six, seven, eight, nine kids without a man in the house. Then there are the delinquents and the criminals who certainly are not apathetic. They are struggling in an antisocial personal activist way. And then again, there is a very small group of the poor who *are* apathetic, so we must be very careful when we talk about the apathy of the poor.

Another aspect of the poverty program that is very important is the way they have bought the idea of the indigenous nonprofessional (Reiff & Riessman, 1964). The indigenous nonprofessional is viewed as a technique, first of all, for reaching the poor and, secondly, as a technique for introducing institutional change. The indigenous nonprofessionals are people who are recruited from the ranks of those we want to help. We've had a lot of experience with that kind of work in Alcoholics Anonymous. Certainly, they are much more successful than psychiatry. We see some programs that appear to be having some success with drug addiction, and this is just one small part of it. The new indigenous nonprofessional is important, first of all, because he serves as a communication link between the middle-class professional and the poor and, secondly, because the nature of his relationship can be different from that of the professional.

Maybe I ought to review this aspect of it because it seems to me significant. It has implications for the training of clinical psychologists. I've had a lot of experience in interviewing psychologists and psychiatric residents for admission to programs. I usually ask, "Why do you want to be a psychologist?" or "Why do you want to be a psychiatrist?" Inevitably, I get the answer, "Because I like to help people." On the other hand, when I talk to the indigenous nonprofessionals and ask them the same question, they also answer, "Because I like to help people." On the surface it appears that the motivation is the same; but if you pursue it further, you find a very interesting difference. The middle-class professional, when he says he likes to help people, means that helping others is a humanitarian principle on which he would like to base his life. He means that he is interested in actualizing himself and that helping others is a means of actualizing himself. That's why he likes to help others. There is an element of noblesse oblige in this concept. On the other hand, the indigenous nonprofessional, when he says he likes to help others, tells you, "Well, why not, some day I might need help. I'll help him today; tomorrow he'll help me." It is a quid pro quo type of relationship, while the relationship between the professional and the low-income person is reciprocal because the professional has an expertise that the low-income person doesn't have. All of which makes for a very important, crucial, difference in the things that an indigenous nonprofessional can do and the things that a professional can do. The indigenous nonprofessional is also important because it's at least a partial solution to the problem of manpower. The poverty movement expects to have some two thousand indigenous nonprofessionals by the end of the year. Frank Riessman and Art Pearl and some of the others who have been working in this area have estimated that there is room in America, if you consider all the human services, for something like three or four million indigenous nonprofessionals.

The use of the indigenous nonprofessional poses some problems for the professional. He must prepare himself to be in a position to supervise, to consult, and to act as an administrator. Administration now becomes an important aspect of a psychologist's function. I would like to tell you about one program at the Lincoln Hospital Neighborhood Service Center. It will illustrate how the indigenous nonprofessional can be used in mental health programs. I think this is the only mental health program in the United States like this. They are opening up Neighborhood Service Centers, that is, store fronts, in the neighborhoods of the poor. The first store is manned by eight nonprofessionals who have been recruited from that neighborhood, and who have gone through a period of three weeks training. The director of the neighborhood service center is a clinical psychologist, and that's the only professional person that ever gets around there, except the visitors from all over the country who come to look at the place. But the indigenous nonprofessionals run the place and do all the work. In the course of six weeks they have had three hundred applications for service. What kind of service? you ask, and some of you, I think, will be surprised because you will find it hard to imagine how this can be called mental health work. I talked to the clinical psychologist in charge and asked her, in preparation for this talk tonight, "How does your clinical background prepare you for what you're doing?" She told me the following:

Here's a case where a woman comes in and asks for help in finding a camp for her six kids. Incidentally, we find out that she has two other kids in the state hospital. Now, I don't know if this is a problem for this woman or not, but my tendency as a clinical psychologist is to sit her down and start exploring this and finding out what we can do. It must be a disrupted family. But, the indigenous nonprofessional says, "No, let's deal with the problem that she presents." And that's what we're doing, and I'm going along with it.

Whether it will be effective or not, I don't know. But the point I am trying to make is that it may turn out that a clinical background in this kind of program may be an impediment. I am coming to the conclusion that clinical training will very much be an impediment unless we are careful. In programs of this kind, in programs of primary prevention, and maybe even in the community mental health programs where secondary prevention is an important aspect, I am concerned about the function of a clinical background.

Recently, I received a letter from a young student in Berkeley who is getting his degree in social psychology in the next month. It was a beautiful letter, an exciting letter. He was interested in devoting himself to the problem of how to bridge the gap between social and individual psychology. I got so excited about the letter, I looked him up when I was in California. I thought I would like to take this man on as an experiment, training a social psychologist without any clinical background in community mental health. And, that's what we're going to do. We're going to experiment with the training of social psychologists. We made it very clear to him that when he's through with our postdoctoral training program he is not going to be a clinical psychologist. He is not qualified to function as a clinical psychologist. He is going to be a community mental health psychologist, and he will function as such.

I have indicated some dimensions we ought to be thinking about in the training of clinical psychologists. I think we have, however, a multiple task; not just the problem of how to train clinical psychologists for community mental health. We have a number of training problems. We have the problem of how to retrain those who are already clinical psychologists, who are functioning and acting as professional people who want to go into community mental health. That's a problem separate and apart from how to train those who are presently students in clinical programs. There is also the problem of how we are going to train the psychologists of the future. We really have three problems here. One of the things we can do almost at once is to begin to plan, to have meetings, to talk to one another—not just clinical psychologists, I mean social psychologists and many other social scientists—about providing an atmosphere of reciprocal professional relationships in the universities, in the field, in the clinics, and so on. We must begin to provide some kind of medium for a reciprocal exchange between those who have a more socially oriented point of view and those who have a more individualistically oriented one. We must create some sort of mechanism. I don't think that the usual graduate university training program is such a mechanism. I'm not sure that it can be. Perhaps we will have to create a mechanism outside of the university.

We ought to do some experimental work before we make any hard and firm decisions. We should train some social psychologists for community mental health work. We ought to do some experimental work on settings; we don't even know what the proper setting for a community mental health program is: Should it be a state hospital? Should it be a clinic? and so on. We have for a long time been talking about the problem of the specialist versus the generalist. I don't really have time to go into this in detail, but I want to introduce the concept of training for versatility. This is not the same as training a generalist but rather a person who is capable of conceptual versatility, one who is versatile in technique and conceptualization; one who can treat middle-class people psychoanalytically, who can treat low-income people by focusing on coping styles, and who can conceptualize the criteria for making the decisions about how to treat whom.

One final note, and that is that I hope that we will not make the mistake of thinking of ourselves as role models for the future psychologist. My guess is that this is the mistake that was made at the Boulder Conference. At that time those who participated were academicians who were moving into clinical psychology. For them personally it was possible to be both an academician, a scientist, and a clinical psychologist, and in this personal image they structured the whole profession of clinical psychology. Now, those of us who are leaders in community mental health are moving from clinical into community mental health. It's possible for us to do it personally, and it may be possible for any other individual to do it personally, but this is entirely different from creating an institutionalized role. A profession cannot be created by decision alone. Certain social forces are operating, which presently are beyond our control, that may make it impossible.

REFERENCES

Goffman, E. *Asylums*. New York: Anchor Books, 1961.
Klein, D. C. Community needs: A challenge for psychology. Paper presented at the annual meeting of the American Psychological Association, September 1963.

Reiff, R. The mental health education needs of labor. National Institute of Labor Education, Working Paper#2, March 1960.

Reiff, R., and Riessman, F. The indigenous nonprofessional: A strategy of change in community action and community mental health programs. National Institute of Labor Education, Report#3, November 1964.

Reiff, R., and Scribner, S. Issues in the new national mental health program relating to labor and low income groups. National Institute of Labor Education, Report#1, June 1963.

Riessman, F. New approaches to mental health treatment for labor and low income groups. National Institute of Labor Education, Report #2, February 1964.

Rosenbaum. M., and Zwerling, I. Impact of social psychiatry on a psychoanalytically oriented department of psychiatry. *Archives of Gen. Psy.*, 1964, 2, 31–39.

Star, S. The place of psychiatry in popular thinking. Paper presented to the annual meeting of the American Association for Public Opinion Research, Washington, D.C., May 1957.

MENTAL HEALTH PLANNING AND MODEL CITIES: "HAMLET" OR "HELLZAPOPPIN"

3

Roland L. Warren

Those who are old enough to have seen the Broadway hit *Hellzapoppin* know that it was a sparkling comedy with great spontaneity that had a way of exploding beyond the confines of the stage and involving the audience in different and unanticipated ways. In a sense, it was a "happening," much like some of the current new theater that is equally explosive and spontaneous and even more sexy. A far cry indeed from the serious, more carefully programmed, much less spontaneous, more introspective, but equally moving production of classical tragedy, perhaps best typified by *Hamlet*.

The mental health drama today, in the states and communities across America, looks a good deal like *Hellzapoppin*; but it is often approached as though it were *Hamlet*. Somehow, it is recognized that the arena of community planning and decision making is a confused marketplace, that the old prepared scripts no longer get one through to the last curtain call, that there is a good deal more audience participation, that one needs to adapt and improvise, that the old rules of the game no longer apply.

The movement of the patient out of the secluded and controlled atmosphere of the mental hospital is paralleled by the movement of the administrator out of this relatively orderly, predictable, and controllable environment, this total institution, this self-enclosed system, into the lively, competitive, uncontrollable, often unpredictable arena of the community, with its conflicting crosscurrents of interest and its competition for scarce resources and the public's attention to "its own thing."

Several issues characterize the current situation. There is, to begin with, the general issue already alluded to: how to develop community mental health services that will be adequate to the needs of people

An earlier version of this paper was given at the annual NIMH Regional Office Staff Meeting, Dallas, October 21, 1969. The author's work was supported by a research scientist award from NIMH. Stephen M. Rose and Hilary Green helped in the preliminary analysis of the mental health data of the Interorganizational Study. Reprinted from *Community Mental Health Journal*, 1971, 7, 39–49. Dr. Warren, a sociologist, is Professor of Community Theory, Florence Heller Graduate School for Advanced Studies in Social Welfare, Brandeis University, Waltham, Massachusetts.

today. That is perhaps the overriding issue, in the face of federal budget cuts and a constant problem of relative apathy at the community level regarding mental health needs.

There is the whole issue of how mental health agencies are to win a greater voice in community-level planning, the underlying challenge of what competencies they offer for such planning, and how pertinent these competencies are seen to be by other, more firmly established interests and competencies in the community planning arena.

There is the constant, elusive problem of coordination of mental health services with each other—whatever coordination is to mean in the mental health context—and of coordination of mental health services with other pertinent human services in the community.

There is the issue of the normative mandate for citizen participation, the lack of clarity as to the appropriate roles for citizens, and the sense of reluctance to relinquish any substantive power in decision making to laymen.

There is the long-standing issue as to whether community mental health should balance its concern for individual mental illness with a concern for a social environment that is more positively conducive to mental health, and whether the responsible mental health professional should become an initiating agent of social change, and, if so, how and in what direction.

There is the dilemma as to whether mental health professionals can maintain a mantle of scientific impartiality while at the same time seeking to influence community-level decisions in health, education, and welfare.

And, finally, there is a whole set of constraints operating on mental health professionals if they seek to expand their role beyond the mere provision of clinical services—constraints that deal with their own limitations in an expanded social action role; public misconceptions about the nature of mental health and mental illness, as well as internal dissension among professionals; constraints of the meager knowledge-base supporting active intervention at the community level, and on through a long list. These issues take on special importance in the Model Cities program.

The Model Cities Planning Process

Most cities of any size have a number of identifiable city-level organizations, whether governmental or nongovernmental, through which decisions are made regarding new developments on behalf of the community. A current research project at Brandeis University is designed to gain information on how these "community decision organizations" behave in their respective spheres of interest and legitimated scope, what accounts for some of the important differences among them, and how they behave with respect to each other, particularly where their interests overlap. The project is predicated on the assumption that, in American society, much of our ability to influence the course of events and the shape of things to come in local communities—however modest this influence may be—takes place in and around such community decision organizations, and, hence, their importance.

A specific cluster of such community decision organizations—or CDO's, for short—has therefore been chosen in nine different cities across the country. The CDO's under study are the board of education, the health and welfare council, the antipoverty community action program, the urban renewal agency, the Model Cities agency, and the relevant organization in mental health, where there is one. The study investigates the interaction of these organizations with each other, especially in relation to the developing Model Cities program in these nine cities.

The Model Cities program has particular relevance to the community mental health field for a number of reasons.

In each city, it presents a live drama of interagency turmoil as specific plans are worked out along the broad scope of concerns including housing, health, recreation, employment, transportation, urban renewal, dependency, crime and delinquency, and so on. To develop a coordinated comprehensive program in all these fields is a gigantic task— perhaps impossible in any meaningful sense. The planning process explodes beyond the usual bureaucratic channels of decision making, as agencies and interests become involved in a highly volatile give-and-take negotiation, often for high stakes.

It also has direct pertinence to the poor people in the community, people who do not relate readily to conventional mental health agencies and who, according to numerous studies, receive differential diagnosis and differential treatment when they do. They are people for whom a vague concept like mental health may be difficult to grasp or take seriously, in comparison with issues like housing, jobs, income maintenance, schools, and so on.

What further complicates the Model Cities planning process is the mandated "widespread citizen participation." Mental health agencies have not been among the leaders in developing innovative ways of affording meaningful citizen participation in major decision making, and the whole concept splits the psychiatric profession.

Again, mental health is somewhat peripheral to the concept of improving the quality of urban life. Or is it? And if it is more than peripheral, what is its role? Significantly, mental health was not mentioned specifically in the basic Model Cities legislation but first appeared under the health category in the implementing administrative guidelines developed by the HUD Model Cities Administration. Since it was not specifically mandated for the Model Cities program in each city, it was therefore an open question as to which cities would include important mental health components in their Model Cities planning, and how and why this would happen, or how and why it would not happen.

In a report in the *Journal of the American Institute of Planners*, an account was given of the planning process for Model Cities in the nine cities under study (Warren, 1969). Briefly, it was found that although various CDO's such as those under study had participated in the initial stages of the planning, they were soon eclipsed by the vigorous struggle that took place in many cities in regard to the respective rights and prerogatives of the residents of the Model Neighborhoods vis-à-vis City Hall, with the CDO's coming back into the turmoil later as priorities emerged and specific program descriptions had to be written up and program components allocated to one agency or another. A rapid, volatile, sometimes cooperative, sometimes conflicting process took place in which decisions were made, priorities set, and programs developed not in anything that would correspond to a model of rational or bureaucratic planning, but rather in a tug-and-haul of conflicting interests, partial information, pressing deadlines, federal and state constraints and inputs of various types, and the struggle of each agency to protect or enhance its domain. Out of this process a series of specific programs emerged in each city that looked more like a laundry list than a comprehensive, integrated program such as had been envisioned in the legislation.

Model Cities is not the only developmental program of importance in the communities today. There will be others tomorrow, one can be sure. But in a sense it is highly representative, symbolic, and important for people operating programs at the community level. It dramatizes, as no other program has yet done, the turmoil, the rivalry, the political finesse, the uncertain publics, the rapid adaptation, the increasing permeability of organizational boundaries, the overlapping interests, the operation, negotiation, and conflict that characterize decision making in the human services field today. So it is pertinent to ask: How did mental health agencies behave in this rapidly moving community planning situation?

Mental Health Agencies and Model Cities Planning

In this phase of the study, adequate data were available from only eight of the nine cities, and so this account is limited to those eight. In only one of these cities the mental health CDO was fairly active throughout the planning stage for the Model Cities program (by "planning stage" is meant the period from May, 1967, to January, 1969).

In five of the eight cities there was virtually no participation by mental health agencies in the planning activities for the Model Cities program.

In these five cities, the project's field research associates reported what might best be termed "organizational reticence" with respect to the Model Cities program, either indicating lack of interest, or a willingness to participate, but only "if asked."

In one city, the Model Cities plan that arose during the period of intensive planning stated that "some hope exists for increased mental health activities provided local Mental Health and Mental Retardation leaders become interested in the Model Neighborhood area."

It should be recalled that mental health was not specifically mentioned in the legislation, and it is easy to understand how a clinically oriented mental health administrator might not think of the Model Cities program as relevant to his immediate concerns. Yet, here was a broad-gauged attempt to enhance the quality of urban life, one that clearly got over into the field of health and social services, recreation, education, and so on. It constituted an opportunity for mental health participation, if the mental health agencies were interested. Whether or not they should have been is perhaps a debatable question.

One thing that caught the attention of the research staff was that the mental health agency officials seemed to be carrying over into the community planning arena a clinical approach to their own role, especially the idea that the "patient" must be the one to take the initiative, to ask for help. Just as they would not go out aggressively seeking patients in private practice, they would not go out aggressively seeking a greater role for mental health in interorganizational planning. This clinical approach to developmental planning constituted a severe constraint on the mental health administrator.

The data indicated that mental health agencies had little political power at the level of City Hall, even as compared with the other CDO's being studied intensively. The Model Cities program is a city-level program, operated under the city's authority and concentrated in a particular designated neighborhood that in most cases does not exceed one-tenth of the city's population. Hence, the two focal levels of decision making are at the city level and at the Model Neighborhood level. Political influence at the City Hall level would seem to depend—as at other levels—on three things: (1) An organized constituency that can be called upon for support at crucial points of contest; (2) a network of interorganizational and political connections, built up over time and out of joint experience in intensive working together—or even conflicting with each other—on numerous occasions in the past; (3) an alertness for the opportunity that can be exploited to advance the purposes the agency serves and a skill in operating effectively in the interagency and political field.

In cities of over two hundred thousand the catchment area concept appeared to place the mental health agencies at a disadvantage in Model Cities planning. To the extent that stress is put on community mental health centers as focal units of planning, it leaves their interrelationship within the city, and their aggregate interest in and participation in city-wide policy making, highly problematic. In the cities studied, the community mental health center catchment areas were typically not organized systematically at the city level for city-level planning. Nor did they correspond to the Model Neighborhood boundaries—so that two, three, or even four catchment areas might extend into part of a particular Model Neighborhood.

The absence of a viable mental health CDO at the city level in practically all of the cities studied has much to do with the relative ineffectiveness of mental agencies in city-level planning. This was encountered early in the field study, when the field research associates in the individual cities rapidly and without difficulty identified and began establishing contact with the board of education, the antipoverty agency, the urban renewal authority, and the health and welfare council, by whatever names they went. But from city after city there came the queries: There is no mental health CDO; how shall we proceed? Or, there are three organizations, each with some claim to being the mental health CDO; which shall I choose?

The project's definition of a community decision organization is an organization that is legitimated for planning and/or program activities in a particular sector of community interest at the community level. To repeat, it was not difficult to find such organizations in the other fields covered by the study. Seldom was there an organization that had the clear mandate to plan for and develop and speak for mental health services at the community level. And where such an organization existed, it often was an integral part of county government rather than city government, thus having little direct administrative relationship to the city government.

Obviously, special organizations with planning and administrative prerogatives governing their geographic jurisdiction cannot be set up for every possible level of geographic inclusion, including the Model Neighborhood level. Perhaps the city level for decision making is not so important in other concerns of mental health agencies. In the Model Cities program, it was crucial.

But again, it was not only a question of the level at which an organization was found that could "speak for" a particular sector of activity with some authoritativeness. It was also a question of the extent to which such decision making was organized within the sector of interest. There was relatively little organization of the various mental health agencies at any level at all; rather, except within a specifically funded community mental health center, the picture was one of a number of independent agencies, each with its own constituency, public or private, each going its own way, serving its own clientele, with little indication of a sense of aggregate responsibility for the mental health of the people of the city.

These remarks, as well as other findings regarding mental health participation in Model Cities, should be taken in the context of a frank recognition that mental health, after all, was not *the* crying issue in Model Cities—though if people occasionally become so desperate and frustrated that they take to burning down their own neighborhoods, it would seem that even a most narrow conception of mental health and mental illness would recognize a pertinence to what mental health agencies are trying to do.

Nevertheless, not only was mental health not mentioned in the original legislation for Model Cities, but even after it was specified as an area of interest and activity in the program guidelines, a study of the priorities given to various possible goals in the Model Cities program indicated that mental health was third from the bottom in a list of ten, being exceeded in apathy only by transportation and recreation. Richard H. Uhlig, the research director of the Model Cities research project, did a special study in which he asked CDO personnel at three different levels—policy-making, administrative, and professional operation—to assign priorities to various goal conceptions of the program. He found that in these cities, as might be expected, employment, education, and housing headed the list (Uhlig, 1969).

Attitudes of Mental Health Personnel

Mental health was given a low priority by almost everyone. But interestingly enough, the relevance of the Model Cities program to mental health was seen differently by top agency executives from different types of CDO's in the cities being studied. Robert A. Porter, a doctoral candidate at the Florence Heller Graduate School for Advanced Studies in Social Welfare at Brandeis University, did a study in ten cities, including the nine cities of the larger study, in which he compared the assessments of Model Cities, the community mental health ideology, and the constraints affecting the efficacy of mental health personnel in a community planning role (Porter, 1970). He examined different responses on these questions among different levels of mental health agency personnel, such as top management, middle management, operating personnel, and policy board. He also compared mental health agency top management personnel with top management personnel of the other CDO's of the study as to their assessments of mental health's relevance to Model Cities, their community mental health ideology, and their conception of constraints on mental health personnel in community planning.

In comparing the five CDO groups in their assessment of the potential of the Model Cities program for reducing the incidence of mental illness, he found that mental health administrators, in aggregate, were somewhat less optimistic than most of the administrators from other agencies. He found that their assessment of the capacity of mental health professionals to contribute to Model Cities planning was just about the same as the assessment by officials of other CDO's. He then took the difference between what respondents felt that the Model Cities program might accomplish in reducing mental illness and emotional disorder on the one hand, and what the mental health disciplines might contribute to planning efforts toward that end on the other. This gave him an indication of the confidence that these officials had in the ability of mental health professionals to contribute to Model Cities planning. On this measure, with one exception, every single one of the other types of organizational officials had more confidence in the mental health professionals' ability to contribute to Model Cities planning than did the mental health officials themselves. The exception to this was the board of education officials, who had less confidence than mental health officials.

We see, then, a group of mental health agency leaders who have less optimism about the Model Cities program's potential for reducing mental disorder than do most of their peers in other CDO's and less confidence in their own ability to contribute meaningfully to Model Cities planning. If we are to return to our analogy—and perhaps we shouldn't—we see here a cast of characters who are more qualified for the Hamlet role, and who show Hamlet's degree of indecision, being pushed unwillingly out onto the stage in the midst of *Hellzapoppin*.

Porter (1970) also asked his respondents to assess a number of constraints, barriers, or other restricting factors that might affect the participation of mental health professionals in a community planning project such as the Model Cities program. He gave them a list of fourteen different possible constraints. The following is quoted from his findings:

> The majority of respondents in all five agency groups are foremost in their agreement that the underprivileged residents of urban

slum areas perceive little relevance in traditional mental health services to their needs, and that major decision makers in the community do not acknowledge or support a very active role for mental
health professionals in community social planning. The majority in all
groups also are in agreement that there *is* an appreciable relationship
between the social problems of the urban ghetto and the incidence of
mental illness; and that the planning of community programs aimed
at the prevention of social stress is fundamentally the same task as
the planning of programs for the prevention of mental illness.

The comparison of mental health agency administrators with administrators of such agencies as health and welfare councils, urban renewal
authorities, antipoverty agencies, and boards of education is enlighten-
ing. Porter developed, tested, and validated a community mental health
ideology scale on which twenty-six different items later discriminated
significantly between mental health agency administrators and the administrators of these other agencies. His scale is made up of a number of
dimensions, some of which are highly pertinent to the present discussion. They provide an indication of the orientation of mental health officials in these ten cities with respect to some of the issues raised earlier
in this paper.

One of the dimensions of his scale assessed the respondents' viewpoint with regard to a stress on bringing about change within the individual patient or bringing about change in the social system. There
were nine items in this subscale. Mental health administrators were
more inclined toward the individual change approach than were most
administrators of these other CDO's. With the exception of the board of
education administrators, all the others—the urban renewal, health and
welfare council, and antipoverty agency administrators—stressed social
system change in mental health more than did the mental health administrators.

Five items went into a subscale relating to degree of politicalization
of the planning process. On these items, exactly the same pattern was
shown, with mental health administrators stressing the political aspects
of the planning process less than most of the other agency administrators.

The other subscales included citizen participation, bureaucratic versus collegial administrative orientation, and interdisciplinary management of mental health centers. All five dimensions were given their
appropriate weightings in the overall "community mental health planning ideology scale." In the responses to this total scale, the same
pattern applied, with mental health administrators being on the conservative side, exceeded only by the boards of education.

Porter's scale, incidentally, was made up from actual substantive statements by acknowledged leaders in the community mental health movement and showed a high degree of validity in discriminating between known groups. There is thus some substantiation for saying that, insofar as these ten cities are representative, most leaders of community decision organizations such as those included in the Model Cities study are more firmly convinced of the community mental health point of view than are the top administrative echelons of the mental health agencies themselves. Returning again to the dramatic analogy it might be said that the *Hellzapoppin* characters are telling local mental health administrators: "Come on out onto the stage; we want you!" while the mental health administrators are standing in the wings, pondering to themselves: "To be, or not to be?"

As a dramatic example of the extent to which this is true, one of the items not finally used in the scale but filled out by the respondents stated: "Community mental health programs should give first priority to broad programs of social intervention and reserve individual treatment for particular instances where these larger approaches fail." "The mental health group [was] on the disagreement side of this issue, while all other agency groups [were] on the agreement side."

As a sideline, the question might be raised as to the difference it makes whether the top administrative staff members are psychiatrists, psychologists, or social workers. Porter found no significant differences between psychologists and social workers in the total score on the mental health ideology scale, but very strong and significant differences between both groups and the psychiatrists. Thus, psychiatrists as a group are much less convinced supporters of the community mental health approach as assessed in the twenty-six items of the scale than are the nonpsychiatric professionals. Since psychiatrists are more numerous among the top administrators, they are the ones who pull the comparative scores down. In this connection, it is also interesting to note that psychiatrists who operate at other levels than top management have higher community mental health scores than do top management psychiatrists. In any event, the group scores of psychologists and social workers are much higher than those of psychiatrists, and, indeed, they are higher than the administrators of all other CDO's except the antipoverty agencies.

The Importance of Model Cities

To be sure, not all people live in cities, fewer yet live in Model Cities, and not all of community mental health is subsumed under Model Cities. There are state and county governments, catchment areas that stretch across the countryside, and a whole kaleidoscope of pieces and parts that relate in one fashion or another to the possibilities for a viable program of community mental health centers and to the larger question of the administration of mental health services.

But two things can be said very specifically in support of the importance of programs like Model Cities and how well mental health agencies muster their resources to consider them and to participate if appropriate.

First, like many such programs, Model Cities is a program in which city-level decision making is crucial. It thus provides an occasion for review of the extent to which catchment area centers and county and other governmental unit planning boards are appropriate for the numerous programs in employment, manpower, poverty, education, urban renewal, housing, and other fields, each with a more or less direct mental health relevance, which are developed and shaped through decision making at the city level.

Second, it represents what is already a widespread situation that may become even more prevalent in the next decade: a planning situation in which fields overlap, in which problems do not sort themselves out by departmental jurisdictions, in which various agencies, services, and interests must find their appropriate place in a mixed process of planning, negotiation, politics, compromise, and pressure out of which program decisions often arise today. The alternative to jumping into this volatile, risky, unpredictable situation is to remain on the sidelines, to be left high and dry, and, possibly, to find one's operational field preempted by other interests and other agencies that are better adapted to the community decision-making process as it takes place in America's communities today.

Citizen Participation

One last item—citizen participation. It is perhaps not necessary to describe how the mental health administrators compared with leaders in urban renewal authorities, boards of education, health and welfare councils, and community antipoverty agencies on their support of citizen participation. They were at the bottom of the list, trailing behind even the urban renewal officials, people who are presumably concerned more with "bricks and mortar" than with social realities.

The research staff's subjective impressions in the study of Model Cities so far are that, to a large extent, the Model Cities programs are developing into long lists of projects that involve the agencies doing essentially the thing they know best how to do. What were to be exciting, innovative programs, intertwined in a manner so as to produce greatest aggregate effectiveness, highly responsive to the expressed interests and needs of disadvantaged citizens, have turned out to be largely more of the same, done by the same people in much the same way. This matter of responding to a problem by doing the one thing one knows how to do best, whether or not it is relevant, is like the traditional concept of "the drunkard's search." The drunkard is on his hands and knees under the lamppost looking for his wallet. "Is this where you lost it?" he is asked. "No," he replies, "but the light's better over here."

If mental health agencies are not to respond like the drunkard, they must be assured that they are not merely doing what they know how to do best, but that their behavior is adapted to the problem at hand. For this purpose they must have a more adequate definition of the problem in disadvantaged areas than a mere indication of agency waiting lists and a table of admissions diagnoses. They must be concerned, if they are serious about community mental health, not merely in expanding this or that cut-and-dried type of service. Rather, they need to know much more about the individual and social situations they are dealing with, so that rather than dictate a cure (which is impossible) they can put their resources at the disposal of the people, to be of aid to them in their search for a better community, including their search for an answer to how they can make the best use of mental health agency resources. It seems difficult to see how this can be done unless a much more meaningful role is developed for citizen decision making regarding mental health facilities.

The Model Cities experience affords an opportunity for reassessment and new approaches to meet new challenges. The next few years will reveal how adequate was the response.

REFERENCES

Porter, R. A. *Community mental health planning ideology of organizational participants in the model cities program.* Doctoral Dissertation, Florence Heller Graduate School for Advanced Studies in Social Welfare, Brandeis University, Waltham, Mass., 1970.

Uhlig, R. H. *Goal conception in the planning phase of the model cities program.* Doctoral Dissertation, Florence Heller Graduate School for Advanced Studies in Social Welfare, Brandeis University, Waltham, Mass., 1969.

Warren, R. L. Model Cities' first round: Politics, planning, and participation. *Journal of the American Institute of Planners,* 1969, 35, 245–252.

THE EMERGENCE OF COMMUNITY DEVELOPMENT CORPORATIONS IN URBAN NEIGHBORHOODS

4

Michael Brower

The most exciting political invention in recent years is the Community Development Corporation, or CDC. In the last few years several dozen CDC's have been created in nonwhite urban ghetto neighborhoods. There are also a few in rural poverty areas, and, more recently, a few have been started in poor white urban areas. Part of the broader movement toward decentralization and local neighborhood control of social and governmental services, the urban CDC is a multipurpose organization, incorporated, usually on a nonprofit basis, and managed and controlled by neighborhood people independently of any municipal or other existing level of government. This paper examines the economic, psychological, and political climate of the urban nonwhite ghettos, concludes that a lack of power in such areas is a fundamental underlying problem, and argues that the CDC is an important and healthy means of creating social and economic benefits and of developing more power in the hands of ghetto residents. A brief account is given of some of the early CDC's, and some conclusions are drawn from their experiences.

The Complex Web of Problems in Low-Income Nonwhite Ghettos

The economic problems of low-income ghettos have received a great deal of study and attention, perhaps because they are the most easily quantified. Unemployment runs twice or three times the national average, and underemployment is much higher; together, these problems

An earlier version of this paper was presented at the March 1970 annual meeting of the American Orthopsychiatric Association in San Francisco. The research was conducted while the author was on the faculty of the MIT Sloan School of Management, part of it with support from the MIT Urban Systems Lab, using funds provided by the Ford Foundation. The author has also benefited greatly from association as a consultant with the staff of the Center for Community Economic Development in Cambridge, which is supported by a grant from the U.S. Office of Economic Opportunity. Reprinted from *American Journal of Orthopsychiatry*, 1971, *41*(4), 656–658. Copyright © 1971, the American Orthopsychiatric Association, Inc. Reproduced by permission. Michael Brower is currently at the Center for International Affairs, Harvard University, Cambridge, Massachusetts.

affect one-quarter to one-half of the ghetto labor force. Thirty-five to forty percent of nonwhite inner-city families had incomes below the poverty level in 1966. Only three to eight percent of Negro males were professional and managerial workers, compared with thirty percent of all employed males in the U.S. (U.S. Department of Labor, 1967, 1968a, 1968b, 1968c, 1969b). Only a small minority of businesses are owned by nonwhites, even in the heart of the ghettos, and these are the smallest and least profitable ones. Capital flows out of the ghettos through white-owned business and banks and white controlled prostitution, numbers, drugs, and other rackets (Clark, 1965; Fusfeld, 1968, 1969). Human capital also flows out if the brightest, healthiest, best educated, most energetic young men leave the ghettos.

Similarly, overcrowded and deteriorating housing has been well documented, as have the low quality and scarcity of health, education, and other social services in ghetto areas (Clark, 1965; Report of the National Advisory Commission on Civil Disorders, 1968).

Recently social scientists have analyzed the devastating psychological impacts of the pressures and conditions of the ghetto, and the compounding, multiplying effects of prejudice and racism. Kenneth Clark (1965, p. 63) wrote:

It is now generally understood that chronic and remediable social injustices corrode and damage the human personality, thereby robbing it of its effectiveness, of its creativity, if not its actual humanity. . . . Since every human being depends upon his cumulative experience with others for clues as to how he should view and value himself, children who are consistently rejected understandably begin to question and doubt whether they, their family, and their group really deserve no more respect from the larger society than they receive. These doubts become the seeds of a pernicious self- and group-hatred, the Negro's complex and debilitating prejudice against himself.

Clark went on to relate the then widespread use of hair straighteners, bleachers, and other ways of trying to make oneself look "whiter," the high rates of homocide, suicide, delinquency, drug addiction, crime, and family instability to these results of injustice, rejection, and enforced segregation.

Black psychiatrists (Grier & Cobbs, 1968; Pinderhughes, 1966, 1968a, 1968b; Poussaint, 1966, 1967) have analyzed the psychological impacts of slavery, racism, prejudice, segregation, and the ghetto environment. Alvin Poussaint in 1966 (p. 420) summed up the then current results:

The most tragic, yet predictable, part of all this is that the Negro has come to form his self-image and self-concept on the basis of what white racists have prescribed. Therefore, black men and women learn quickly to hate themselves and each other because they are Negroes. . . .

Poussaint goes on to point out, as do other students of poverty (U.S. Department of Labor, 1969a), that low social class and income levels alone have important negative psychological effects, independent of race. But:

. . . being a Negro has many implications for the ego development of black people that are not inherent in lower-class membership. The black child develops in a color caste system and inevitably acquires the negative self-esteem that is the natural outcome of membership in the lowest stratum of such a system. Through contacts with institutionalized symbols of caste inferiority such as segregated schools, neighborhoods, etc., and more indirect negative indicators such as the reactions of his own family, he gradually becomes aware of the social and psychological implications of racial membership. He may see himself as an object of scorn and disparagement, unwanted by the white high caste society, and as a being unworthy of love and affection. Since there are few counter-forces to this negative evaluation of himself, he develops conscious or unconscious feelings of inferiority, self-doubt, and self-hatred.

From that point in early life when the Negro child learns self-hatred, it molds and shapes his entire personality and interaction with his environment. In the earliest drawings, stories, and dreams of Negro children there appear many wishes to be white and a rejection of their own color. They usually prefer white dolls and white friends, frequently identify themselves as white, and show a reluctance to admit that they are Negro. Studies have shown that Negro youngsters assign less desirable roles and human traits to Negro dolls. One study reported that Negro children in their drawings tend to show Negroes as small, incomplete people and whites as strong and powerful [1966, p. 420].

And Oscar Lewis, after lengthy studies in Mexican, Puerto Rican, and Puerto Rican–American slums, reported:

. . . there is a hostility to the basic institutions of what are regarded as the dominant classes. There is hatred of the police, mistrust of government and of those in high positions and a cynicism that extends to the church . . . a strong feeling of fatalism, helplessness, dependence and inferiority [1966].

These problems are all related to the fundamental underlying fact that these ghetto residents lack not only income but also status and power. To be a complete, healthy man in our society has traditionally meant being powerful and productive, exercising power, and being respected for one's power. But black men, unemployed or underemployed, unable to provide adequately for their women and children, or to protect them from the violence of criminals or the racism and brutality of police and other authorities of white society, feel impotent and powerless, and this penetrates to the core of masculine self-esteem, identity, ambition, and hope. Ghetto residents who have no savings and own no property have no reserve power for emergencies, no potential for becoming wealthy, or to even feel some degree of financial security. They lack the basic currency of respect and authority determined and measured by a capitalistic society. As one black ghetto resident said:

> A lot of times, when I'm working, I become despondent as hell and I feel like crying. I'm not a man, none of us are men! I don't own anything. I'm not a man enough to own a store; none of us are [Clark, 1965, p. 1].

In the words of Lord Acton's famous warning, "Power tends to corrupt and absolute power corrupts absolutely." White middle- and upper-class Americans have been preoccupied with these dangers for centuries, blindly and blissfully unaware that it can be equally valid that a *lack of power* tends to corrupt. The psychological effects described above are the form of corruption that overtakes human beings and communities when they suffer from the lack of power over the basic forces and decisions that shape their lives. They develop, in the words of Poussaint, "conscious or unconscious feelings of inferiority, self-doubt, and self-hatred," and feel, as Lewis reported, "hostility, hatred, mistrust, fatalism, helplessness, dependence, and inferiority."

And if a lack of power is corrupting, then total lack of power is *absolutely* corrupting. The person totally lacking in power escapes into a world of complete apathy or fantasy, or he may erupt into violence, unlimited by any fear of consequences. Writing of the 1964 Harlem riot, Clark wrote:

> The Negro seemed to feel nothing could happen to him that had not happened already; he behaved as if he had nothing to lose. His was an oddly controlled rage that seemed to say, during those days of social despair, We have had enough. The only weapon you have is bullets. The only thing you can do is to kill us [1965, p. 16].

Collectively, as well as individually, the ghetto residents lack power. They have, or had until recently, no control or even influence over the schools that provide "death at an early age" (Kozol, 1967) for their children. Police protection is often nonexistent or blatantly (and sometimes violently) discriminatory against them. Murders go uninvestigated. Dope pushers operate openly, as do numbers runners and pimps. Nonwhite ghettos are unable to procure their fair share of other basic city services, including trash and garbage removal, and street repairs and cleaning. Fire insurance was, until recently, impossible to obtain for many ghetto-owned businesses; theft insurance still is. Playgrounds are scarce and littered with broken glass, their equipment broken and unrepaired.

White middle-class society has traditionally blamed all of these problems more on the black morals, or lack thereof, than on their true causes—poverty, discrimination, prejudice, and the lack of black power. This sentiment is sometimes shared by middle-class blacks, such as the woman who urged Harlem mothers to organize a community group to buy brooms and sweep the filthy streets. Kenneth Clark (1965, p. 56) correctly wrote about this woman:

She did not understand that it is not the job of the people to sweep the streets; it is the job of the Department of Sanitation. It had not occurred to her to advise these women to organize to gain these services to which they were entitled. In a middle-class neighborhood, the people see to it that government does provide services. To lecture the miserable inhabitants of the ghetto to sweep their own streets is to urge them to accept the fact that the government is not expected to serve them. But to force the government to provide sanitation and care is an effort beyond their capacity, for, in such ghettos, people are so defeated that their sense of powerlessness becomes a reality. They are immobilized against action even in their own behalf.

The Creation of Community Development Corporations

Over the past decade or so, local leaders in dozens of ghettos have become increasingly aware of these complex interrelated causes and have arrived at some or all of the following conclusions about cures for their problems, although they would not necessarily phrase them in these terms or this order:

1. A solution to the problems of ghettos and the underlying white racism cannot be found through the escape of a small proportion of the most successful blacks into integrated middle-class communities, leaving behind the vast majority of ghetto residents.

2. The treatment of the economic needs and psychological problems of individual ghetto residents, important though it is, can never bring about a cure for the basic underlying social problems. When the vast majority of residents of an area suffer similar problems, the pathology is social, not individual, and it must be treated as such.

3. Ghetto residents need to wield power, both for what that power will secure in rights and services and for the enhancement in pride, stature, dignity, and self-confidence that comes with wielding power. These changes among blacks and the wielding of power by blacks will in turn confront, contradict, undermine, and reduce white prejudice.

4. Individuals acting alone cannot obtain or wield much power unless they have great wealth or great charisma. Organizations are needed in the ghettos to develop, consolidate, wield, and enhance power.

For these reasons, during the early years of the 1960s (and in some cases ten or twenty years before that), ghetto leaders built organizations to attack a variety of the social needs and problems of their neighbors. But usually these organizations sought a single objective or a very few objectives, such as blocking urban renewal, fighting gouging landlords, boycotting selected stores or businesses, or seeking jobs. Sometimes these organizations survived and added new purposes, but often they folded after winning or losing their original objectives.

Then in the latter years of the 1960s two other ideas began to achieve widespread support:

5. To attack successfully the many interrelated problems of ghetto poverty it is necessary to make coordinated attacks on several basic parts of the problem at once. This requires multipurpose development organizations controlled by ghetto residents.

6. Outside funding for ghetto organizations, whether from government or foundation sources, is temporary and uncertain at best, always subject to outside influences and pressures from donor agencies and likely to be cut off whenever the organization begins to challenge traditional power relationships. Consequently, these ghetto organizations need to develop some permanent sources of income under their own control.

So it was that evolving out of earlier, simpler forms of organizations, because of ideas and understanding such as these, there was born the Community Development Corporation, or CDC. Under a variety of names and organizational forms, the CDC's usually, although not always: (1) are organized by leaders in a neighborhood with a specific geographical area and a specific ethnic (sometimes white) community as a base; (2) are set up as nonprofit corporations; (3) have a variety of economic and social objectives, with the underlying more controversial goal of building power implicit, less openly expressed, and perhaps at times unrecognized; (4) have provisions for considerable local participation in the management and ultimate control; (5) develop and maintain a number of economic enterprises in which the CDC starts with 100 percent ownership and maintains at least a strong minority position, in part to promote development of the community and in part to provide funds for the CDC when profits develop sufficiently.

Structures and Activities of Community Development Corporations [1]

East Central Citizens Organization (ECCO), Columbus, Ohio (Kotler, 1969a, 1969b; Miller, 1969)

ECCO, perhaps the first of the neighborhood CDC's, was set up in 1965 as a nonprofit tax-exempt corporation to serve an area of about one square mile with over 6500 residents, about 70 percent of whom are black. It received a donation of a settlement house from a local (formerly white) church, assistance from the National Council of Churches and the Stern Family Fund, and, beginning in 1966, federal Office of Economic Opportunity (OEO) grants that to date have totalled about $750,000.

ECCO's membership is open to anyone in the area over sixteen, of whom there are about 4200. Total membership is said to be about 1500, of whom 100 to 200 turn out for the annual assembly. ECCO is governed by a council of thirty community people, fourteen elected by the annual assembly (of whom four must be teenagers), and four elected from each of the four neighborhood clubs that founded ECCO.

The early activities of ECCO dealt with social services and mild pressures on the municipal government: daycare, equipment for a tot lot, reprimanding a policeman, better sanitation services, legal services, more foot patrolmen, family planning information, and a Youth Civic Center (YCC) for teenagers. Besides offering recreation facilities, YCC runs job training and placement and remedial education programs. Then, in 1968, the ECCO Development Corporation was set up to promote housing and business developments programs, which are now getting under way.

---

[1] This section is based primarily on extensive field trips and personal interviews. Other sources were newspaper articles, annual reports, and other unpublished materials from the CDC's, as well as the published sources cited. Especially useful is the descriptive CDC directory published by the Center for Community Economic Development (1971), 1878 Massachusetts Ave., Cambridge 02140. Since this paper was written, the Twentieth Century Fund has published a book by Geoffrey Faux (1971) that is now the best single source of information available about CDC's.

The Bedford-Stuyvesant Corporations (Bedford-Stuyvesant Restoration Corporation and Bedford-Stuyvesant D & S Corporation, 1969; Inner City Development Corporation 1969; Kennedy, 1967; Tobier, 1968)

The biggest of the CDC's, and among the most successful, Bedford-Stuyvesant is also one of the most conservative. Set up by Robert Kennedy in the spring of 1967, it has two side-by-side nonprofit corporations that operate out of the same set of offices in the nation's second largest black ghetto. The white organization, D & S Corporation, has a blue chip Wall Street board and is run by former Assistant Attorney General John Doar. The black organization, Bedford-Stuyvesant Restoration Corporation, has a chairman, State Supreme Court Justice Thomas Jones, and a President, Former Deputy Police Commissioner of New York Franklin Thomas, generally considered to be solid citizens of the establishment.

Financed by a variety of foundation grants and by the largest of the OEO Title I-D Special Impact grants totalling nearly $20 million by 1970, the Bedford-Stuyvesant corporations have an impressive list of accomplishments to their credit:

1. An economic development program had assisted forty-three individual Bedford-Stuyvesant businesses in obtaining $4.3 million in financing, with job creation of 1160 by the end of 1969.

2. IBM set up a new computer cable factory in an old warehouse, which employs over two hundred people. According to one news account, many of these employees were formerly employed and were not hard-core unemployed.

3. The exteriors of 1466 row houses on thirty-five blocks have been renovated at an average cost equivalent (if done by outside contractors) of $450 per house, with property value increases as high as $1000 per house, but with a charge to the homeowner of only $25. Previously unemployed residents, 2235 of them, were trained in painting, carpentry, masonry, and landscaping for this work, and about 70 percent have gone on to other permanent employment. Homeowners, to qualify for renovation, had to organize a block association, in which 50 percent of the residents on the block agreed to participate. A total of 275 blocks did so and applied for renovation—about one-half of all the blocks in Bedford-Stuyvesant. The lucky thirty-five blocks were chosen by lottery from among the 275 applicants.

4. Eighty Manhattan banks and financial institutions have been persuaded to set up a mortgage pool of $100 million for home mortgages in Bedford-Stuyvesant. By the end of 1969, 578 people had applied and 286 loans had been approved for a total of $4,468,000—an average of $15,600 per loan. An additional 102 loans were in process for a total of $1.6 million more.

5. Four run-down homes have been purchased for rehabilitation and sale to area residents, and there are plans for rehabbing as many as two hundred more.

6. Two "Superblocks" have been created—one completed and dedicated—by closing off a street and putting in terraces, benches, and playgrounds where cars formerly ruled supreme.

7. The corporation has purchased 25,000 square feet of land and secured financing to put up a fifty-two–unit six-story apartment building.

8. An abandoned dairy plant was purchased and converted into an attractive modern community center, office building, and headquarters for the Bedford-Stuyvesant corporations. A shopping center–village will be developed around it.

9. The corporations have run a sizeable Opportunities Industrialization Center (OIC) for training of the formerly unemployed.

Other activities have included training Community Planners, running a TV series for half a year, and planning for a community college, which plan has apparently fizzled for lack of funds.

Despite all of this, and more in the planning stage, questions are still raised about this CDC. The results are impressive but very small compared to the size of the task. Bedford-Stuyvesant has 450,000 people in 635 blocks, with unemployment of 6.2 percent and underemployment of 28 percent in 1969; both are surely much higher today. Forty-three percent of the families had incomes under $4000 per year (U.S. Department of Labor, 1968b). The scale and clout of what is needed to cope with such a massive ghetto boggle the imagination, and the twin corporations have certainly not yet turned the area around. And most of the tangible benefits so far have fallen to the middle-class home owners of the area, with very little benefits except for some training and jobs going to the vast lower class. Then, too, the organizational structure of these corporations is anything but democratic. Senator Kennedy himself chose and named the men to serve on both boards—not just the board of white financial bigwigs but also the board of the black corporation, which supposedly represents the community. New board members are not elected by the community; they are named by the present board or its chairman. There is thus built in little direct community participation and absolutely *no* accountability to anyone—except to government grant donors and individual consciences.

The West Side Community Development Corporation
(Ellis, 1969; Miller, 1969b)

Out on the west side of Chicago, in a ghetto including the infamous Ward One, base of both the Mafia and Daley's machine, five grass roots organizations banded together in 1968 to form the West Side Community Development Corporation, or WSCDC. In contrast to Bedford-Stuyvesant, neither the WSCDC nor its member organizations were set up by any white establishment figures. Nor have they any white parallel corporation helping to raise funds or provide services. Barely tolerated originally, they are now under fire from the Daley machine. But they do have one terribly important and impressive thing going for them: They are run by men who represent people of the streets, the poorest, and perhaps the angriest, people of the community.

The WSCDC was formed by five constituent community organizations, several of which are, or operate as, CDC's themselves. There is the Conservative Vice Lords, the outgrowth of a once greatly feared youth gang, which now owns two frozen custard franchises, an ice cream parlor, a pool hall, the African Lion fashion shop, and which promotes a police–community relations program and a black culture and history program. There is the Cobras, two thousand strong in 1967 as a tough street gang, but, by late 1968, also oriented towards business development. The West Side Organization (WSO) started in 1964 and since then has placed over one thousand constituents in jobs, organized a militant welfare union, and claims to have successfully processed 1300 welfare grievances. The WSO publishes a regular newspaper; it runs a Christmas food program, a drug addict program, a community mental health center, and a very successful filling station and McDonald's hamburger franchises. The WSO has a four-man paid staff, large numbers of volunteer workers, and appears to command broad support from the people of the area. The other two constitutent organizations in WSCDC, both born in 1967, are the Student Afro-American Group and the Garfield Organization, which includes neighborhood block groups, high school student groups, and church organizations. The Garfield Organization owns a holding company named Go Forth, Inc., which operates a Midas Muffler franchise, a supermarket, and a couple of restaurants.

With a loan of $250,000 from the Chicago First National Bank, the combined WSCDC has bought an old truck terminal and some new trucks and equipment. WSCDC has a long-term guaranteed price contract for the supply of baled waste paper to the Container Corporation, which is also providing management and technical and moral support. Half the truck terminal will be used for collecting and baling paper; the other half will be used for promoting distribution of black products. If WSCDC can get the contracts, despite Daley's efforts to block it, WSCDC would like to run a newspaper distribution agency. Other projects are being planned; all depend on raising investment capital.

In an area where a direct effort to wrest political power from the machine may be worth a man's life, these tough people of the streets are trying to build instead a base of economic and organizational power with which to better the lives of their people. They are working in an area of twenty square miles, with a population of 400,000 people. This is almost as large as Bedford-Stuyvesant, and the WSCDC leadership appears to be more directly representative of the vast mass of the people in their ghetto than is the management of the Bedford-Stuyvesant Corporations. Yet, so far, they have received little or no government support and only occasional sprinklings of church and corporate aid, except for that of Container Corporation. So, survival and growth are constantly jeopardized by a lack of adequate funding.

The Hough Area Development Corporation (HDC) of Cleveland

HDC operates in one of the poorest ghettos in the nation. Its area is about 2.5 square miles with a population of about sixty thousand. Open unemployment in Hough and other Cleveland black slums went up from 13.7 percent in 1960 to 15.5 percent in 1965, while it was dropping in the rest of the country. At 15.5 percent, it was six and one-half times the rate for Cleveland as a whole, and it is surely higher today. Beyond that, as many as one-half of the people in Hough are subemployed, according to the Labor Department survey (U.S. Department of Labor, 1968a). Median family income dropped 16 percent from 1960 to 1965, while it was rising in Cleveland and the nation as a whole (U.S. Department of Labor, 1967).

HDC was set up in 1968 and received the first Title I-D Special Impact grant from OEO; it later received a second grant for a total of over $3 million.

HDC created Community Products, Inc., (CPI) a wholly owned injection rubber molding plant, that sells to the big auto companies, IBM, and other corporate giants. CPI was not expected to start turning a profit until late 1970 or early 1971 during its second year of operation, at the earliest. But the product is of high quality, the market potential is good, the contracts are coming in, and the outlook seems promising. Half the employees are former welfare mothers. When the operation is profitable, HDC plans to sell part of the stock to its employees and part to local community residents.

HDC's biggest project will be the Martin Luther King, Jr., Plaza, combining a street-level shopping center containing a supermarket, a branch bank to be sold eventually to blacks, and a variety of other black-owned stores, with a project of rental town houses for low-income families above the center. Other HDC programs include the Handyman's Maintenance Services (HMS), which trains hard-core unemployed men and sends them out on maintenance and landscaping jobs, a credit union soon to open, and two McDonald's hamburger franchises. When it becomes profitable shares in HMS will be distributed to its workers.

HDC was started by a black preacher–community leader, DeForest Brown, and the head of Cleveland CORE, Franklyn Anderson, together with forty other outstanding local leaders. On its large board sit representatives of most major community organizations in the area. HDC's achievements to date are real, but still partial, with the full promise yet to be realized. Its experience shows that it takes a long time to put projects together, get them underway, and see them begin to show a profit. But, nevertheless, HDC had earned enough support and power by 1970 to weather a storm of nasty criticism launched by one Cleveland newspaper and to come out with strong backing from diverse elements in Cleveland and a renewal of their federal government grant, after passing through a whole series of searching investigations.

Other Community Development Corporations

For lack of space, I will only mention here a number of the most exciting and promising of the other CDC's. There is the empire of organizations and activities constructed by Reverend Leon Sullivan in Philadelphia (Llorens, 1967; Sullivan, 1969), which grew out of the contributions of ten dollars per week over thirty-six weeks by seven thousand parishioners in his and related churches. Sullivan's projects now include a magnificent shopping center plaza, an apartment house, a garment manufacturing company, an electronics and metals working factory, a nation-wide chain of Opportunities Industrialization Centers for training hardcore unemployed, a program of part-time courses for local businessmen, a training school for black economic development organizers from around the country, and an organization for promoting shopping center development in other cities. There is FIGHT, in Rochester, (Northwestern University School of Business 1967; Ridgeway 1967), with its subsidiary manufacturing organization and other economic projects. FIGHT was founded with help from organizer Saul Alinsky, and it is militant and grassroots controlled—it has had a series of tough political campaigns in which leadership passed to younger hands in fiercly fought open community elections. The Woodlawn organization in Chicago (Brazier, 1969; Silberman, 1964), also organized with Alinsky's help, once militant in fighting the University of Chicago, urban renewal, and slum merchants and in pursuing employment for residents of the area, is now turning towards capital ownership and economic development as goals. Operation Breadbasket in Chicago, led by Jesse Jackson (Ewen, 1968; *Playboy* Interview, 1969), perhaps not, strictly speaking, a CDC, is a nonprofiit organization with many similar objectives to the CDC's and is enjoying tremendous local participation and support for a wide range of economic and social activities. The Real Great Society in Spanish East Harlem is combining community organizing, housing rehabilitation, street schools for high school drop-outs, and the development of a new clothing business. Operation Bootstrap in Los Angeles (*Business Week,* 1967) is run by former civil rights activists who will have no part of federal funds and strings, and who are rapidly building up, besides their other projects, Shindana Toys, with considerable help from Mattel, Inc., the giant toy makers. Shindana proudly announces that its goal is to overcome Mattel's million to one lead and put it out of business. And there are many, many more of these CDC's and CDC-like organizations, in Chicago and Boston, St. Louis and Baltimore, Washington and Roanoke, Seattle and Detroit, and a dozen other cities at least.

Lessons from Experiences with the Community Development Corporation

Some important lessons from this brief experience are:

1. The CDC is a workable, viable form of organizing in the ghetto to promote economic and social development and to some extent to develop political power.

2. These organizations can and do vary tremendously in size and in the area of their constituency. At their largest, in Bedford-Stuyvesant, for example, they could hardly be said to be operating in a single neighborhood. The neighborhood impacts of the Bedford-Stuyvesant Corporations, however, can be seen in their Superblock developments and in their promotion of block organizations in one-half of all the blocks in Bedford-Stuyvesant. For such a large area, perhaps it would be better, as proposed by Rosenbloom (1969), to have a single, large Urban Development Corporation for the area of the city or even the state, and much smaller Local Development Corporations for neighborhoods.

3. It takes a long time to build up a staff of competent people, let them gain experience, study projects, secure financing, find or construct facilities, hire and train employees, find markets, and begin to operate a new ghetto manufacturing operation. From the beginning date of production, it takes two or three years before a solid profit can be expected (Brower, in press; Brower & Little, 1970). Simpler projects and services can get underway in only a year or two; shopping centers, on the other hand, take longer. On the whole, the CDC will probably not generate a significant flow of its own income during its early years.

4. Most CDC's will need sizeable amounts of outside, probably largely governmental, financing for at least five to ten years and perhaps even longer in some cases. So far, only a fraction of the support necessary for significant success has been made available, and this to only a minority of all the CDC's.

5. Success must be measured by a wide range of criteria, difficult though this is, and not just by some simple economic numbers such as amount invested, or number of projects generated, or numbers of employees hired or placed, or profits generated. All of these are important. But since the goals are to promote the general economic, social, and human development, and, ultimately, the total power available in a ghetto, the methods and attacks must be multiple to accomplish this, and so too must be the criteria for measuring success or failure (Brower, 1972).

6. There are very real problems involved in obtaining a high degree of local participation in planning, organizing, managing, staffing, and controlling a CDC. The existing CDC's range from being very strongly involved with the grass roots to being practically isolated from them. And there is probably considerable conflict between emphasizing sophisticated economic and management analysis and leadership on the one hand, and emphasizing continuing participation and involvement of uneducated poor people of the area on the other hand. The former is obviously vital; yet, as Roasbeth Kantor (1968) has warned, without meaningful participation part of the basic purpose of the CDC will be lost, and there is a risk that the CDC will become just another big bureaucratic business out of touch with the alienated people. She has suggested that all employees of the CDC should be members of it, that broad-scale community participation perhaps should be valued above financial profitability, that common community activities involving a great many people should be sought and carried out, and that in larger areas decentralized sub-CDC's might be used. It seems to me important that these and other ideas be tried out because meaningful, continuing, widespread community participation in the activities and control of the CDC is one of the most important needs and difficult challenges the CDC's (and, on a larger scale, all of our institutions) face today.

7. The CDC's alone cannot provide more than a tiny fraction of the employment and the funds for public purposes needed in the ghettos. The ghettos need, as does the rest of the country, a national full-employment policy, adequate national funding for housing, education, and health, and an income floor for every family in the country. Without these programs, no CDC can turn a ghetto around and make it soar, and ghetto development is doomed to failure.

8. Even with highly successful federal programs of full employment, family income support, and funding for social needs, ghetto development will *still* fail unless these and other public and private programs provide adequate support for, plan and carry out programs together with, and channel resources and operations through, indigenous locally controlled neighborhood organizations whose underlying fundamental

purpose is to increase the power exercised by the ghetto residents themselves.

REFERENCES

Bedford-Stuyvesant Restoration Corporation and Bedford-Stuyvesant D & S Corporation. *Annual report 1968.* Bedford-Stuyvesant Restoration and D & S Corporations, Brooklyn, N.Y., 1969.

Brazier, A. M. *Black self-determination: The story of the Woodlawn Organization.* Grand Rapids, Mich.: Eerdmans, 1969.

Brower, M. The criteria for measuring the success of a Community Development Corporation in the ghetto. In S. Doctors and S. Lockwood (Eds.), *Minority economic development: A revolution in the seventies.* New York: Holt, Rinehart and Winston, in press.

Brower, M., and Little, D. White help for black business. *Harvard Business Review,* May–June, 1970, 48(3), 4–16, 163–164.

Business Week. A self-help program stirs a Negro slum. March 25, 1967.

Center for Community Economic Development. *Profiles in community-based economic development.* Cambridge, Mass.: Center for Community Economic Development, 1971.

Clark, K. B. *Dark ghetto.* New York: Harper & Row, 1965.

Desiderio, R. J., and Sanchez, R. G. The Community Development Corporation. *Boston College Industrial and Commercial Law Review,* Winter 1969, Vol. X, No. 2, 218–264.

Ellis, W. W. *White ethics and black power: The emergence of the West Side Organization.* Chicago: Aldine, 1969.

Ewen, G. The "green power" of Operation Breadbasket. *Commerce, Chicagoland Voice of Business and Industry,* April 1968.

Faux, G. *CDC's: New hope for the inner city.* New York: Twentieth Century Fund, 1971.

Fusfeld, D. R. Anatomy of the ghetto economy. *New Generation,* Summer 1969, 51(3).

Fusfeld, D. R. The basic economics of the urban and racial crisis. Ann Arbor: University of Michigan, Department of Economics, Working Paper No. 2, Research Seminar on the Economics of the Urban and Racial Crisis, November 25, 1968.

Georgetown Law Journal. From private enterprise to public entity: The role of the Community Development Corporation. 1969, 57, 956–991.

Goodfaster, G. S. An introduction to the Community Development Corporation. *Journal of Urban Law,* 1969, 46(2).

Grier, W. H., and Cobbs, P. M. *Black rage.* New York: Bantam Books, 1968.

Hampden-Turner, C. Black power: A blueprint for psycho-social development? In R. Rosenbloom & R. Marris, (Eds.), *Social innovation in the city, new enterprises for community development.* Cambridge, Mass.: Harvard University Press, 1969.

74   The Politics of Defining Deviance

Harvard Law Review. Community Development Corporations: A new approach to the poverty problem. January 1969, *82*(3).

Kanter, R. M. Some social issues in the "Community Development Corporations" proposal. Waltham, Mass.: Brandeis University Department of Sociology. Unpublished mimeograph, 1968.

Kennedy, R. F. *To seek a newer world.* New York: Bantam Books, 1967.

Kotler, M. *Neighborhood government.* New York: Bobbs-Merrill, 1969. (a)

Kotler, M. The road to neighborhood government. *New Generation,* Summer 1969, *51*(3). (b)

Kozol, J. *Death at an early age.* Boston: Houghton-Mifflin, 1967.

Lawrence, P. R. Organization development in the black ghetto. In R. Rosenbloom & R. Marris (Eds.), *Social innovation in the city, new enterprises for community development.* Cambridge, Mass.: Harvard University Press, 1969.

Lewis, O. The culture of poverty. *Scientific American,* October 1966, *215*(4).

Llorens, D. Apostle of economics. *Ebony,* August 1967.

Miller, K. H. Community capitalism and the Community Self-Determination Act. Cambridge, Mass.: Harvard Student Legislative Research Bureau, *Harvard Journal of Legislation,* May 1969, *6*(4), 413–461. (a)

Miller, K. H. Community organizations in the ghetto. In R. Rosenbloom & R. Marris (Eds.), *Social innovation in the city, new enterprises for community development.* Cambridge, Mass.: Harvard University Press, 1969. (b)

Northwestern University School of Business. *Eastman Kodak and fight.* Intercollegiate Case Clearing House Case No. ICH 12H68, 1967.

Pinderhughes, C. A. Pathogenic social structure: A prime target for preventive psychiatric intervention. *Journal of the National Medical Association,* November 1966, *58*(6), 424–429.

Pinderhughes, C. A. The psychodynamics of dissent. In *The dynamics of dissent.* New York: Grune & Stratton, 1968. (a)

Pinderhughes, C. A. Understanding black power: Processes and proposals. Preliminary prepublication copy of paper presented at American Psychiatric Society Meeting, Boston, Mass., May 15, 1968. (b)

Playboy. Playboy interview: Jesse Jackson. November 1969.

Poussaint, A. F. The Negro American: His self-image and integration. *Journal of the National Medical Association,* November 1966, *58*(6), 419–423.

Poussaint, A. F. A Negro psychiatrist explains the Negro psyche. *The New York Times Magazine,* August 20, 1967.

Report of the National Advisory Commission on Civil Disorders. New York: Bantam Books, 1968.

Ridgeway, J. Attack on Kodak. *The New Republic,* January 21, 1967.

Rosenbloom, R. S. Corporations for urban development. In R. Rosenbloom & R. Marris (Eds.), *Social innovation in the city, new enterprises for community development.* Cambridge, Mass.: Harvard University Press, 1969.

Silberman, C. E. *Crisis in black and white.* New York: Random House Vintage Books, 1964.

Sullivan, L. H. *Build, brother, build.* Philadelphia: Macrae, 1969.

The Inner City Development Corporation. *Virginia Law Review,* 55(5), 872–908.

Tobier, A. Bedford-Stuyvesant after Kennedy. *The New York Advocate*, 1968.

United States Department of Commerce, Bureau of the Census. *Trends in Social and Economic Conditions in Metropolitan Areas*, Current Population Reports, Series P-23, No. 27, February 7, 1969.

United States Department of Labor. *Social and economic conditions of Negroes in the United States*. Bureau of Labor Statistics Report No. 332, 1967.

United States Department of Labor. Subemployment in the slums of Cleveland. (Multilith, no date.)

United States Department of Labor. Subemployment in the slums of New York. (Multilith, no date.)

United States Department of Labor. Subemployment in the slums of Philadelphia. (Multilith, no date.)

United States Department of Labor. Perspectives on poverty. *Monthly Labor Review*, February 1969. (a)

United States Department of Labor. Employment situation in poverty areas of six cities, July 1968–June 1969. Bureau of Labor Statistics Report No. 370, 1969. (b)

United States Department of Labor. The employment situation in urban poverty neighborhoods: Fourth quarter 1969. 1970.

Virginia Law Review. The Inner City Development Corporation, 1969, 55(5), 872–908.

A SYSTEMS APPROACH TO THE DELIVERY OF MENTAL HEALTH SERVICES IN BLACK GHETTOS

5

Richard H. Taber

In our attempt to develop new and more effective models for the delivery of mental health services to children in a black lower socioeconomic community, we have found the concept of the ecological systems approach extremely useful. Using this model, we have explored the ecology of our community in order to define naturally occurring systems of support within the community—systems that, when utilized as a target for special types of intervention, could maximize the impact of our work.

This paper will focus on the rationale for our selection of two small natural groups: a partial social network composed primarily of mothers of highly disorganized families with young children, and a peer subsystem of fourteen- to seventeen-year-old boys. The ecological framework provided significant direction to our attempts to approach and work with these indigenous systems in such a way that members of the natural groups were given mental health services without being required to perceive themselves as patients.

The Rebound Children and Youth Project is jointly sponsored by the Children's Hospital of Philadelphia and the Philadelphia Child Guidance Clinic. It is charged with providing comprehensive health, dental, mental health, and social services to children in the area adjacent to these two institutions.

The community is a black ghetto in which 47 percent of the families have incomes below $3,000 and "only 38 percent of the 1131 children covered in our survey are growing up within an intact family unit" (5). The project enjoys a positive image in the neighborhood because of the involvement of the community in ongoing planning and the sensitive work of indigenous community workers as well as the provision of much-needed pediatric services on a family basis.

We began this project with the view that many children in the black ghetto live with several pervasive mental health problems, primar-

Presented at the 1969 annual meeting of the American Orthopsychiatric Association, New York, N.Y. Reprinted from the *American Journal of Orthopsychiatry*, July 1970, 40(4), 702–709. Copyright © 1970, the American Orthopsychiatric Association, Inc. Reproduced by permission. Richard H. Taber is currently at the Philadelphia Child Guidance Clinic, Philadelphia, Pennsylvania.

ily poor self-image and the concomitant sense of powerlessness. There are three ways of conceptualizing this problem. One is the individual psychological approach, which would identify early maternal deprivation as a primary cause. This factor can be identified in numerous cases we see clinically. Many children in this population have experienced early separation, abandonment, or maternal depression.

A second is the sociopolitical point of view, which directs attention to the systematic oppression and exploitation of this population by a predominantly white power structure. It also identifies historical and current influences that have undermined the family structure in the black ghetto and points to white racism as the source of black feelings of inferiority.

The ecological systems approach, the third way, directs our attention to the transactions and communications that take place between individual members of the poor black population and the systems within and outside of their neighborhood—that is, what actually goes on between the individual and his family, the individual and the extended family, the individual and the school, the individual and his job, the individual and the welfare agency, and so on. Our exploration of these transactions, or "interfaces between systems," shows that most of the transactions that take place are degrading and demoralizing, and are experienced by the ghetto resident as "put-downs."

When the problems of poor self-image and sense of powerlessness are approached from the concept of ecological systems, pathology is seen as the outcome of transactions between the individual and his surrounding social systems. Because no one element of these systems can be moved or amplified without affecting other elements, the ecological approach to the delivery of services requires exploration of the ways in which "the symptom, the person, his family and his community interlock" (2).

As an example, to plan effective services for a fifteen-year-old boy we must explore not only the boy as an individual but also what takes place at the interfaces between the boy, his family, the school, and other formal institutions, and at the interfaces with peers, adults, and other representatives of the larger society. Chances are that his family expects little of him that is positive except that he stay out of trouble. He may often hear that he is expected to turn out to be a no-good bum like his father. At the interface with adults in the neighborhood, he meets with open distrust and hostility. If he should wander out of the ghetto into a white area, his blackness, speech, and dress quickly cause him to be labeled as a hoodlum and treated with suspicion. He sees the police or "man" as a source of harassment and abuse rather than protection. If he is still in school, he has become used to not being expected to learn (3).

He may not know that the curriculum was designed with someone else in mind, but he is certainly aware that his style of life and the style of learning and behavior expected in school do not mesh (8). If he is in contact with a social or recreational agency, chances are that its program is designed to "keep him off the streets" and control his behavior. Competence is not expected from him and cannot be demonstrated by him. However, his peer system, usually a gang, does give him an opportunity to demonstrate competence. He is needed by the gang in its struggle to maintain "rep" and fighting strength. Gang membership offers him structure, a clear set of behavioral norms, a role and opportunity for status—all essential elements in the struggle toward identity. He is, however, then caught up in a system of gang wars and alliances that he has little or no control over and that limits the availability of role models.

Adults in the ghetto neighborhood have similarly limited opportunities for self-definition as persons of worth and competence. For reasons that have been dealt with elsewhere (6), a mother may not perceive herself as able to control her children's behavior outside of her immediate presence; yet she is expected to do so by a whole series of people representing systems within her neighborhood—her neighbors and relatives, the school, and so on—and outside her neighborhood—the attendance officer, the police, and so on. Her transactions with people representing formal social agencies and other social systems are usually experienced as destructive. In the interface with welfare, legal, medical, and other services, she receives attitudinal messages that are critical or punitive or, at best, patronizing. If she goes for therapy or counseling in a traditional psychiatric setting, she must accept another dependency role— that of patient. One of the conditions of receiving such help is usually that she admit to a problem within herself. She may also perceive the therapists's interpretations of her behavior as robbing her of any expertise about herself. What may hurt her most are the verbal and nonverbal attacks she receives from moralistic neighbors.

One source to which she can turn for acceptance and support in dealing with personal and interfamilial crises is her social network of friends, relatives, and neighbors. An important function of the network is to offer her guidance in her contacts with external systems. A friend or relative may accompany her to an appointment. Often after an unsuccessful encounter at an interface, the group will offer sympathy from collective experience and suggestions for avoiding or coping with the system the next time the need arises.

Having identified the existence of these two social groups in our community (the social network and the gang), we began to wonder how to utilize our knowledge so as to intervene in these systems in a way that would maximize their natural mental health functions. Unlike members of an artificial group, members of a natural group have day-to-day contacts and ongoing significance in each others' lives. The effects of therapeutic intervention in them should be able to transcend a one-hour-a-week interview and reverberate through the ongoing system. Also, intervention with natural community groups fits with our point of view that the answer to the problems of ghetto residents must come from the emergence of self-help groups within the community. Sources outside the community will never be willing or able to pour enough resources into the ghetto to solve the problems there. And our recognition of the value of local self-help organizations brings us to a point of substantial agreement at the interface between our project and emerging black awareness and black nationalism.

We sought to work with natural systems without requiring that the people perceive themselves as patients. The intervenor sought to define his role as that of advisor, rather than leader or therapist. We felt that this model would prove most effective for the promotion of indigenous leadership and help establish the self-help system on a permanent basis. Through successful task completion, people would have concrete reason to see themselves as worthwhile and competent.

In order to avoid making people patients, we chose to focus attention on transaction and communications at strategic interfaces rather than on individual problems. We find that this focus is more syntonic with the point of view of our target population, because members of the disorganized lower socioeconomic population tend to see behavior as predominantly influenced by external events and circumstances rather than intrapsychic phenomena (5, 8).

One advantage of an approach that does not require that people perceive themselves as patients is that the natural group and the intervenor's involvement are visible. This increases the potential of the group for having an impact on other individuals and systems in the community. And the individual, far from being shamed because he is a patient, feels the pride of being publicly identified as a member of a group that enjoys a positive image in and outside the community.

The "C" Street Network

The social network we choose to work with was one of highly disorganized family units that had been observed in the course of an anthropological study of families in the neighborhood (4). The families that formed the core of this network lived on "C" Street, a street which has a reputation in the neighborhood as a center of wild drinking, promiscuous sexual and homosexual behavior, the numbers racket, and gambling.

The approach to the "C" Street network was planned by a project team that included a pediatrician and two indigenous community workers. Our plan was to seek to improve child-rearing practices and parent–child communication by raising the self-esteem and effectiveness of the parents. The indigenous community workers played a key role in introducing the mental health intervenor to members of the network and have played important ongoing roles as linking persons in the interface between network members and the white middle-class social worker.

Our approach to the system was through one couple in the network who in response to a survey question had indicated interest in participating in a discussion group on neighborhood problems. The worker introduced himself as a person interested in working with neighborhood discussion groups. It was agreed that such a group might be most effective if it were limited to people who knew each other well or who were related. Despite the expressions of interest by the network members, it was several weeks before the group began meeting formally. Before the members could trust the intervenor and before they could feel that meeting together might really accomplish something, it was necessary for the social worker to have many contacts with the members in their homes or on the street. In addition to discussions of members' ideas of what could be accomplished by meeting together, these contacts were social in nature since it was necessary for the members to see the intervenor as a person who was sincerely interested and was not turned off by clutter, roaches, and so on.

Initially we wanted to let the network define itself, but we were also committed to including the men of the community in our intervention program. Because of the sex role separation in this group, however, we had limited success in including men in formal group meetings, although the intervenor did have other contacts with the men in the network.

One critical step in the development of this program was that the network members, assisted by the community workers, needed to help the intervenor unlearn some of the antiorganizational principles of group therapy and to recognize the importance of ordered, structured communications. In other words, the group itself had to push "to stop running our mouths and get down to business." Once officers had been elected and rules had been developed for conducting meetings and a dues structure had been set up, the group became task-oriented. The format was that of an evening meeting in the home of one of the members, the formal business meeting followed by a social time during which refreshments including punch and beer were served. The first main areas of concern were more adequate and safer recreation for the children and improvements in housing. Through group and individual activity, houses were fixed up and the street beautified. Recreation for the children included children's parties and bus trips, planned and executed by the mothers, and the sponsorship of a play-street program.

One of the community workers is now working more closely with the group as the social worker begins to step back. The group plans to run its own play-street program this summer, as they are convinced that they can do a better job than the community house that ran it last year.

The Nobleteens

The other natural group that we began to intervene with was a subsystem of the local gang. The boys initially contacted were still in school, although far behind; they did not have major police records. The intervenor discussed with them the idea of getting together with other boys to discuss what it's like to grow up black in a ghetto community. They were asked to bring their friends.

Letters and personal reminders were used for the first several weeks. The intervenor was frequently out on the street, available for informal encounters. Unlike the adult network, where almost all our contacts have continued to be in the group's neighborhood, the boys have had their meetings in the clinic from the outset. They still stop by almost daily to see their advisor.

The initial ten-meeting program was focused on current relationships with school, police, and community, on vocation and the development of black pride and awareness, on sex and parenthood. Use was made of movies such as "The Lonely One" and "Nothing But a Man" and dramatizations of written material such as *Manchild in the Promised Land.*

At an early meeting of the group one of the more articulate members referred to the tape recorder and asked if this was to be like a study of ghetto youth. The intervenor said that that was not the purpose but that one project that the boys might be interested in would be to make tape recordings about life in the ghetto to educate "dumb white people." The group picked this up enthusiastically as an opportunity of showing people outside the neighborhood some of the positive things about themselves since they thought that the papers usually talked about the bad things. The passive process of having discussions that were tape recorded turned into the active process of making tape recordings. From his position as a learner from a white middle-class background, the intervenor could ask questions and promote reflections. It became possible to highlight and underline examples of positive coping. The group became for the boys a place in which they could express the most positive aspects of themselves.

After the initial period, the group decided to become a club, and the intervenor's role was then defined as that of advisor. (One of the club president's functions is to be a "go-between" between members and advisor.) The group structured itself and took a more active task focus —throwing dances, starting a basketball team, starting an odd-job service (which has since involved contracts to move furniture), writing articles for the *Rebound Newsletter*. Carrying on their "thing" about educating people outside their system, the boys made presentations to the staff and agency board of directors, spoke on a "soul" radio station, and wrote articles about themselves. Maximum use of these experiences was made by the intervenor in promoting recognition and development of individual assets and skills.

As a result, new opportunities for role experimentation and contact with role models has been made available to the boys. Through successful completion of tasks the group has won a "rep" in the neighborhood and gets positive reinforcement from adults. One development is that the Nobleteens have "quite the corner." As they became involved in the Nobleteens and began to see themselves as valuable people with futures, the boys spent less time hanging out with the gang and reduced their delinquent activities. This affected the fighting strength of the gang in the balance of power with other gangs, and so they challenged the Nobleteens' existence by beating up several members. The next day, a member of the gang happened to be stabbed, but when a runner came to enlist the Nobleteens for revenge, they refused to fight.

A black male community worker is now co-advisor to the Nobleteens. His focus with the group will be to further promote positive black identity through involvement in activities such as a Black Holiday marking the date of the assassination of Malcolm X. He will also be helping the boys take on a business venture of benefit to the community. The present intervenor hopes to develop a program in which a subgroup of the club will be hired as big brothers to younger boys who have been clinically identified as needing a relationship with an older black male.

The Role of the Intervenor

Because the intervenor or advisor is in frequent contact with group members, often on a social basis, he enters into and can influence the social context on their behalf. He also stands in a unique position in the group in that he is conversant with external systems. He can therefore provide a linking function by bringing the systems together, promoting what is hopefully a growth-producing transaction for the group member and an educational one for the representative of the external systems. In terms of communication he can act as a translator for both sides. Because accommodation has taken place between him and the group members, he is better able to use their language, and they, his.

Several examples here may illuminate the therapeutic possibilities of the intervenor's role in the interface between the natural group and the external system.

Example 1

In the first several months of the Nobleteens, Rick, a fourteen-year-old boy, visited, as a guest, a cousin of a member. He was known by the nickname "Crazy" because of his impulsivity and lack of judgment. He impressed the worker as a depressed, nonverbal youngster. He then stopped coming.

During the summer the advisor was approached by Rick's mother to act as a character witness. Rick had been arrested for breaking into a parking meter, and she was panicky because he had already been sent away once. The advisor talked with Rick while they cleaned paint brushes. Rick convinced the advisor that he really didn't want to be sent away again, and the advisor convinced Rick that it wasn't going to be as easy to stay out of trouble as Rick pretended it would be. They finally agreed that the advisor would recommend Rick's inclusion in the club and would report his impressions to the court.

Rick was known to the boys in the Nobleteens but usually hung out with a more delinquent subgroup. When the advisor recommended his inclusion in the club, one of the members (who happened to be retarded) questioned why Rick should have preference over the boys who were waiting to get in. He then recalled seeing the advisor coming down in the elevator with Rick's mother, realized that it was about the trouble Rick was in, and quickly withdrew his objection.

Beyond this there was no discussion of Rick's problem, but the message was clear. The club members included him in their leisure activities and protected him when trouble was brewing. Eventually the charge was dropped, and he has not been picked up for delinquent behavior since that time. He has responded positively to the feeling of group inclusion, appears noticeably less depressed, and is more verbal. The payoff came for Rick when he was unanimously elected captain of the basketball team.

Example 2

A well-known child psychiatrist was brought to a Nobleteen meeting to consult with the boys in writing a speech for influential people in the health and welfare field. His goal was to argue for more flexibility on the part of youth-serving agencies. The intervenor's only role was to bring the two together. The psychiatrist was familiar with the boys' language, and they were experienced in discussing topics that focused on their relationships with external systems. Tape-recorded material from the meeting was included in the speech, and the boys gained a great sense of competence in verbalizing their concerns and points of view.

Example 3

At one meeting of the "C" Street network club, two members informed the advisor that Mrs. White, the club president, was having an extremely severe asthma attack. The group discussed this informally and came to the conclusion that it was really her "nerves" and that she should go into the hospital. Mrs. White had been hospitalized several times previously and was diagnosed as a borderline schizophrenic. Mrs. White's main supports, her sister and her closest friend, were extremely anxious, their own fears of death and separation coming to the surface. This placed them in a real approach–avoidance bind. The advisor agreed to a visit Mrs. White after the meeting.

Mrs. White was lying on the couch coughing in uncontrollable bursts. The advisor soon labeled the coughing (which was panicking her and the other two women) as a "good thing" and encouraged it. He sympathetically listened to Mrs. White recount her dramatic collapse on the hospital's emergency room floor and her subsequent hallucinations. While she talked, the two network members busied themselves cleaning up the house and attending to the children. Once the advisor had listened, he began exploring areas of stress with her. The most recent crisis was that she was being threatened with eviction for nonpayment of rent. She had contacted her relief worker, who had promised to contact the landlord. The advisor promised to talk to the relief worker. He also learned that in desperation she had gone to a different hospital. She had confidence in the treatment she received there, but did not see how she could go back for an early morning clinic. The advisor agreed that Rebound could provide her with a cab voucher.

Then the three women and the advisor sat and discussed the events of the club meeting. Mrs. White's coughing subsided, and she became calmer as she related to outside reality. The friend's and the sister's anxiety was also reduced. They could then respond in ways that reduced rather then heightened Mrs. White's anxiety.

The significance of this intervention lies not so much in the availability of the professional to meet the immediate dependency needs and to manipulate external systems on the woman's behalf but in his being in a position to repair her system of significant supports. A member of her own system would thenceforth be able to remind her that her rent was due when she got her check and remind her about the attendance officer if she became lax in getting her children off to school. The program continued to meet her dependency needs and support her medical care through the cab vouchers. Initially the vouchers were obtained for her by the professional; later she took responsibility for reminding him about getting them; eventually she went to the clinic's business office to get them herself. She has not suffered a severe attack or psychotic episode since the intervention.

Our commitment was to develop models for the delivery of services that multiply our therapeutic impact by bringing about change in existing systems. By focusing on competence and mutual support rather than on pathology, we have experimented with a model for the delivery of services to people who do not wish to perceive themselves as patients.

REFERENCES

1. Attneave, C. 1969. Therapy in tribal settings and urban network intervention. *Fam. Proc.*, 8:192–211.
2. Auerswald, E. 1968. Interdisciplinary vs. ecological approach. *Fam. Proc.*, 7:202–215.
3. Clark, K. 1965. The dark ghetto: Dilemmas of social power. Harper & Row, New York.
4. Leopold, E. 1969. Hidden strengths in the disorganized family: Discovery through extended home observations. Paper presented at meeting of Amer. Orthopsychiat. Assn.
5. Leopold, E. 1968. Rebound children and their families: A community survey conducted by the Rebound Children and Youth project. Mimeo.
6. Malone, C. 1966. Safety first: Comments on the influence of external danger in the lives of children of disorganized families. *Amer. J. Orthopsychiat.*, 36:3–12.
7. Minuchin, S., et. al. 1967. Families of the slums: An exploration of their structure and treatment. Basic Books, New York.
8. Minuchin, S. 1969. Family therapy: Technique or theory. *In* Science and Psychoanalysis, J. Masserman, ed. *14*:179–187. Grune & Stratton, New York.
9. Minuchin, S., and Montalvo, B. 1967. Techniques for working with disorganized low socioeconomic families. *Amer. J. Orthopsychiat.*, 37:880–887.
10. Rabkin, J., et al. 1969. Delinquency and the lateral boundary of the family. *In* Children against the Schools, P. Graubard, ed. Follett Educational Corp., Chicago.
11. Speck, R. 1967. Psychotherapy of the social network of a schizophrenic family. *Fam. Proc.*, 6:208–214.
12. U.S. Department of Health, Education, and Welfare. 1968. Report of the President's Advisory Commission on Civil Disorders.

A PSYCHIATRIC CONTRIBUTION TO ALLEVIATING HARD-CORE UNEMPLOYMENT

6

John S. Visher,
M. Robert Harris

Exciting innovations in traditional psychiatric services resulting from the community mental health "revolution" are being matched by the development of new methods in the prevention of emotional disorder and the amelioration of disabilities that have derived from severe emotional deprivation, social isolation, segregation and minority group membership, and poverty. One method is mental health consultation offered to those in the community who are community agents or "caretakers." These individuals, in their vocational or avocational roles, are in strategic positions, contacting people who are in crisis or are confronted with complex and difficult problems directly or indirectly affecting or relating to their mental health.

Caplan has aptly described how, with the support and understanding that mental health professionals can sometimes contribute, community caretakers are often able to work more effectively with their clients, helping them to accomplish their immediate goals and thereby promoting the mental health of both the client and the community (1).

This paper describes the work of mental health consultants from the Langley Porter community mental health training program with eight youth and adult opportunity centers (2, 4) of the California State Department of Employment.[1] These special employment offices are physi-

Read at the 123rd annual meeting of the American Psychiatric Association, Detroit, Mich., May 8–12, 1967. Reprinted from *The American Journal of Psychiatry*, 1968, *124*, 1505–1514. Copyright © 1968, American Psychiatric Association. The authors are with the community mental health training program, Langley Porter Neuropsychiatric Institute, 401 Parnassus Avenue, San Francisco, Calif. 94122, where Dr. Visher is staff psychiatrist and Dr. Harris is director. They are also with the department of psychiatry, University of California School of Medicine, San Francisco, Calif., where Dr. Visher is assistant clinical professor and Dr. Harris is associate clinical professor.

[1] The authors wish to express their appreciation for the cooperation of Miss Eunice Elton, Mr. George Jarrett, and Mr. William Appleby, as well as the other staff members, managers, and supervisors of the California State Department of Employment who have assisted them in offering this consultation experience to their trainees.

86

cally located in the poverty sections of San Francisco. In each office there is a small staff of six to ten employees with training and experience in job placement and vocational counseling, under the direction of an office manager. Their responsibility is to provide intensive employment services to applicants from the neighborhoods in which they are located.

These services include job placement, vocational counseling and testing, special job development for specific applicants, and evaluation and recruitment for training courses and camps. They also offer numerous other services directed toward the goal of obtaining employment for applicants who have been unsuccessful in obtaining jobs, often desperately needed, through usual channels.

Center staff members have been especially selected and have had training courses to prepare them for their work. They are usually young, intelligent, and enthusiastic college graduates with considerable idealism, and they are often naturally inclined and strongly motivated to help overcome some of the social problems of our times. Their supervisors encourage them to develop and use all possible means for helping applicants to find jobs and retain them, rather than serving in a more traditional employment service fashion merely as intermediaries between employers and job-seekers.

The Applicants

The applicants for employment present many serious problems that have interfered with their efforts to find jobs. They are from minority groups, predominantly Negro, and their families are often on welfare and living in extreme poverty. Educationally, the applicants are usually school dropouts who have fallen behind their classmates and have been unable to obtain satisfactions and rewards from ordinary school situations. Fifty percent of applicants in one typical center tested below the seventh grade level, and 75 percent have dropped out without completing high school. They have minimal skills and job experience, and they often lack rudimentary knowledge of how employers expect them to behave, how to take preemployment tests, or how to discipline themselves to be punctual and responsible in their work performance. As a result, they are low in self-confidence and fearful of contacting employers.

Their physical appearance often discourages employment; their clothing, hair style, speech, and physical mannerisms, as well as skin color, mark them as outsiders in any middle-class employment situation. In addition, an individual who grows up in a socially deprived environment often has a police record for either minor or major offenses, and this too is often an important obstacle to employment. Applicants may have serious and uncorrected health problems. Fifty to 80 percent report using drugs, as well as alcohol, and most have long histories of failure in jobs, marriages, and social relationships.

Riessman, Pearl, Cohen, and Hartog, among others, have vividly described the impact of a culture of poverty upon its inhabitants (3, 5, 6). Some case examples of typical applicants graphically demonstrate further problems and emphasize the hopeless and frustrating characteristics that are frequently apparent.

Case 1

A twenty-year-old girl applied for help at a youth opportunity center. She was a tall, slender, and attractive unmarried woman with two preschool children. Since dropping out of school five years previously, she had held three jobs, each of which had lasted less than five months. Her aptitude scores qualified her for a vocational nurse training course, but she was dropped because of absenteeism and another pregnancy. She was unable to apply herself in a consistent manner to vocational planning, saying, "Why should I? I've been waiting all my life."

Case 2

A nineteen-year-old young man was uncommunicative, wary, and defensive on his first visit, but with further contact he became pleasant and alert. A staff member helped him to plan to attend a vocational training class, but he soon dropped out and moved from his parents' home to live with another boy. Subsequently he was arrested and put in jail for overdue parking tickets, and following release he had an accident in a car he was driving, which caused $3,700 damage and injuries to a girl passenger. A requirement of probation was that he find a job and pay for the damages.

Six months later he was arrested for driving without a license and for possession of narcotics. He held five temporary jobs, obtained with the help of the center, but failed to follow through by taking a civil service exam when he had a chance for a permanent position. When last seen, he had no apparent source of support but was thought to be living on income from illegal activities.

Case 3

A seventeen-year-old girl was suspended from school and a year later was referred for employment services by the school probation officer. She was the unwed mother of a month-old daughter and was living with her mother and six siblings. The family was on welfare and living in public housing in a segregated area.

She initially said she wanted to return to high school to get her diploma, but, after taking aptitude and achievement tests, she eventually agreed to a training class for telephone operators. Her attendance at the class was poor, and she blamed this on trouble with her mother and nine-year-old brother, who, she said, was abusing her baby. She feared that, if she left home, the child would be taken from her and placed in a foster home.

Finally, after four different staff members had tried to help, she was picked up by police. An examination showed that she was six months pregnant and had a venereal disease. Next she disappeared from home and was again arrested after spending a week in Los Angeles with a suspected procurer twelve years older than herself. A final interview with a staff member revealed that she was interested in a job that would be exciting and glamorous but not in training or working at something routine.

Case 4

In contrast, there was a twenty-year-old youth who may turn out to be a success story after many hours of interviewing and effort on his behalf by staff members of a center. He dropped out of school in the ninth grade, where he had learned to read prolifically, developing an extensive and astonishing vocabulary, but failing to learn how to write. The staff member helped him to pass a test that provided him with the equivalent of a high school diploma and also persuaded him to enroll in college part-time.

The staff member also convinced him to change his appearance as well as to accept a menial and unrewarding job that would support his educational efforts. But the rewards of a college education seemed remote, while his contacts in the poverty community offered immediate rewards in the form of money and prestige as a successful narcotics hustler. The current problem is how to sustain his interest in the nebulous rewards of a college education.

Consultation Arrangements

How did it happen that such employment centers were established and mental health consultation became a part of the program? In 1963 an opportunity center was opened in a segregated public housing area of San Francisco, supported by the Ford Foundation, for the purpose of exploring the utility and feasibility of providing special employment services to applicants from poverty areas who had severe employment and other problems (7). In a short time it became obvious that many of the job applicants had emotional difficulties that were interfering with their search for jobs and affecting their employability.

The staff of the pilot program found that they were in need of help in understanding and dealing with the problems presented, and a request for mental health consultation was made to the Langley Porter community mental health training program. This training program offers both basic and advanced training experiences in community mental health for psychiatrists and psychiatric residents, clinical psychologists, predoctoral psychology students, social work students, and medical students (8). After negotiation of appropriate arrangements, a consultant who was a trainee in the program began regular consultative sessions with the staff group. No charge was made for this service. He in turn discussed his consultation experiences and received supervision from the staff of the community mental health training program.

After the expiration of the pilot project grant, the opportunity center program was expanded with the assistance of new federal grants administered by the state Department of Employment. Eventually eight centers were opened in poverty areas of San Francisco, four for youths twenty-one years of age and under and four for adults. Group mental health consultation was requested for each of these centers and was again provided free of charge by trainees from the community mental health training program on a regular weekly or bi-weekly schedule.

The trainees were from each of the three professional disciplines—psychology, psychiatry, and social work—and were assigned for the duration of their experience in the program, which varied from six months to one year, either half- or full-time. Each consultant was responsible for one or two centers and had opportunities to discuss his experiences with staff members of the program at regular intervals.[2] The managers of each of the centers met monthly with a program staff member to discuss the uses of consultation and some of their own work problems. Wherever possible, the managers were also encouraged to participate in the group consultations in their own centers. As consultants finished their training experience, they were replaced from a new group of trainees.

A primary goal of consultation in each of the centers was the opportunity for the consultees to present and consider problems and issues arising from their work with their clients. The consultant usually acted as a facilitator of group discussion, encouraging the consultees to look at

[2] The following staff members and trainees of the community mental health training program have participated in or supervised the employment center consultations: Dr. Robert Anderson, Dr. Egon Bittner, Dr. Jean S. Bolen, Dr. W. Reed Brockbank, Mr. Arthur Cobb, Mr. John Davis, Dr. Raymond Fidaleo, Dr. M. Robert Harris, Dr. Joseph Hartog, Mrs. Edna Hilty, Dr. Laurel Jones, Miss Rosalie Jones, Dr. Betty L. Kalis, Dr. Gilbert Lewis, Dr. Lawrence Lurie, Mrs. Helen Perry, Dr. Gerald Resner, Dr. Arthur C. Roberts, Miss Lida Schneider, and Dr. John S. Visher.

the various problems presented and to clarify the problems of the job applicants as well as their own difficulties in understanding and working with them. He helped the group to focus on their work problems and did not encourage them to dwell on personality factors of other staff members or administrators. In fact, we generally discouraged reference to personal problems or difficulties that were unrelated to the task of the center.

In his comments and questions, the consultant attempted to clarify problems in layman's terms, not advocating a particular psychiatric theory or technique. Insofar as possible, the consultant was a discussion leader, avoiding the role of an authority with "all of the answers." He encouraged the group to recognize their own expertise about employment planning and to respect their own ability to cope with most problems in satisfactory ways. The consultant seldom suggested or encouraged referral to mental health clinics or other traditional psychiatric facilities, stressing that such facilities do not have "the answers" either. Often someone who has a contact or relationship with the client can do more to help than can a stranger who lacks information and rapport.

Characteristically, after a period of orientation to the consultation situation, patterns of use of the experience emerged. In retrospect these could be specified as concern on the part of the consultees with three general types of subject material. The "personality" or "style" of each center varied considerably, as did the use of consultation. It should be emphasized that the consultation "style" was not consistent and varied from one session to the next, depending on what was uppermost in the minds of the consultees at the time.

Examples of the use of consultation will be given under three general headings: (1) discussion of individual applicants and problems in working with them; (2) staff-oriented discussions of work-related problems, including relationships within the office; and (3) informational discussion of mental health, referral resources, and cultural characteristics of applicants with relevance to employability.

Case-Centered Consultation

Group consultation centering on the problems of individual clients was infinite in variety, as indicated in the following examples:

In one session, a case was presented of a man who entered the office with a chip on his shoulder. He angrily shouted his feelings about being sent from one office to another: All he wanted was the name of an employer who had jobs available. He emphatically did not want to sit down and talk with anyone, and when he was finally persuaded to do so, he refused to discuss any subject that would give the interviewer information that could be used to assess his abilities. He was especially reticent regarding a twelve-year period of his life.

Because his shouting and antagonistic manner caused discomfort in the interviewer, it was quickly arranged to transfer the applicant to a counselor who presumably was more skilled in interviewing techniques. However, the new counselor was equally uncomfortable and described in the consultation how he had conveyed the impression that he was eager to be rid of the applicant. He told the applicant that if he was unwilling to give information, he could not be helped. The applicant himself seemed to know that he frightened people with his bombastic manner and to enjoy the effect he had on them.

The consultant helped the group to discuss the handling of this problem, using such techniques as sympathetic listening and not pushing for information early in the interview when the applicant was obviously reluctant to give it. It is necessary to establish rapport before significant material can be discussed. It was suggested that the applicant be given subsequent appointments to facilitate the development of a working relationship. In a later consultation session, it was reported that the applicant had returned and was less demanding and antagonistic. He seemed more accepting of explanations of the inability of the staff to meet his requests immediately without obtaining more information.

In another consultation session, a staff member brought up the case of a Chinese woman who felt she was being discriminated against by a supervisor. She worked in the accounting department of a large firm and had recently been transferred to another type of accounting work at her request. Her new supervisor was critical of her language ability and, according to the client, advised her that she would lose her chance for a bonus and vacation if she did not take some special language lessons that cost $50. The client came back to the employment service to discuss her problem with her placement worker.

During the discussion, the staff, which was primarily of Chinese ancestry, reacted strongly and identified with the woman, whom they felt was being discriminated against. There were hostile expressions toward her supervisor, and a suggestion was made that the woman be encouraged to bypass him and go to someone higher up with her complaint. With further discussion, however, the group began to consider the possibility that the woman was distorting something in the situation and that there was a need to look behind the facts of the story as she gave it—to find out more about what was really going on. Perhaps the supervisor had merely "suggested" the lessons, possibly in a rough manner, so that it seemed like an ultimatum to a person who was already sensitive to being an outsider and expecting discrimination because she was an immigrant. Others wondered if it would be appropriate to contact the supervisor and get the other side of the story or take some action with the Fair Employment Practices Commission.

Finally, a feeling was expressed that perhaps it might be helpful if the applicant had an opportunity to discuss her problems with the staff person at regular intervals for a time. She could then discharge some of her tensions as well as explore more fully the alternatives open to her, such as talking again to the supervisor or getting another job. The group seemed proud of its ability to work through this situation and then moved to discuss tendencies to overidentify with Chinese people who have job problems and difficulty with the English language as they themselves had had. One group member confessed that he had been trying for years to get rid of his own accent.

Staff-Centered Consultations

Those staff groups that appeared to be more comfortable with feelings and a lack of structure in their involvement with the consultant tended to prefer to use the consultation time to discuss staff relationships and to express feelings about administrative problems. Although the consultants kept the discussion limited to problems of the work situation and did not permit personal references to unconnected activities, the groups nevertheless frequently participated in a therapeutic manner, with successful working through of many difficult problems and feelings.

One staff group used the consultation sessions to discuss their feelings about communication within the office. Many staff members had apparently felt slighted or left out when they did not hear of new programs or policies that were continually changing, or the cancelling of regular staff meetings. The custom of communicating with the staff through the use of memos that were supposed to go from desk to desk was not effective: Memos were buried on desks instead of being passed on. New people who joined the staff were often not introduced.

In consultation, feelings were expressed about these topics. It was possible to explore why meetings were cancelled, for example, when the manager explained that he had not wanted to have meetings unless there was something important to call to the attention of the staff. The staff made it clear that they felt a need to meet whether or not specific topics were on the agenda. The staff also resented not having personal contact with each other and with the managers.

Changes were introduced in the procedures of the office in order to meet the expressed objections, and over a period of time some of the problems disappeared. Staff meetings were held regularly after the manager understood the importance of the meeting to his office staff, and an effort was made to keep everyone better informed of new policies and new additions to the staff. In addition, some practical changes in inter-office memos were made so that one memo could be posted while the others circulated. The staff learned to know one another and were more comfortable once feelings were out in the open.

A significant event that occurred during one of the consultations was several days of rioting in segregated sections of the city. The staff discussed their varying reactions and used the event to become aware of their feelings of ambivalence toward the rioters. On the one hand, they felt that the importance of their own work with Negro youth was emphasized and that this might make it easier to obtain funds to support the centers; on the other hand, there was much uneasiness expressed. The staff discussed the motivation of the young people who had rioted, their difficulties in finding a masculine way of behaving when they could not find work, and the reaction of Negro boys to female staff. They wondered if they were regarded as "the enemy" by the rioters. Perhaps the discussion of these anxiety-laden issues made it possible for the office to remain open and to continue to function effectively during the riot period.

Improving Staff Morale

In one instance, a consultant was asked to meet with a staff group that had very poor morale. The office had been newly opened, and there were many complaints about the lack of understanding supervision and particularly about the demands that the staff felt were being made for tangible evidence of successful performance as measured by the number of jobs obtained for job applicants. The personnel in the office felt pressured and unable to devote what they regarded as adequate time to each applicant. It was clear that a gap existed between the expectations of the manager as understood by the employment personnel and their actual performance. As a result, there were feelings of guilt, inadequacy, and failure, as well as anger, which were directed at the unreasonableness of the supervisors and the whole system in which they were working.

The consultant felt that he could be helpful if he could assist the group to modify its perceptions of the demands, thus narrowing the gap between expectation and performance. Their clients were especially difficult, and if even a small percentage could obtain jobs, the result could be considered most worthwhile. He agreed to continue to meet with the staff to help them ventilate their feelings and work on this and other factors responsible for the morale crisis in the office.

On one occasion a consultant noticed a clipping on the bulletin board of the group with which he consulted reporting the death of a woman who had been the manager of the opportunity center program. She had been expected to return from a year's sabbatical leave. The manager of the office spoke to the consultant, expressing personal sorrow about the loss and saying, "She was like a mother to us all." When the consultation session began, however, the subject was not mentioned and was finally introduced by the consultant. This made it possible for the staff to discuss and express their feelings.

Some of them were upset because they had learned about the death in an impersonal way from the newspaper clipping. All felt a sense of loss. One person spoke with tears in his eyes about how important the manager had been to him and how he had looked forward to showing her the progress they had made in developing her plans and ideas while she was away. With further discussion, it became apparent that there were also feelings of anger related to losing in death a person they cared deeply about.

The consultant helped the group to express their feelings. A sense of cohesiveness in the group began to replace the individual reactions as they worked through their feelings in a manner that probably would not have been possible without the consultation opportunity. A normal grief reaction developed and with it a noticeable decline in the tension and isolation of the consultation group members from each other.

A common problem presented to the consultants by all the center staffs is one that derived from the nature of their work and their tendencies to become deeply involved with applicants whose problems are extremely serious and frustrating. Staff members tend to care deeply about their work, and those who are most successful are often the ones who care most. With experience they find that the culture of poverty from which the applicants come has produced infinitely more complex and involved situations than they are prepared to cope with. Often they have the experience of investing hours of time and much effort and energy in helping a young person, only to have him fail to keep a job interview appointment or even to disappear for months. They have learned that a frequent defensive pattern of the disadvantaged youth is to blame adults and society and "bad luck" for his troubles. But when opportunities are opened for him, he is often frightened about putting himself to the test.

With frequent failures, the staff members experience feelings of futility and personal inadequacy, and those who are the most sensitive feel them most strongly. They question whether they are really helping, and they ask, "Why are we here?" Tensions and hostilities engendered by these feelings are often expressed in the form of anger at "the system," the higher-ups in the employment service, or fellow employees. No one except them understands how difficult things are in the ghetto, professors of sociology do not seem to care, and the government is not doing enough to help the poor.

Consultation sessions gave staff members an opportunity to explore such feelings and to share them with colleagues and an understanding consultant, who helped them to be more objective and to comprehend the reasons behind their reactions. They learned that failure in dealing with an applicant's problems is to be expected and that successes are the exception to the rule. In short, they learned to be more realistic and objective and thus more effective in their difficult and demanding jobs.

Informational Uses of Consultation

A third type of use of the consultation was educational in nature, with a focus on general concepts of mental health, sources of referral, and the like. Since this use of consultation is self-evident, examples will not be given. However, discussion of cultural characteristics of applicants also proved helpful, as indicated in consultation sessions at a center located in a Chinese section of the city, which was staffed in part by Cantonese-speaking Chinese–American employees. The discussion there frequently concerned the subject of the cultural characteristics of the Chinese and their effect on employment problems. The reaction of the United States–born Chinese to the immigration of large numbers of foreign-born Chinese was discussed. Immigrants were willing to work for lower wages and displaced American-born workers with higher standards of living.

Another cultural problem discussed was that of the isolated Chinese man who long ago had left his family in China to come to America in order to make his fortune, only to meet with disappointment and frustration. These lonely men, living in flophouses or flea-bag hotels, represent a "population at risk" from a mental health point of view. Language is another and constant problem; virtually no Chinese person is employed outside Chinatown unless he is fluent in English. Those who cannot speak English are limited to very low-paying jobs under sweatshop working conditions in the garment industry or in restaurants where they do not have the benefit of unions or minimum wage scales. Chinese people are frequently passive, and they would "rather switch than fight," partly because of fear of legal action or deportation if they become visible in the community—many are in the United States illegally.

As the staff of the center discussed these and similar issues, they seemed to become more aware of their own cultural backgrounds and, through achieving some distance and objectivity, were better able to understand the reactions of their clients and themselves. The staff realized that they tended to overidentify with Chinese clients who were facing problems the staff people themselves had struggled to solve. Non-Chinese staff members also achieved greater insight about their Chinese colleagues and clients through these discussions.

Discussion

We will first discuss the skills and training of the mental health professional that are important in his contribution to the solution of a difficult social problem in the community. We will also consider the reactions to the consultation experience of the trainee consultant, the employment center staff members, and the center managers and supervisors. And finally, we will discuss the problem of validation and evaluation of consultation as one example of indirect mental health services.

In his role as consultant each trainee utilizes his knowledge of personality dynamics and relationships in social systems to help the consultees deal more effectively with their clients. While it is important to stress that the trainee does not make interpretations or attempt to produce therapeutic insights through his interventions, his knowledge of human beings and their modes of coping with problems often helps him to understand the behavior of job applicants and consultees. His training contributes to his ability to be comfortable, sympathetic, and understanding during discussions of difficult behavioral problems. Familiarity with group dynamics deriving in part from work with therapy groups also is useful, although the novice consultant is likely to perceive the group in therapeutic terms. The consultant also finds applications for his knowledge of social systems and community organization.

As a consultant, each trainee benefits from exposure to nontherapeutic situations in which he can learn about the similarities and differences in groups and some of the dynamics that account for the differences. He learns what kinds of leadership contribute to the optimal functioning of small groups. He learns how to alter his leadership techniques according to the needs of each group. Most importantly, he obtains a vicarious understanding of and contact with the backgrounds and problems of the poor and unemployed in a setting that is totally different from that of the clinic or the hospital. He learns that unemployment, poverty, and other social problems do exist, and that there are many people who are never able to find solutions. He develops greater understanding and appreciation of the contribution of untrained individuals and recognizes that they often have much to offer toward the solution of difficult problems.

The employment center managers differed in their reaction to the consultation. Sometimes they expressed their anxiety as patients do in individual therapeutic relationships by forgetting sessions, experiencing difficulty calling the group together on time, or dominating the consultation sessions with discussion of routine office business. On other occasions they would limit free discussion by directing members of the staff to prepare cases for presentation to the consultant or asking him to present a didactic lecture. Some managers appeared to fear that permission for freedom of discussion in consultation sessions might lead to rebelliousness and less tractability and compliance by staff members. But most managers were genuinely appreciative of the sessions and felt that they and their staffs had been greatly helped by them.

Just as the managers varied in their reaction to the consultation sessions, the staff members differed also. Some would eagerly look forward to the sessions, while others would find excuses to be absent. Some preferred all of the sessions to be didactic, with discussion limited to one topic selected in advance and presented by one of the group members. They would ask the consultant to give lectures on such subjects as mental illness, resources in the community to which clients could be referred, and what to do about applicants who had previously been hospitalized. These staff members were most often those who tended to be less open and more afraid of discussing their own personal feelings and their involvement with clients. Others wished to use the group for personal therapeutic purposes and had to be restrained from doing so by the consultant or other staff members.

As always in our work, we face the problem of measuring the changes, if any, that have resulted from our professional intervention. The multitude of possible variables in each situation makes such evaluation extremely difficult. Our subjective impression, however, is that most if not all of the staffs to which we provided mental health consultation have benefited in terms of relaxation of tension, the discovery of more effective ways of working together, increased confidence in their ability to be of help with their clients, and greater understanding of emotional problems. Whether any applicants have found jobs that they would not have found without our assistance is not possible for us to say. But the general response of the employment staffs has been enthusiastic, and they usually wish to continue the consultation experiences. Our consultants report that they have found the experience to be a challenging and rewarding one as they become familiar with a new professional role.

REFERENCES

1. Caplan, G.: Principles of Preventive Psychiatry, New York: Basic Books, 1964.
2. Guidelines for Youth Opportunity Centers. Department of Labor, Bureau of Employment Security, Manpower Administration, 1965.

3. Hartog, J.: Problems of the Poor, unpublished paper.
4. Kranz, H.: The Youth Opportunity Centers of the Public Employment Service. New York: New York University Graduate School of Social Work, 1966.
5. Pearl, A., and Riessman, F.: New Careers for the Poor. New York: Free Press (Macmillan Co.), 1965.
6. Riessman, F., Cohen, J., and Pearl, A.: Mental Health of the Poor. New York: Free Press (Macmillan Co.), 1964.
7. Valdez, A.: San Francisco Experiment in Juvenile Delinquency Prevention, Employment Service Review (Department of Labor), May 1964.
8. Visher, J. S.: Methods of Training in Community Mental Health, *Calif. Med.*, 106:117–119, 1967.

Discussion

Paul V. Lemkau

Years ago at the last APA annual meeting in Montreal we had a banquet speaker who chose as his topic "Caries in the Ivory Tower." He gave a wonderfully humorous address in which he exposed how completely the life of the world was passing the university by. This paper by Drs. Visher and Harris is evidence that at least one university training center, and certainly it is far from the only one, has opened its "ivory tower" to experience and data that can lead to improved community services through new forms of using skills and knowledge.

While there linger in the paper some of the old shibboleths about referral that have become so very trite in the literature, there is also the statement, contrary to the theory of a few years ago, that often more can be done to help by someone who has a contact or relationship with the client than by a stranger who lacks information and rapport (implying "regardless of level of training"). The authors might have added that by avoiding a referral the irritation the client experiences in telling and retelling his dreary story, often with incidents that embarrass him and affirm his own low opinion of himself, is also avoided. They probably also have come to realize, as we have in Baltimore in consulting with VISTA workers, that the giving of direct service is often both feasible and productive in changing patterns of functioning, particularly when approached without the preconception that it won't work.

Changes can become established without any verbalized insight whatever. I recall an old, true story recorded by Ruth Fairbank in 1933. It was in reference to a seventeen-year follow-up study of a group of retarded girls (1). They had turned out far better than the psychiatrist who had examined them originally had predicted they would. One of the girls was asked how it happened she hadn't done such things as being promiscuous and having illegitimate children. Her answer was simple: "Miss Persis told me not to."

Dr. Lemkau is a physician in Baltimore, Md.

Miss Persis was the powerful but deeply sensitive and loving principal of the school the girls attended. Rapport and example obviously counted more with the girls than insight.

The authors comment upon the variability of the groups consulted with, particularly in cultural differences, and the differences that existed between the office managers in their acceptance of or resistance to the consultative procedure. They seem, as I interpret it, to ascribe the differences in styles of consultation to these two factors. Perhaps it was restriction of time and space that prevented them from discussing the third factor, the consultant. It is hard to believe that these trainees did not themselves have different styles of working that affected how the groups accepted them and their help, or that all were equally successful. I am certain the authors have knowledge on this point, and I hope they will share it in the future. What I am asking is: "Can you tell us some things not to do wrong?".

I should also like to know whether any senior staff who supervised the consultant trainees themselves took groups in the field. In Europe, particularly in England, the proportion of senior staff men who are active in home visiting, for example, is impressive. Duncan Macmillan, director of the famous Mapperly Hospital, was doing home visiting with geriatric patients up to the day he retired—he was a model for all the rest of the staff. In this country we seem too often to leave the field work to the trainees, the paramedical personnel, often those of lesser experience, being content ourselves to stay a bit back of the "phase junction" between the helping professions and the public they serve.

It seems to me that if the model of consultation is to work, senior as well as junior members of staffs must take part in it. Since the venture we heard about in Drs. Visher and Harris' excellent paper was successful, I predict that we will hear that they and their senior colleagues have first done the job themselves, and probably continue to do it, while supervising their trainees.

REFERENCES

1. Fairbank, R. E.: The Subnormal Child—Seventeen Years After, Ment. Hyg., 17:177–208, 1933.

PROGRAMMING FOR PREVENTION

7

Frank Kiesler

I live in a community that five years ago began to tax itself to buy a mental health program. Convinced by the earnest salesmanship of a public school superintendent, a general medical practitioner, and a county welfare director, the taxpayers envisioned a typical psychiatric clinic, and perhaps even a few psychiatric beds, to serve the sixty-eight thousand people living in three rural northern Minnesota counties.

Here was an area, almost the size and shape of the state of Massachusetts, with no mental health specialists whatsoever. Some parts of the most northern county on the Canadian border were two hundred miles from the nearest private psychiatric help. The state psychiatric hospital serving the region was even farther from this border county. More happily situated was the southern-most of the three counties. Its county seat was only sixty miles from the state hospital. The apparent need was for psychiatric services within more reasonable distances.

In the five years since 1959, the mental health program has not developed in these three counties as originally visualized. There is still no psychiatric clinic, and there are no psychiatric beds in any of the local hospitals. The three professional staff members hired during 1959 and 1960 had other ideas about how the mental health needs of such an area might best be met. With increasing acceptance and implementation of these ideas by key people in these three counties, another pattern of mental health services has evolved.

In 1959, when our three counties appointed a nine-member community mental health board to organize and operate a mental health center, it was assumed by most people that a psychiatric clinic providing direct diagnostic and treatment services would solve the community's most pressing mental health problems. Also, many had very specific goals in mind. Busy doctors wanted to turn the care of certain trouble-

Presented on February 5, 1965 as part of the John W. Umstead Lecture Series of the North Carolina Department of Mental Health at Raleigh, N.C., and published in the North Carolina *Journal of Mental Health*. Reprinted here by permission. This article was written as a summary of the author's experience from 1959 through 1964; the years since that time have brought further development. Dr. Kiesler is Director, Northland Mental Health Center, Grand Rapids, Minnesota, and Clinical Associate Professor of Psychiatry, University of Minnesota School of Medicine.

some patients over to a psychiatrist. School administrators needed the services of a psychologist for IQ determinations. The juvenile court hoped that psychiatric treatment might answer the question of what to do with youthful offenders. Wives of alcoholics hoped their husbands might be brought under better control. PTA program chairmen anticipated lots of speeches to help fill their program schedules. Almost everyone was found to have his own special expectation. Rapidly it became clear that somebody would have to enunciate some overall task definitions so that truly community-serving patterns could be evolved, particularly since tax money was going to pay for what was done. A few people recognized that the community could not afford to have the mental health center become the captive of any one problem-bearing group, no matter how needy and deserving.

In any community, in any population, two kinds of health tasks can be defined. One of these is the care of existing and emerging casualties, the clinical task. The other is the task of reducing the numbers of new casualties, the preventive task. Medicine generally has steadily become more proficient in meeting both tasks. Where do we stand in mental health? Probably the best medical analogy is cancer control. With both mental disorder and cancer we have become better at early diagnosis and treatment. In neither field do we as yet have anything akin to primary prevention through immunization.

In our three counties, budget limitations made it clear that within the foreseeable future only three professional staff members could be employed by the mental health center. What, then, were to be the functions of one psychiatrist, one clinical psychologist, and one psychiatric social worker in relation to the mental health problems existing and emerging in a widely and thinly dispersed population of sixty-eight thousand persons? How could the capabilities of these three be put to work for the most people? How could their efforts best be addressed to both clinical and preventive tasks?

When we three arrived in the area, there was one obvious answer. We weren't alone. Although we were the only mental health specialists in the three counties, we were certainly not the only source of help for mental health problems. It was obvious that before we came, someone had taken some kind of responsibility for helping those with mental health problems. Not every troubled person had been packed off to Duluth or to the Twin Cities or to Moose Lake State Hospital for specific psychiatric services. Systematic inquiry showed that our three counties had a professional manpower pool of over three hundred persons who had been having various kinds and degrees of influence on the mental health of troubled people. These were the doctors, the lawyers, the clergymen, court-services personnel, school administrators and counsellors, the welfare case workers, and the public health and school nurses.

Since these firing-line professionals knew the community and its mental health problems, we reasoned that we could best concentrate our efforts on learning how they had been doing their jobs so that we could find how we might most effectively join our capabilities with theirs. We began by deciding that it was absolutely essential that none of them be permitted to turn his mental health business over to us. We were convinced that, if the community were to meet its clinical task, firing-line professionals would not only have to continue to take responsibility for mental health problems, but they also would have to increase their proficiency in doing so. We concluded that systematic approaches to the preventive task would have to wait until experience with the clinical task had taught all of us much more about the mental health problems and resources in the community. Besides, it was clear that the clinical door was the only one open. We had to use it.

When we explained our ideas about the necessity of keeping the clinical base in the community itself—with the firing-line professionals —most listened attentively and politely agreed that we had described a most logical approach. There were some scattered anguished howls of protest, and a few denounced us as impractical dreamers who would only waste the taxpayer's money. In fact, a few doctors decided we were the entering wedge of socialized medicine—a fifth column—and concluded that to traffic with us would be unethical and perhaps even dangerous. One doctor almost cost us a substantial chunk of our budget support one year by giving a local merchant, the president of the Taxpayer's Association, the impression that all of the doctors thought the mental health center should be run out of town. It took a public county board hearing to set the record straight, and it was set straight by the testimony of doctors.

Despite our attempts to describe a broader concept of mental health center operation, almost every firing-line professional went right on trying to use us in the only really familiar way—as a psychiatric clinic. When referrals came, we immediately engaged the referring professionals. We talked with them on the telephone or saw them anywhere or at any time convenient for them. We asked for information, not only about prospective patients and their families, but also about the realities of professional practice in this area. In all sincerity, because all three of us had come to this area as strangers, we literally asked them to be our teachers—to help us become more usefully oriented. When firing-line professionals talked about how they had been trying to solve the mental health problems that had come to them, we began to find that their reasons for requesting help from the mental health center tended to fall into either of two general categories.

In one category, help was requested in reaching specific professional decisions. Probate judges wanted help in deciding whether or not psychiatric hospital care really would be appropriate for some of the persons brought to commitment hearings. Doctors wanted help in deciding how to appraise and deal with people who cut their wrists or took overdoses of medication. Doctors also wanted advice about how best to use new psychotropic drugs. Sheriffs needed to decide whether prisoners in jail were showing signs of mental illness or "just acting up." In paraphrase, the most common question was, "Is this to be treated as sickness, or dealt with as a behavior problem?" Generally, most hoped it would turn out to be sickness and, therefore, a problem for the psychiatrist. Most diagnostic errors were in the direction of labeling immature and misbehaving people sick. Only infrequently was mental illness either missed or dismissed. All firing-line professionals wanted to know if it was appropriate for them to continue to try to take responsibility for some kinds of problems, or if they should be transferred to the mental health center or to a psychiatric hospital for specialty help.

In the other category, help was requested because some kinds of problems were making firing-line professionals uncomfortable. Aside from difficulties caused by certain personal sensitivities or biases, most discomfort appeared to stem from feelings of professional inadequacy. Most often it was stated directly: "I don't know what else to do," or, "I'm too busy to struggle with this kind of problem," or, "This woman is calling me all the time and driving me nuts!" or, "I've done these things, but maybe the mental health center can do what is really needed."

As mutual experience in interprofessional consultation grew, and with it, mutual acquaintance and confidence, it more frequently was mutually concluded that firing-line professionals were either doing all that could be done or that other suitable ways of solving problems were available at the local level—and that direct intervention by us would accomplish no more. As time went on, we were more often asked to confer about problems than to see patients. More than once at two in the morning the phone rang, and there would be a doctor 140 miles away on the Canadian border, saying, "I've got a problem, and I want to see what you think of what I'm doing about it." Within three months our waiting list for direct clinical service had permanently disappeared. By the end of 1960, seven of every ten families about whom we were asked to consult were continuing in the care of local professionals without having had direct contact with us. Currently we see less than two of every ten families about whom we consult. We see families ourselves when specific psychiatric opinions are required, or, when evaluation by us will lend needed weight to conclusions or recommendations, and when we can deliver brief therapeutic services not available from other sources in the area.

Some interprofessional clinical consultations are one-shot, five-minute curbstone sessions. Others require several contacts, sometimes with the inclusion of other local professionals. The doctors have found that many acute crisis reactions can reverse rapidly if handled in the local hospitals on the regular wards. We may give them a hand with some of these, but we have no hospital patients of our own, nor do we write prescriptions. We are on the move too much. We need to keep the local doctor in the driver's seat as far as consistent medical responsibility is concerned. If psychiatric hospital treatment should be required, we often assist in arranging for it elsewhere. We know that if there were a privately practicing general psychiatrist in our area, fewer people would have to go elsewhere for specific psychiatric care. We have been trying to recruit one.

We've done some crude analyses of the costs of the various things we do. When we describe our two kinds of clinical work (direct service and clinical consultation) in cost terms, we find that seeing families ourselves for direct clinical services costs the mental health center budget ten times as much per family as does consultation with firing-line professionals. Our average total cost per family seen by us at the mental health center is $245. Our average total cost per family consulted about and not seen is $25. Analyzed another way, we have found that, per unit of our professional time, we can influence nine times as many families through Clinical Consultation as we can through Direct Clinical Service. Since this trend became apparent in 1961, we have progressively increased our consultative assistance to other professionals and decreased our direct service time to what appears to be an irreducible minimum. With only 10 percent of our time currently spent in direct clinical contact with patients, we do not consider ourselves to be operating a psychiatric clinic. Our pattern of consultation activities has also shifted from its original totally responsive one to more regularly scheduled visits to doctors' offices, welfare departments, schools, clergymen, and others. For example, with only thirty-nine doctors in the three counties, and those grouped almost entirely into three hospital staff groups in the three county seats, we can literally see most of them regularly.

The fact that more than eight of every ten families about whom we consult are never seen by us does not mean that we have set up family doctors, clergymen, sheriffs, social workers, and a host of others in an imitation of psychiatric practice. These people are not interested in stepping into other professional roles than those they already have. Our experience shows that most troubled people in our area obtain no better results with our help than they do with local professional help. One of our working hypotheses is that the earlier the problems of adaptation can be defined by firing-line professionals, the better the results that can be obtained from relatively simple straightforward corrective approaches. We have a major research program going to test this and related propositions.

Illustrating what can happen with straightforward approaches is the experience of a general medical practitioner in our area, a big burly Irishman who pitched bush league baseball to help put himself through medical school fifteen years ago. Five years ago, when he found he would have to continue to take care of many patients he had hoped to send to the psychiatrist who was coming to the new mental health center, he grumbled, but agreed that the logic of the mental health center operation demanded that he "do psychiatry" whether he wanted to or not. Throughout these five years he has continued to grumble. He has also worked hard at increasing his proficiency. He has learned a lot about when to listen and when to take action. Besides talking with us about patients, he has several times arranged for me to sit with him, as his guest, in his office or at the hospital while he sees his people. (At first he tried to maneuver me into taking over, but I refused, saying, "These are your patients—you are the doctor—I'm your guest!") He has helped to organize some series of formal seminars on diagnostic and therapeutic principles useful to family doctors in our area. He has also become involved with us in community mental health planning. (Parenthetically, I should say that he is not alone in becoming involved in all of these things; other doctors are too.)

The other day, he told me that he now regularly schedules patients who need to talk through some of their problems for the last half hour in the afternoon and charges them ten dollars for it. He said that he had put off doing this for a long time because he feared people would protest about the larger fee. When he finally went ahead, he was delighted to find that his patients simply put their ten dollar bills on the desk as they left. He said, "You know, after fifty-three patients in an afternoon, it's kind of nice to take your time with the last one, and feel like it's worth something." Then he added, "I saw one last night, though, that I just couldn't charge."

He described having been called out into the county to a miserable shack to see a woman who was acutely reacting to the death of one of her twelve children. She stood in one corner, mute and unresponsive, seemingly catatonic. He was able to walk her over to a chair and put her in a sitting position, but there she remained, immobile and staring into space. He began to talk to her about losing her child. When he said, "You have to realize she's dead," it was like pulling a trigger, and suddenly the woman burst forth with screaming that seemed completely out of control as it went on and on. He waited, and when she finally stopped and lapsed into sobbing, she was completely accessible to comforting by her husband and children, and he left them that way clinging to each other in full mutual expression of their grief. When I remarked that there was more than professional satisfaction in his voice as he told the story, he turned to me and said, "But I still don't like to do psychiatry!" My answer was, "That sounded more like the practice of medicine to me."

I want to describe now how large numbers of professional and lay persons throughout our three counties have been collaborating in educational activities, community planning, and research, all with the objective of finding approaches to the task of prevention. This is where our real hope lies. The adaptive casualties we have, and will continue to have, must be cared for with increasing ingenuity and continued devotion. But we cannot afford to delude ourselves into thinking that better patient care will be sufficient answer for the mental health problems of communities. Until we can find how to bring about actual reduction in the numbers of adaptive casualties of all kinds in populations, we will have only begun to scratch the surface of our mental health problems.

In our section of northern Minnesota, we have committed ourselves to the long-range task of assisting a three-county community of sixty-eight thousand persons to mobilize and deploy its mental health–influencing resources so as to improve the effectiveness of all kinds of measures, both clinical and administrative, for identifying, sorting, and handling existing adaptive casualties and for developing preventive programs—all with the objective of finding out if doing this will produce significant reduction in the prevalence and incidence of casualty behavior in the total population. Our general hypothesis is that this can be accomplished.

Toward the end of the first year, in the course of clinical interaction with all varieties of professionals, we more deliberately began to turn attention, in terms related to their own areas of concern and competence, to the necessity of utilizing more than clinical approaches if the mental health picture in the whole community was to change. We began actively to sell our convictions that appropriate mental health programs must include more than concern with the already sick and handicapped, more than work with individuals or even individual families—but, also, organized efforts based on public health principles and carried out in the community at large as community functions.

A natural outgrowth and extension of interprofessional clinical consultation has been organized education for professionals. As professionals were helped with clinical problems, they began to ask for more systematic presentations aimed at enabling them to become more proficient in diagnostic and treatment techniques. From the beginning, both in clinical consultation sessions and in accepting referrals, our staff has emphasized the desirability of focusing upon the whole family rather than upon single individuals. When we were asked for more formal systematic presentations, we continued with the family focus. In this context we have been able to foster a transition from disorder-centered evaluation and assistance toward an interest in health maintenance and promotion.

In consultation regarding families where the apparent initial reason for professional attention was disorder in one member, it has been possible to stimulate interest in formulations that include planning not only for correction or management of disorder but also for protection and enhancement of the mental health of others in the family group. These are concepts well known in both medicine and social work, but we have found they need repeated restatement and reclarification in the mental health context. Further, so that total professional effect could be exerted over a broadened base, it was possible to foster a shift in orientation toward the value of employing only bolstering or holding actions for those with unalterable handicaps, while using sharply focused brief techniques to assist those most capable of change.

Reciprocally dependent upon each other are the remaining two sectors of our Public Health Functions. These are community planning and research. From successful development of clinical consultation, there was a gradual transition to administrative and program consultation with school and welfare administrators who were concerned about how their policies and programs were affecting the functioning of their organizations and the groups of people for whom they had responsibility. Shortly, these people began to ask us to join with them in appraising the meaning of the masses of data accumulating in their files and in determining from it what directions they might take in various aspects of their own program planning.

From the beginning we had been building into the structure of the mental health center the machinery for consistent quality control research on our own activities. From the beginning we had also hoped to become able to facilitate the development of an apparatus for continuous measurement of changes in the adaptive health of the whole population of our area in relation to changes in the deployment and utilization of all mental health–influencing resources. As we became active in program consultation, key administrators very quickly began to talk with us about their needs for systematic program appraisal methods, and very soon it became clear that we were engaged in the preliminary stages of community-wide epidemiologic research program development. Since

1961, we have been fortunate in having become able to set up an entirely separate research organization to design and put into action a comprehensive, continuous, community epidemiologic study in our area.

If an epidemiologic study is to have practical value, appropriate items must be counted. For example, an attempt to use the base rate for schizophrenic reactions as a criterion in a given population immediately "comes a cropper" on the problem of what to count because of serious disagreements about the proper criteria for diagnosis of schizophrenic reactions. On searching for less equivocal and more useful items to count in establishing base lines from which to measure change, it is possible to conclude that certain events, symptomatic in nature to be sure, but reasonably readily countable, can be used. These are bio-psychosocial events to which the community attaches significance, generally because people in the community think it would be better to have fewer of these events. A few of these are marriage failures, school dropouts, juvenile court hearings, mental hospital admissions, and accidents of various kinds. If we examine marriage failures, for example, we immediately see many kinds, and several possible causal sequences are suggested. In our area we have become particularly concerned about one particular kind of marriage failure because of its apparently high frequency in the group in which it occurs. We have become concerned, also, because it has provided the opportunity for demonstrating to the community one way in which preventive programs may be put into action.

Early in the history of the mental health center, our attention was taken by a rapidly growing roster of marriage failures among couples not yet out of their teens, or, at most, only in their early twenties. In addition, these marriages all had one fact in common in that they had occurred because of pregnancy and that, by the time of failure, there had been born, not just one child, but usually two, three, or even four children. At the time of failure, the marriage partners were bitter and discouraged and felt cheated. They were completely fed up with marriage and children. Our concern about these marriages arose not just because many pairs of teenagers had made a mistake in trying marriage and parenthood before they were ready, but also because there were regularly at least two children involved. Similar concern about this problem has been voiced in many parts of this country in recent years.

Our research organization is now obtaining accurate local data on the annual incidence of such marriages, the incidence of failure, what happens to these families after failure, and what may be the differences between those that fail and those that do not. Meanwhile, however, in order to have a preliminary basis for deciding what might be done about these families, we early obtained estimates of the frequency of failure from those sources we considered best able to provide such information. These were the family doctors. We chose family doctors because they diagnose pregnancy, deliver babies, and supply medical care to young families, and because they are generally in at both the beginning and at the end of such marriages. The doctors' estimates of failure rates for such marriages in our area ranged between 50 and 100 percent, with estimates averaging at about 80 percent.

When the whole sequence leading to failure of these marriages is inspected for points at which preventive activity might become effective, it becomes redundantly obvious that the ideal solution should ultimately come from more adequate preparation of children for handling adolescent relationships so that there would be fewer pregnancies propelling teenagers into premature marriage. However, on looking for something with the possibility of faster pay-off, we concluded that there was one point at which the sequence of pregnancy, marriage, child bearing, and marriage failure might most readily be interrupted. Because almost invariably these marriages had been arranged by parents to solve the problem posed by pregnancy, and because practically all of these marriages had been performed by clergymen, it occurred to us, as it has to others, that clergymen might hold the key. If clergymen could become convinced that the long-range results for everyone concerned would be better if marriage did not occur, they would be in an ideal position to counsel pregnant teenagers and their parents toward another kind of solution.

By not performing marriages carrying such apparently high-failure risk rates, clergymen could become key people in setting into motion a train of preventive events. Instead of allowing marriage to be used as the only alternative, clergymen could offer help to teenagers and their parents in working out plans that might have more of a chance of correcting than of compounding the mistake. If not permitted to marry, teenagers might be helped to use opportunities to finish growing up and preparing for mature marriage. If suitable for adoption, the children to be born of these pregnancies could have the opportunity to start life in stable families. Further, without marriage, second, third, and sometimes fourth children would not be born while their parents were least prepared to be adequate parents.

This, then, is one of the preventive formulations professional persons and the general public in our area have been slowly translating into changes in community attitudes and practices in the hope of reducing the incidence of disorder arising from this particular source. Taking the lead have been one of the county mental health associations and some of the clergymen. We have served as resource persons. In one of our larger towns we found that the Roman Catholic priest had independently come to the same conclusions and had already announced to his congregation that he would perform no more pregnancy-propelled teenage marriages. His reason was that he expected those he married to stay married, and these people were not remaining married.

Two Mental Health Association sponsored workshops on "Finding Better Solutions for Problems Resulting from Teenage Pregnancy and Marriage" for clergymen, school administrators, school counselors, school nurses, doctors, welfare caseworkers, attorneys, justices of the peace, and others, were well attended and were thoroughly reported in the local newspapers. Civic organizations, parent groups, and youth groups have asked for information. The general reaction has been one of relief that someone has finally talked about this in public. But, more than that, it has mobilized a ground swell of serious interest in family and community responsibility for better preparation of all children for eventual marriage and parenthood. Thus far, those who are asking the most questions appear to be the most healthy members of the community. We hope their interest will provide a portal for study of adaptively successful families. We hope to become able to describe the epidemiology of mental health in this area, as well as that of mental disorder.

Each year more of our professional time and effort are allocated to assisting in community programming of various kinds. We are convinced that the avenue to reduction in prevalence and incidence of casualty behavior is not professional service to individuals but changes in community attitudes and practices.

2

The Politics of the Emerging Professions

The redefinition of the concept of mental health discussed in Part 1 has led to a redefinition of what sorts of people should deliver mental health services and how they should conduct themselves. Two trends will be explored here. Section 1, "The Paraprofessionals," contains papers concerned with the role of the specially trained mental health worker, the "new careerist," and the role of a non–mental health professional, namely, the police. Section 2, "The New Breed of Professional," contains papers that call for dramatic changes in training programs with the hope that these changes will produce a new breed of professionals that are at home in the community. A final paper is included to illustrate the sort of ethical and political dilemmas that this new professional is likely to face.

SECTION
1

The Paraprofessionals

The lead article by Christmas, Wallace, and Edwards sets down the basic philosophy guiding the new careers movement. The authors clearly want something more than more jobs for the poor. Rather, they are demanding that explicit career ladders be established and that the new careerists transform the mental health delivery system so that it becomes part of a total movement for radical social change. The impact such a program has upon the people trained in a center imbued with this radical point of view can be seen in the article written by Mrs. Hines, a nonprofessional mental health worker. The training obviously liberates and politicizes the trainees. Mrs. Hines does not take a detached, neutral attitude toward mental illness but rather sees the causes and cures for mental illness in terms of social–political events.

The new careerists are much more apt to reach out to potential clients and are much more likely to function in a preventive way. They do not sit in their offices waiting for clients but go into the homes and communities of the people they are committed to help. Yet, as Liberman has shown, about 50 percent of the patients and families from a large Eastern city use the police as *the* community resource. His research indicates that people turn to the police because conventional resources that are available are reluctant to deal with the recalcitrant individual. Thus, if the police are so heavily involved in the life of the mental patient, it would certainly make good sense to provide law enforcement personnel with special skills for handling the potentially dangerous mentally ill person.

Sullivan describes such a program developed by Dr. Morton Bard in which eighteen volunteer patrolmen were assigned to a Family Crisis Intervention Unit. The success of this unit should have an impact on the training of all policemen. And, of course, changing the police attitudes toward mental patients will inevitably lead to transforming their role in society. A police force actively concerned with the mental health of the general population is a force for political and social change.

NEW CAREERS AND NEW MENTAL HEALTH SERVICES: FANTASY OR FUTURE?

8

June Jackson Christmas
Hilda Wallace
José Edwards

For six years the Division of Rehabilitation Services, Department of Psychiatry, Harlem Hospital Center, has been engaged in developing sociopsychiatric rehabilitation services for persons with chronic psychosis and in training and using men and women from the Harlem community in new mental health roles. Service, training, and research programs of Harlem Rehabilitation Center, its community-based facility, are directed toward training and use of paraprofessional specialists who are vitally needed not only in inner-city ghettos but in innovative sociopsychiatric and socioeducational approaches to human services in general. The salient feature of these programs is that members of the community whose potential for productive service to others has not been fulfilled are enabled, through special educational experiences, not only to contribute to the development of others but to realize their own resources more fully.

The implementation of the concept of new careers at the center involves employment of persons in entry-level positions, acceptance of life experiences as a requirement for employment, performance of dignified and competent labor for compensation commensurate with duties, opportunities for upward and lateral mobility, continuing education, meaningful participation in the provision of human services, modification and improvement of services, and institutional and social change. In this

Read at the 125th anniversary meeting of the American Psychiatric Association, Miami Beach, Fla., May 5–9, 1969. Reprinted from *The American Journal of Psychiatry*, 1970, *127*, 1480–1486. Copyright © 1970, the American Psychiatric Association.

The authors are with the Harlem Rehabilitation Center, Division of Rehabilitation Services, Department of Psychiatry, Harlem Hospital Center, 121 W. 128th St., New York, N.Y. 10027, where Dr. Christmas is chief, Mrs. Wallace is a psychiatric rehabilitation technician, and Mr. Edwards is a staff development specialist. Dr. Christmas is also a research associate, Department of Psychiatry, Columbia University College of Physicians and Surgeons.

This work was supported in part by Public Health Service grant MH-14844 from the National Institute of Mental Health and by Social and Rehabilitation Service grant RD-1922-G from the Rehabilitation Services Administration.

117

concept, paraprofessionals are not seen primarily as a bridge between poor patients and alien professionals, or as aides to overburdened, scarce professionals, or as nonprofessionals doing the unattractive low-status tasks that professionals avoid. Rather, the aim is the development of new professional, paraprofessional, and patient–client roles and new rehabilitative services to meet the needs of chronically mentally ill persons more effectively, to broaden the mental health field, and to alter the conditions that may themselves have been among the determinants of mental disorder.

New Careers in Mental Health

Applications for positions as psychiatric rehabilitation trainees were sought from men and women over thirty who lived in the ghetto, could understand and articulate the needs of community people, and showed evidence of compassion, commitment, and ability to develop work competence. Recruited through block and tenants' associations, welfare and employment agencies, parole offices, lodges, churches, poverty programs, and by word of mouth, these individuals had a variety of life experiences as school dropouts, parents, ex-offenders, domestic and factory workers, and welfare recipients (1).

Successful applicants gave evidence, in a series of group interviews, of being able to relate to chronically mentally ill persons and to others and of being expert in knowing how to maneuver social systems of the ghetto successfully and knowledgeable and appreciative of the life styles of low-income black communities. Other criteria for selection were a seventh grade reading and writing level, no prior employment in health, no education beyond high school, and no current mental illness that would interfere with work performance. In addition, the applicant must have been unemployed or underemployed.

For permanent employment as a psychiatric rehabilitation worker, the requirements included successful completion of the designated work-training period as a trainee, a reading and writing level of the ninth grade, and fulfillment of the other criteria for trainee level as well.

Implicit in new careers is training appropriate to develop attitudes and skills effective in human services, a reevaluation of current educational approaches, and the use of techniques compatible with the learning styles of those ordinarily screened out by the educational process.

During a month of full-time orientation, the experienced paraprofessional and professional staff used a number of socioeducational approaches. These included self-evaluation, participant-observation, development and use of community surveys, field trips, role playing, audiovisual aids, log books, feedback sessions, interaction groups, and team teaching.

The group experiential focus remains upon in-service training, continuous with the work experience. This includes several hours weekly of (1) *core knowledge* (human growth and development; social forces, issues, and the human condition; an overview of human services; how groups operate; the community; human service techniques); (2) *workshops* (principles and practices of sociopsychiatric rehabilitation; the therapeutic use of oneself as a change agent; the therapeutic community; black identity and the rehabilitative process; group approaches); (3) *techniques of rehabilitative services in specialized areas;* (4) *self-development as a rehabilitation worker* (peer group conferences; sensitivity training and self-development; remedial skills development); (5) *individual and group supervision;* and (6) *supportive services.*

A staff of more than thirty psychiatric rehabilitation workers either function as generalists or specialize, according to assignment, in sociotherapeutic activities, vocational evaluation and training, case services, community services, or health service expediting.

They are the primary rehabilitative agents. They play many roles in crisis intervention and ongoing therapeutic relationships, as leaders of rehabilitative activities, groups and meetings, as teachers, counselors, trainers, expediters, advocates, providers of assistance, and recorders of observations; they serve as role models and catalysts for the development of leadership potential in member–clients and perform numerous other change agent roles in the rehabilitative process.

Interdisciplinary professional staff provide indirect service as program and service coordinators, program planners, consultants, administrators, supervisors, and trainers. They also function as part of the rehabilitative team, providing direct service requiring professional skills.

New Mental Health Services

As developed in this center, new mental health services have included the approaches of sociopsychiatric rehabilitation. Sociopsychiatric rehabilitation involves the use of multiple, comprehensive, coordinated, interdisciplinary interventions related to intrapsychic, interpersonal, and social factors. These interventions are directed toward aiding individuals to achieve productive social, psychiatric, educational, and vocational roles, within the limit of their capacities and potentialities, with recognition of their disabilities. The range includes, but is not limited to, therapies, activities, services, assistance, education, training, self-development, self-help, advocacy, and individual and group social action.

Center services are organized into three rehabilitative programs: the psychiatric program, which is sociotherapeutic in emphasis; the vocational program, emphasizing vocational training; and the continuing program, with a socialization focus (4). Each program also provides social and community services and medical and psychiatric health services. The basic rehabilitative staff in each are trained paraprofessional new careerists.

The elements essential to sociopsychiatric rehabilitation are social, therapeutic, educational, and environmental (2). In the social aspects, planned activities and personal contacts are directed toward socialization, resocialization, and the development of meaningful interpersonal relationships. The sociotherapeutic features include therapeutic relationships and activities, psychopharmacological therapies, crisis intervention, and health services directed toward psychosocial and interpersonal adaptation, social learning, and physical health. The socioeducational focus emphasizes social learning, skills development (avocational, prevocational, and vocational), and the acquisition of knowledge. The socioenvironmental features relate to control over decisions affecting one's life, control of the environment, and the development of potential for constructive action in the social environment.

Planned change interventions occur in social systems at the level of individuals, the therapeutic dyad, small core groups, and larger, more peripheral groups, including transactions between individuals, institutions, and significant sectors of institutions.

The therapeutic community is a vehicle for rehabilitation with member-clients and staff at all levels engaged in the decision-making and implementing process. Group approaches are used as rehabilitative techniques and forces. A rehabilitative continuum is developed through graduated stress and graded tasks.

Acknowledgment is given to the *potential* for health, growth, and autonomy of individuals and groups. Attention is paid also to such characteristic *disabilities* as dependency, deficiencies in social knowledge, psychopathological behavior, ineffective coping mechanisms, lack of marketable skills, and other manifestations of chronic mental illness, institutionalization, deprivation, and racism.

Creative use is made of the community base, of the strengths, stresses, and culture of the community, of social action, and of other transactional relationships to enhance, support, and assist the rehabilitative process or to serve as the intrinsic rehabilitative force (3).

The human needs of marginal men who are poor, black, and ill are given attention by the development of programs relevant to and effective in meeting their needs.

Progress and Problems

The evaluation of the new careers and new mental health services programs awaits the findings of current center research. Impressionistically, community-linked rehabilitation services, provided primarily by trained paraprofessional staff from the local community, appear to affect favorably the course of rehabilitation of persons with severe, chronic mental illness. But progress in the development of new roles and programs is not without problems, influenced by the institution, the field, and the wider social context.

Mental health has traditionally been low in the priorities of poor communities caught in a struggle for existence. Thus, there was an initial tendency among paraprofessional staff to minimize personality factors and focus purely on the social forces—bad schools and housing, poor nutrition, unemployment, racial discrimination, and power politics, denying any but social determinants of mental illness. It took time for the staff to see both the reality of social factors and the individuality of each person in his inner and outer worlds (5).

Life experiences of patients and staff from the ghetto may lead to scars as well as strengths, evidenced at times in staff by a facade of indifference, hostility, and dependency or by absenteeism and "beating the system." In addition, there are the realities of disruptive home life, frequent needs to attend to personal business during working hours, problems with child care, and personal bouts with alcoholism, family conflict, and financial stress (4).

Understanding the social and psychological factors contributing to these problems, the staff decided to provide supportive services of confidential short-term counseling to deal with the negative and positive influence of personal life on work.

In the beginning of the program, rivalry existed between some professionals and paraprofessionals. Some of the former hid behind the mask of professionalism, jargon, or authority. Others feared that paraprofessionals might usurp their roles or do successfully what professionals had been unable to do alone—to rehabilitate poor black people with chronic schizophrenia. A few others were jealous of administrative attention to the development of career ladders. Cooperative work, joint sensitivity training, and experiences as functional teams helped to decrease this distrust (6).

Rivalry also developed between clerical and paraprofessional staff. Service careers had been conceived for those without skills, thus excluding the clerical staff, who had been hired with skills, work experience, and, in some instances, advanced education. Clerical staff viewed the program as supportive of paraprofessional needs and not theirs and described paraprofessionals, when a career ladder was adopted, as undeserving of high salaries and training. This was accentuated by the service emphasis of the program and the higher value seemingly placed on patient care than on supporting services. This problem has not been resolved, although progress was made in the inclusion of clerical staff in sensitivity training and in more active roles in center planning.

For most staff a four-step career ladder, recently instituted, has manifested itself mainly in retroactive grade titles and in very significant increases in salary, well above their former level. A senior staff member, one of the two paraprofessional coauthors of this paper, has been promoted to the third grade as a psychiatric rehabilitation technician, in a position of greater status and authority as supervisor of the continuing rehabilitation program. The grades enacted to date are those of trainee, worker, technician, and specialist. Each grade contains three levels. Movement within grades is achieved upon satisfactory completion of a year's work. Movement from grade to grade is promotional. Most of the staff currently employed are workers, grade II.

The definition of other needed service roles requiring greater skills (either in specialties or generically) is currently needed so that there are opportunities for more staff to move up the ladder. Efforts will also be made to develop the projected four additional steps, each requiring higher education plus in-service training and work experience.

Meanwhile, lateral mobility is restricted. The only likely grade to which transfer might be made in the hospital is equivalent to the worker grade, but there is little incentive to move to a position with less pay and a traditional aide title and role, even though the work is less demanding. Efforts are being made to legitimize the psychiatric rehabilitation worker positions in city institutions. Civil service has permanency, but it also has a tradition of acceptance of work laxity, personnel abuses, and a rigidity of roles. Yet, unless such positions are established from the lowest to the highest grade, there may be little chance of permanency or of influence on the nature of public mental health services. If hospitals or civil service adopt this system, they will have to drop requirements of a high school diploma for entry-level positions. Such recommendations have been made to the city and state officials seeking center advice on mental health service staffing..

Relationships with trade unions have worked well. Local 1199 of the Hospital and Drug Workers Union encouraged the development of career ladders, accepted the job titles created, and was instrumental in getting agreement on a jointly financed (union and employer), combined work—study program for selected union members. It also agreed to extend the probationary period for psychiatric rehabilitation workers to six months rather than the customary two for aides; this period was considered essential for evaluation of trainees for permanent employment. Discussions have begun among officials of District 37, State, County, and Municipal Employees Union, center staff, and city administrators in regard to the creation of permanent hospital staffing patterns incorporating these new positions.

One of the problems in developing a relationship with a formal educational institution has been the lack of relevant educational programs. A number of institutions have expressed an interest in linking their programs with those of the center but have not indicated by their curricula or attitudes that they are in tune with the educational needs of youth, poor people, black people, or the changing mental health field. Before colleges move into this field they need to be revamped rather than to improvise makeshift training programs with old courses and new names.

Appropriate educational experiences need to be further defined. For example, there are areas of knowledge not provided currently in center training that will be needed if paraprofessionals are to play a role of greater power, along with professionals and consumers, in developing and administering programs. These are in the areas of organization, program planning, development, analysis and evaluation, fiscal management, and legislation, as well as techniques of functioning as board and community corporation members. Staff training has focused on advocacy, assistance, and relationship roles successfully. With the direction of health services toward decentralization and community control, these other organizational, policy planning, and administrative skills must be developed by both professionals and paraprofessionals.

Meanwhile, accreditation and certification still bear fruit, both financially and in terms of status. The hope has been expressed by some staff that center training will qualify them not only for the high school equivalency diploma as planned but also that it will be accepted for entry into community colleges or serve as the equivalent of certain college courses with credit. Hopefully, as new persons in traditional places, they will be productive forces for change in these institutions. They have already begun to influence the mental health field through their work, where they have been agency consultants, conference panelists, and community activists fighting for better health services.

Dire predictions have been made, generally by middle-class white professionals, that black ghetto residents, once employed at mediocre salaries, often in temporary jobs, will forget their poverty-stricken backgrounds and become professionalized and identified with the Establishment, losing the sensitivity and awareness for which they were chosen.

The professional staff of the center did not hold such fears or unwittingly work to see these prophesies fulfilled.

Such predictions did *not* come true. Perhaps this was because the center stands actively against that part of the Establishment responsible for underfinanced health budgets, insufficient staff, and the resultant second-class services that mark the game of Russian roulette played with the lives of the poor. Perhaps the closeness of professional staff to their own ghetto backgrounds—whether middle-class or slum—and, most important, their identification with black people, allow them to appreciate the strengths of ghetto workers and patients, as well as their own, without idealizing or devaluing either one. Perhaps the workers' continuing struggles to improve the quality of their own lives help them to enrich their life experiences with skills and still retain the identity and humanity that they brought to their work. At any rate, mutual respect and work as colleagues have led to growth on the part of all staff, with each gaining from the other as they successfully join in service.

Implications

New careers programs in mental health are rare. They need to be developed to meet needs specific to various mental health problems, to different age groups, and to populations where transactions between men and the social context should determine the nature of services.

New careers programs in human services can be conceptualized on five levels. Most current programs fall in the first two levels. The center programs lie somewhere between levels three and four.

The first level is that of *tokenism*. Quantitative change takes place with increased use of paraprofessionals as assistants or aides to traditional professionals, in temporary or dead-end jobs. The keynote is *more jobs*.

The second level is that of *reorganization*, characterized by the entry of paraprofessionals into traditional systems in numbers significant enough to effect change in the personnel pattern, by the use of new personnel in old roles (for example, the role of research aides), or by the use of new persons in new roles (the role of teacher aides). The keynote is *new jobs* on a permanent or temporary basis and limited reallocation of manpower resources.

A third step is *reform in existing systems*. Innovative programs take place that have a limited or moderate effect upon the total system. A pilot program is initiated and discontinued when the trial is over, or innovative programs are continued but seen as deviant, avant-garde appendages to the basic traditional programs. These may involve the use of new persons in new roles (both professional and paraprofessional) in limited areas and with limited power. Included in this level may be credentials and licensure for new categories and positions and the entry into traditional professional tracks of those formerly excluded and/or underrepresented—new entrants into old careers. This is structural change. The keynote is *limited new careers*.

The fourth level is that of *redesign of systems of service*. Here are the beginnings of qualitative change. Planned, instigated, controlled interventions take place. Strategic innovations and new models for the delivery of services occur. New professional and paraprofessional categories are developed. New multidisciplinary professions develop. New professional roles are played by those who formerly played more traditional roles. New professionals develop from the ranks of those who were formerly paraprofessionals. Paraprofessional career ladders are instituted, not necessarily ending in old professions but in new professions as well, such as that of the specialist in sociopsychiatric rehabilitation. New roles develop and new coalitions with community social systems take place. This is a level of institutional change with a keynote of *new career ladders and improved services*.

The fifth level is the level of *radical change*. New models for the delivery of services are extensive, systematic, and radical. Instigated social change takes place in large social systems. The development of community health, mental health, rehabilitation, education, and social and welfare systems is interdisciplinary, integrated, and linked to social change, both as a cause and effect. New systems of service include various community social systems—professional, paraprofessional, lay, and consumer—receiving, planning, providing, administering, and controlling new social structures, institutions, and processes. Services are numerous in quantity, widespread in allocation, and relevant and effective in meeting human needs. On this level, the keynote is *new careers—a movement for radical change*.

The Future

The critical need is threefold. The need for relevant and effective human services for people who are black, poor, and ill is great: With admission rates from black inner-city areas to state psychiatric hospitals being among the highest in the city, the need is striking for rehabilitative services for chronically ill persons who are discharged from hospitals unready and unable to return to full life in their community. With unemployment disproportionately high, the need for work is greater still. But a third need is even greater—the need and desire of people to participate in meaningful ways in efforts that contribute to removing the negative conditions of their lives and to gaining power and control over

126 The Politics of the Emerging Professions

their lives. The imperative is to meet these needs without further waste of human resources.

Although late in articulation, the demands of planners, practitioners, and consumers for modification and improvement in mental health and other human services are urgent, insistent, and necessary. New careers could contribute to a redefinition of institutional and human service goals, and to their implementation, through developing its potential link with local community institutions and utilizing its potential for creativity. But this is dependent upon conceptualizing and implementing new careers as a dynamic force for improved services rather than as a static slogan with the form and not the substance of change. It will require facing such issues as professional resistance, institutional vested interests, racist social policies and practices, community demands that exceed community cohesion, paraprofessional satisfaction with a larger slice of the status quo, and the limitations of knowledge of the mental health field.

New careers, in its broadest connotation, has the potential for being a dynamic force for such constructive change in human services. These efforts at individual and group rehabilitation, along with those of many others in the black community and in other deprived communities, may forge an essential link between service and social change and thus contribute to the solution of these critical problems.

REFERENCES

1. Billingsley, A. Black Families in White America. Englewood Cliffs, N.J.: Prentice-Hall, 1968.
2. Christmas, J. J. Sociopsychiatric Rehabilitation in an Urban Ghetto: Conflicts, Issues and Directions, Amer. J. Orthopsychiat., 39:651–661, 1969.
3. Prigoff, A. Service or Self-Help as Therapy in the Ghetto, Journal of Current Social Work Thought, 1:5–8, 1968.
4. Richards, H., and Daniels, M. Sociopsychiatric Rehabilitation in an Urban Ghetto: Innovative Treatment Roles and Approaches, Amer. J. Orthopsychiat., 39:662–676, 1969.
5. Riessman, F., Cohen, J., and Pearl, A., eds. Mental Health of the Poor. New York: Free Press of Glencoe, 1964.
6. Wallace, H. V. The Role of the Mental Health Aide in a Socially Deprived Community, read at the 44th annual meeting of the American Orthopsychiatric Association, Washington, D.C., March 22–25, 1967.

A NONPROFESSIONAL DISCUSSES HER ROLE IN MENTAL HEALTH

9

Laura Hines

My name is Laura Hines; I am a forty-one-year-old black woman with a family. At fifteen years of age, I came out of school to go to work to help my family. Most of my twenty-six years of employment I have spent as a waitress, not staying on a job long enough to get a vacation. Before I came to the center to work I had also been trained through the state employment office to be a sewing machine operator. This was a boring job to me because you were required to sit at a machine all day. I only lasted on this job for three months.

There were many jobs being created by different agencies that were listed in the antipoverty offices, so I thought I would apply for a job. After being interviewed there, they sent me to the little neighborhood schools. I was hired as a home and school coordinator. This job was temporary and lasted only three months.

After the job terminated. I returned to the antipoverty office to see if there were any more openings. They told me that the community mental health center was going to conduct a survey of the North Philadelphia area and that they were going to hire people to work as census takers. I applied at the center, was interviewed and hired. On October 10, 1966, training began. Training consisted of interviewing techniques. We spent two weeks of training and then the frustration began (census taking).

I had to get used to going in and out of different neighborhoods and had to adjust myself to different kinds of personalities. Most people in the survey area were very reluctant about answering questions. They were tired of answering questions and having promises made. It was hard to tell people that you were from Temple University because of the feelings that people had about Temple. Some people thought that you were spying for other agencies. It was difficult: being polite to people when they in turn were rude, seeing people who were hungry, seeing

Read at the 125th anniversary meeting of the American Psychiatric Association, Miami Beach, Fla., May 5–9, 1969. Reprinted from *The American Journal of Psychiatry*, 1970, *126*, 1467–1472. Copyright © 1970, the American Psychiatric Association. Mrs. Hines is a mental health assistant, Temple University Community Mental Health Center, 1531 W. Tioga St., Philadelphia, Pa. 19140.

people who were jobless, seeing family after family without a father and the mother trying to survive on her welfare grant, seeing all these things and nothing being done about them. Some people's attitudes were almost unbearable. But I worked, knowing how people felt, feeling that what we were trying to develop would be a good place for the community, hoping that some pressures would be removed. I grew a lot with the survey; I was not aware that there were starving people living only blocks away from where I have lived all my life.

Learning To Be a Mental Health Assistant

In early 1967, I moved from census taking to mental health assistant I. I had ten weeks of full-time training that consisted of seminars dealing with psychiatric and social concepts. The training consisted of lectures, reading, and paper work. It was given by professional staff from the center—psychiatrists, a psychologist, a social worker, and a nurse.

My knowledge of mental health or mental illness was very limited when I first came to the center, limited to the extent that all people in the community who acted queerly or whose behavior was not as I thought it should be, I thought of as crazy. After being in class for a short while, I saw that people who were not able to function were not crazy but people who needed help. Being directly from the community that the center was going to serve, and wanting to help people, and hoping that I could, I was willing and hoping that I could learn what was about to be taught at the center. I was hoping that with this teaching I could be very effective in my community.

Learning to become a mental health assistant was a frustrating experience for me. It was made as simple as possible, but I still had a tough time getting adjusted. There were nights that I hardly slept, thinking of tomorrow when class would resume. It was hard for me to adjust because I never liked school anyway, and I had been out of it for so long. But I was able to adjust with the help of the training director, who was nice but stern. For example, each week she insisted upon your learning to use ten words that were unfamiliar to you. I had to learn how to pronounce them, spell them correctly, and use them in a sentence (which I thought was very useless). It proved to be quite useful in work when talking with different people in other agencies about patients who were in some way connected with their agency.

The director of the program also was a very stern person but one who made every effort to make his teaching as simple as possible for all the trainees: describing symptoms, problems, medication, colors of medication, effectiveness, and so on. Some days I came away from class feeling like a medical student, and some days I came away from class feeling like a social worker. I had to take this learning, put it together, and make it work.

There are still ongoing training programs in the center, and it is very important that the mental health assistant have this opportunity.

I have been in our psychosocial clinic on a part-time basis for nearly one and one-half years and have seen about 150 people. My case load has never been over 50 cases at one time. I have been able to work with people making most of my own decisions about how I work with a patient.

During my clinical work I have been supervised at different times by a social worker, psychiatrist, or a psychologist. My supervision by the social worker was quite rewarding. His supervision also included formal teaching such as group therapy concepts and family dynamics. We exchanged experiences and gained knowledge and also techniques involved in working with other agencies. In contrast to this social worker, most professionals, I think, have not listened to people such as myself, mostly because they do not understand what we are saying: More sensitive people are needed to work in the poor sections. Workers are needed who will put their hands on people and can make some changes in their lives.

Having been taught all I know about mental illness by a psychiatrist, I felt as though any psychiatrist could teach and support people with less education than they. But I learned how different psychiatrists could be when I started in our psychosocial clinic and had a psychiatrist for a supervisor. He made me feel less important and needed than I had felt from the beginning of my training. My ideas were not accepted as good ideas but as useless thoughts. He did not realize that if we worked together and worked hard, we would be able to be effective and do a great job together for the people that we serve. He should not have let differences in theories or methods prevent him from working with me. Together we could plan and maybe initiate the needed change in our area and also try to create solutions to some problems. But as I worked on, my perception of professionals changed some from my first thoughts. To some extent some professionals still relate to you on a professional–nonprofessional level and do not want to learn your ways of thinking.

Clinic Work and Home Visits

All patients are given an appointment by the receptionist, and a mental health assistant is then assigned to the patient. Whether in the clinic or on a home visit on my first contact, an intake is done. This consists of obtaining social and clinical data and getting any other information that is available from other agencies or other family members. I record all information in patients' charts. I also notify referring agencies that the person has reached us. In other words, I am responsible for the patients' care. I also make periodic home visits; I check on patients' medication, and I make home visits to people who do not attend the clinic regularly. I also help people to secure welfare, help them in getting housing, and arrange for psychiatric evaluation, psychological testing, social work consultation, and so on. I record all contacts, visits, and phone calls. I discuss and determine with my supervisor termination of patients, and I am able to make some very good decisions about how I am going to work with them.

One factor that contributes to rapid patient service is my approach; that is, when people come into the clinic, I try to pinpoint the problem and get right to work on it. That way the problems get solved and my case load does not build up. There are many problems in this area that may be related to mental health but are more social. These factors are often diagnosed as mental illness when this is not the case. It has been proven through the center and the mental health assistant that a person diagnosed as psychotic has been able to function in the community with follow-up care. People who have been confined in institutions for many years have been able to come home to live with their families or in some cases to live in boarding homes where they must to some degree be able to take care of themselves.

My first patient had been interviewed by a psychiatrist and by a social worker. I was then assigned to do the follow-up. The patient had been diagnosed by the psychiatrist as being borderline psychotic. The diagnosis was not too clear to me since in the back of my mind I thought she was definitely schizophrenic and wondered why the psychiatrist had not seen this. I was very reluctant about telling my supervisor what I had discovered, but as I continued to work with the case, the symptoms of schizophrenia became clear to both of them.

Groups for Children and Patients

I am the primary therapist with three groups. One group consists of six preadolescents, all boys who spend from one hour to an hour and one-half one day a week in the group. The first half hour consists of play therapy. The other hour is spent in discussing their relationships with each other and with their parents (which is a very big issue) most of the time. Most of the sessions are taped, and these tapes are used only for supervision. Most preadolescents are never heard or really ever listened to. We first talk about their reasons for being in the clinic; the reasons are often different than what the school referral has stated.

One patient, who is eleven years old, had always screamed and yelled when he became upset, even fighting his other brothers and sisters for no reason. He had at one time gone into the basement where all the canned food was kept and opened every can in the pantry, just because his parents would not let him go outside with the other children. He never had a nice word for anyone but became much different after coming to the group for a month. His parents became quite upset when the patient began to say what he did not like. He began to tell the teacher that other children were bothering him. He also began to ask questions in school by raising his hand instead of becoming withdrawn as he had been. His parents could not tolerate the change, and that is when I decided that I would have to try something else.

I decided that I would then start a parent group and called the parents together to tell them about my plans. They all agreed to be part of the group for a trial. Well, this has worked out fine. The parents are really interested in the future of their children and the attendance is good. Each week all of the children and the parents are there, staying sometimes longer than the time we had planned.

Working with youngsters in groups as a therapist is something new for me. I took it upon myself to form these groups, realizing that I was not able to relate to the children on an individual basis, but also thinking how well youngsters relate to each other. On an individual basis youngsters always tell you what they think you want to know, but when they talk to each other, it is much different. I am happier working with children than with anyone else. If there is a diagnosis from some other agency, I can work with the youngster with a different thought in mind, not letting the diagnosis have any influence on my goal or treatment plan. I have my own style of working, and I am enjoying it.

I have also developed a group for adolescent girls that also meets once a week. Most of these girls, when they first came to us, were having problems relating to their parents and teachers. In some way most of these girls have shown more interest in themselves since being part of the group. I do not think that these youngsters have ever had anyone who would listen to them. Most youngsters have many fears and concerns about themselves but are afraid to talk about them. All of them have similar problems. They share experiences and in some cases provide good solutions for each other.

With each case that I am assigned, I make a home visit at least once. With some assigned cases home visits are the only answer to people being seen, especially older people who are senile or some people who are psychotic and not able to travel alone. They get more follow-through with home visits than other patients. I do not only go to see about their medication, but I also go to see about their personal needs. Besides working with children I find great rewards working with older people.

I have found that youngsters do better mentally and put forth greater effort under a spirit of approval than under criticism. This is the way that I work with the youngsters, sometimes approving of behavior that is said to be bad by others.

Neighborhood Outreach

One question that always comes up is does a mental health assistant do therapy? I feel that, when a person comes into the office to sit and talk with me, that in itself is therapeutic. As my case load began to climb, I became aware of my ability and was able to make diagnoses, recommend treatment, and also set up goals for the person that I was seeing. Here I was with five months of formal training, and functioning as though the training had been longer, feeling very important and very needed.

There are people who do not like to work in their own neighborhood, but I do. My neighbors in many cases have come to me for some kind of information. There was a neighbor who had been in a private sanitarium for some five or six years, who returned home only to find out that her daughter, who was twenty-three years old, had a tumor on the brain and had to have an operation. After the operation, the mother was in a state of depression, not doing anything for herself, not even combing her hair. The minute you began to talk to this woman she would burst into uncontrollable tears and cry for at least ten or fifteen minutes. After she stopped crying, she would want to talk about her children and her husband not getting along with each other.

I took it upon myself to become her therapist, and, using my training and my clinical experience, I began to work with this woman and her family in the evening. I was able to spend at least two hours with this family and to sit and talk with them. I took this family all the way back to when they had gotten married and was able to bring them up to the present date. During the sessions I wondered if I was doing the right thing because at times it was interesting and sometimes it was frightening. This had not been a happy marriage, but the woman never had revealed this to her mate. It was a matter of days before I could see any progress in what I was attempting to do. The woman was able to come out of this depression, began to take care of her husband, and also was able to visit her daughter in the hospital. Since this breakdown, this woman has been able to survive and function very well, with her daughter having to go into the hospital for five more operations.

After the daughter was discharged from the hospital, she also was very depressed. I talked to the neurosurgeon, told him that I was a mental health assistant and that I worked at the community health center. I told him how important it was that she be seen by someone, that until this point I had played a very important part in this family's life, and that I would like to continue. He thought this was a very good idea. I spent many tearful days with this young lady. One night we sat up most of the night just talking about her and her life and how she had been mixed up from school days. I also was able to use my homemaking skills with this family. I would help this mother plan her day, because she had a lot to do in one day with a twenty-three-year-old who came home almost a vegetable. Now the mother is able to take care of her daughter, husband, and do her household chores without any help from me. The daughter has gone back to work, and the mother looks forward to my stopping by every Friday evening.

Homemaking Services

During the survey I was almost shocked to see how some people kept their homes and their children, and I wanted to do something about this. I brought this back to the center, and I was given the responsibility of developing a homemaking service. There are a few agencies that use the service in the needed way, but most agencies are afraid to really deal with the "nitty gritty" of the problems that exist in the poor areas. They do things that only create more problems. Rehabilitating houses and not rehabilitating people is a most unrealistic thing. They are only building more ghettos. Also there is no service available to people who are in a depressed stage or even going through a crisis, not able to take care of their family. We do not have any kind of service to keep this family together.

When a mother comes into the crisis center, maybe to be admitted to some psychiatric setting for a week or ten days, her family (children) in most cases have to be separated by placing the children in a sheltering agency or foster home. The children then become emotionally upset, and the mother may not respond to treatment. The children are placed in separate homes, different schools, with different playmates, but most of all with different parents. Then the child begins to act out in school.

Also, older people who are able to function but are not able to cook or do their own errands (pay their bills) can become even less able to function when these kinds of pressures remain. I have a patient who is seventy years old who through her lifetime has had only trouble. She had five children who were physically and mentally normal but had a child during her menopause who was born retarded. Right after the child was born, her husband died. This woman kept her child with her because she was alone. The other children had begun to marry and were leaving home. This child has never been in school, but yet she is a wonderful housekeeper. The mother has had several breakdowns and has been hospitalized on several occasions. She is now incapacitated, and her daughter is going downhill. With my visits it makes things different. There seems to be only one answer, and that is to put this woman in a home or to hospitalize her. But my answer is that, if there was a service available, such as homemaking, for this family, they could be kept together. At this point, we consider two people as constituting a family, mother and daughter.

I did not receive any help at first in developing the homemaking service. The director of the program, who has always been a busy man at the center, helped me with it and gave me all the moral support that he could. And this was all that I had to keep me going. Other people who were able to help just did not. There were people (professionals) who even told me to forget it because I would not be able to write such a proposal. There were also agency people who communicated freely with me until they found out I was a nonprofessional. And there were professional people who tried to discourage me because they had previously submitted similar proposals and had been rejected. But through the frustration and tears I have finally written a proposal that I think has very good content and value, and one that I think will work. At this point, now that they (professionals) have seen that I was not giving up, they are beginning to support me. Although most of them are late getting involved, I am still very happy to have their support. I think that my effort and desire to complete what I had been assigned to do has in some way influenced the professional people in the nonprofessional's capabilities.

"Total Community" Services

I guess you are wondering if my training affected me as a person and if it affected my home life. Well, it has had an awful lot to do with the reason that my family is together. My husband helped me a lot during training. As time went on and people in my neighborhood were coming to me for all kinds of help, he saw some positive results and also became proud of me. I have all kinds of contacts in my area, from the police to the man who will drive people to the hospital during emergencies.

I think that at this point the mental health center has been good for the community. It has taken people from the community, such as myself, and trained them to help others in the community. I feel as though my role is a good role for people who are in the community. But, by the same token, people in the community think the center should be doing more, such as coping with agencies that seem to create mental health problems (schools, welfare, and so on). This is where I become confused about mental health centers and their responsibility to the community. I do not believe that mental health centers can take care of all of society's problems.

I do believe that the center provides good care for people in the community who are mentally ill, but it should do more than this. It should try to change some of the agencies to make them less harmful to people. From my understanding of the mental health legislation, the centers have to be too clinically oriented. I do not think that this should be the direction for mental health centers operating within areas deprived socioeconomically. In view of my own experiences, I am led to believe that much more emphasis should be placed on higher quality education and vocational training for the hard-core unemployed. We should also work toward providing more adequate housing and consumer education, both of which could be provided through our homemaking service. We should improve medical care offered to the poor, both in attitudes and quality. There should be an emphasis placed on better police–community relationships in the poor area. There should be more community people involved in the operation of stations in their own communities.

I recognize that these are the needs of the total community, not only of patients. But if they could be resolved, then many problems presented in clinics would not appear. If centers do not concentrate on these goals, and if they cannot see what is really creating mental illness, then there is no relevance for them to mental health. Unless all mental health centers try to provide the kinds of "total community" services that I have mentioned, legislators will never understand and appropriate the kind of funds that such an approach demands.

POLICE AS A COMMUNITY MENTAL
HEALTH RESOURCE
10
Robert Liberman

The research reported here is addressed to the question: Why do the police play such an important part in the care of the mentally ill? The
prominence of the police as an agent in the handling of the mentally ill
is found in most communities around the country (Glasscote, 1966).
Statewide surveys made in 1959 and 1963 in Indiana found that 1258 patients spent an average of seven days in jail during these two years.
Most of them were in jail awaiting disposition to psychiatric treatment
facilities. During 1964 in Virginia, just under 1600 persons were held in
jail awaiting commitment to mental hospitals. A spokesman for the
Texas Department of Mental Health estimates "that over half of the
mentally ill patients in Texas who are awaiting diagnosis or commitment and are considered incompetent or dangerous spend at least a
few days in a local jail." A similar situation is found in Florida where
mentally ill people spend from ten to fourteen days in jail awaiting
competency hearings (Glasscote, 1966). The states mentioned here are
presented as examples of a nation-wide situation.

In San Francisco the police referred one-fifth of the patients at the
psychiatric service of the public hospital (Bittner, 1967). Hollingshead
and Redlich (1958) found that, in the lowest socioeconomic class, more
than half of psychotic patients are referred to psychiatric facilities by
the police. In Baltimore, the site of the present report, nearly half the
residents admitted to state hospitals in 1957 came from police stations
where they had been arrested and detained as prisoners (Maryland Association for Mental Health Report, 1961). The majority of these patients either come to the police themselves or are apprehended following
a complaint by a family member or relative. Most of the "police pa-

This study was performed when the author was associated with the Department of
Mental Hygiene of The Johns Hopkins University School of Public Health and Hygiene. The research was financed by the Henry Strong Denison Fund for Medical Research. The author appreciates the encouragement of Professor Paul V. Lemkau and
the technical assistance of Mrs. Mary Grotefend, R.N. Reprinted by permission from
the *Community Mental Health Journal*, 1969, 5(2), 111–120. Dr. Liberman is a psychiatrist currently associated with Camarillo State Hospital of the California Department of Mental Hygiene.

tients" in Baltimore are held in custody until a brief mental-status examination is performed by two physicians, who are usually not psychiatrists. If deemed sufficiently ill, the person is committed to a state hospital from the station house. Almost half of these patients, in 1957, were kept behind bars for more than twelve hours before being admitted to a hospital.

The present research approaches the police–mental patient involvement from the point of view of the patient and his family: Why do some people take their behavior and psychological problems to the police, while others turn to what would appear to be more functionally appropriate medical and psychiatric facilities?

Methods

A comparison was undertaken between those white, first admission patients from Baltimore who used the police ($N=17$) and those who used medical or psychiatric resources ($N=35$) for entry into the state mental hospitals. Details of the sample population and the selection process are given in other publications (Liberman, 1965, 1967). Interviews were conducted with each patient and a key family member within one month of admission. From the initial interview with the patient and from the patient's record it was determined who was responsible for the *decision to seek help from that community resource that led to the hospitalization.* This person was defined as the *decision-maker.* For the police cases, sixteen of seventeen decision-makers were close relatives of the patient; one patient came himself to a police station for help. Among the medical–psychiatric cases, twenty-two of thirty-five decision-makers were relatives; the remainder were the patients.

The interviews were semistructured and covered six areas that were conceptually relevant to the process of seeking help from community resources: (1) demographic background characteristics; (2) ways of recognizing and labeling the deviance (Schwartz, 1957); (3) ways of dealing with the problem prior to obtaining formal, outside help; (4) immediate situational factors surrounding the decision to seek help from community resources; (5) influences on the actual decision-making process; (6) accessibility to and attitudes toward different community resources. In addition, detailed information was obtained from the patients and their relatives on the actual community resources used, leading to hospitalization. Because both patients and relatives were interviewed, data on the consensus between them could be ascertained for the variables above. The results of the study will be presented in terms of this multiple variable model of the pathway to the mental hospital taken by police and medical cases.

Results

Some typical reactions of police patients to their experiences are presented here.

My neighbors certainly wouldn't want to associate with me after seeing the police taking me away in a patrol wagon. It was a poor (sic) down, degrading thing to do. I'd be very embarrassed in church or anywhere.

The plice came to our house and surprised me. My mother thought she was doing the right thing. It was terrible being taken away by the police, but I went willingly.

Six policemen and a policewoman came and picked me up. They took me to the police station and I stayed in the bleak, awful cell for three hours. I felt shamed to my heart. I knew it wasn't the place for me. . . . It's a place for a criminal. I felt I was under judgment by the world.

(Told by a patient's daughter.) They put her in a cell and she was screaming and climbing on the bars to see if we had left yet. . . . We had to go back there several times to calm her down.

I spent one night and a day in the police station. It was unpleasant. . . . I couldn't sleep . . . just sat on a bench and stared at the wall. . . . They put me in handcuffs for the trip to the hospital.

How much damage is done to the therapeutic process by the jailing of prospective patients is hard to say, but it obviously delays the onset of treatment and adds another trauma to the individual. Over 70 percent. of the police patients claimed they would not again use the police if they had a choice, but over 90 percent of their relatives who actually made the decision to call the police said that they would do so again if the opportunity arose.

Background Factors: Police versus Medical Cases

The people who decided to call the police for help were significantly older than those who decided to use medical or psychiatric resources. However, the ages of the two groups of patients did not differ. Social class was determined arbitrarily for comparative purposes from education and rent. Individuals with both a high school education or more, *and* rent of $80 per month or more, were placed in the "upper" class (25 percent of the sample). Those with either a high school education or more, *or* rent of $80 per month or more, were considered "middle" class (40 percent of the sample). "Lower" class individuals had less than a high school education *and* paid less than $80 per month rent (35 percent of the sample). The police patients tended to come from the "lower" class (65 percent), while the medical patients more often belonged to the "middle" class (66 percent), which is significant at the .05 level. However, social class did not differentiate key family members or decision-makers in the police and medical groups. No differences between the two groups were found for marital status, sex, religion, church attendance, or residential mobility.

The distribution of admission diagnoses given the patients in the police and medical groups is shown in Table 1. A significantly greater proportion of police patients were diagnosed as schizophrenic (all paranoid type) or as having personality disorders, whereas the medical patients were more often diagnosed as neurotic or depressed. The differences in diagnoses between the two groups parallel the differences in attitudes of the patients toward getting help as will be shown below.

Recognizing and Defining the Problem

A striking difference between the police and medical patients is seen in their degree of willingness to define their problem as "mental" or psychiatric. Denial of mental illness is made by 94 percent of the police patients but by only 29 percent of the medical patients. The relatives of the patients in these two groups did not show this difference. Over 90 percent in both groups viewed the problem as "mental."

Three indexes of *tolerance for deviance* were derived from the time elapsing between (1) recognition of the problem and defining it as "mental," (2) recognition of the problem and seeking help from the first community resource, and (3) defining the problem as "mental" and seeking help from the first community resource. No differences emerged between the police and medical cases on these indexes of tolerance for deviance, either for the patients or for their family members. Similarly,

Table 1
Admission diagnoses of police and medical cases to state hospital

DIAGNOSIS	POLICE CASES		MEDICAL CASES	
	%	No.	%	No.
Schizophrenia	58	10	26	9
Personality disorder	24	4	14	5
Neurosis	12	2	28	10
Depression	6	1	23	8
Involutional melancholia	0	0	9	3
Total	100	17	100	35

$p < 0.05$, chi square, for differences between police and medical cases in schizophrenia and personality disorders versus neurosis and depression and involutional melancholia.

Table 2
Patients' definition of their illness or problem at the time
of hospitalization

	POLICE CASES		MEDICAL CASES	
DEFINITION	%	No.	%	No.
"Mental" or psychiatric	6	(1)	71	(25)
Denial of "mental" label	94	(16)	29	(10)
Total	100	17	100	35

$p < 0.001$, chi square, difference between police and medical cases.

there was little or no difference between patients or family members of the two groups on such important variables as *causation* imputed to the illness, *seriousness* attributed to the illness, *duration* or *acuteness* of the problem, or patient–family member consensus on these variables. These findings contradict the assumption made by Hollingshead and Redlich (1958) that families who call the police for help with a disturbed member are unsophisticated in their perception and definition of the disturbed behavior, and more tolerant of deviance.

The key members of the patient's family were asked whether they thought the patient was to blame for his problem or whether he was just a victim of circumstances beyond his control. The resulting moral judgment passed on the police patient was significantly negative, that is, blameworthy, more often than for the medical patient.

The attitude of the patient toward getting help—his *readiness for help*—as seen by the patient himself and by the key family member clearly differentiates police cases from medical cases. Tables 2 and 3

Table 3
Readiness for getting help from formal community resources

	POLICE CASES		MEDICAL CASES	
PATIENTS' RESPONSES	%	No.	%	No.
Never wanted help and didn't think it was necessary	71	(12)	11	(4)
Knew help was necessary but didn't want to go for it	12	(2)	9	(3)
Realized need for help and wanted or was persuaded to get help	17	(3)	80	(28)
Total	100	17	100	35

$p < 0.01$, chi square, police versus medical cases.

show that the police patients are significantly more reluctant to see a need for professional help and less willing to go voluntarily to the state mental hospital. There was marked consensus between the patients' stated attitudes in these matters and the attitudes ascribed to them by their key family members.

Informal Ways of Dealing with the Problem

Did the police cases cope with their problems differently from the medical cases before seeking formal assistance from community resources? The interviews revealed that patients and their relatives in both groups used, to about the same extent, such coping mechanisms as prayer, social withdrawal, displacement behavior (for example, "I tried to keep busy doing other things"), and informal, nonprofessional sources of help and advice, such as other relatives, friends, and co-workers.

Precipitating Factors

The police cases could not be differentiated from the medical cases by factors in the immediate situation surrounding the decision to seek help from community resources. A majority of decision-makers in both groups claimed that some event precipatated their acting to seek formal assistance. This event could be a sudden worsening in the patient's symptoms; his actual or threatened violence to self, others, or property; or situational factors extraneous to the patient's behavior. An example of extraneous situational factors in the case of the husband of a chronic schizophrenic woman who developed tuberculosis himself and had to enter a sanitarium. For many years he had sheltered and protected his wife without outside assistance. He realized that she could not live at home alone, and so he brought her to the Visiting Nurse Association. They could not provide treatment or hospitalization, and the husband subsequently called the police for help. Another example in this category is the patient who was hospitalized by his brother with whom he was living. This was precipitated by the marriage of the brother's daughter and her needing the patient's room when she moved in with her husband.

Personal Influences on Decisions To Seek Help

Sixty-three percent of the decision-makers in the total sample were directly influenced in their choice of the specific resource leading to hospitalization by another person. Elaboration of this *direct* personal influence can be found in another publication (Liberman, 1965). In terms of *indirect* personal influence, almost half of all decision-makers reported that they knew of other cases that had used the same kind of resource they had chosen. Less than one-third of the decision-makers indicated

142   The Politics of the Emerging Professions

that the mass media played a part in making them aware of their chosen resource.

Accessibility to Community Resources

An individual's accessibility to community facilities is a complex outcome of (1) evaluative attitudes toward the facilities, (2) knowledge of their existence and availability, and (3) previous contact with the facilities. From responses to questions tapping these variables, an "accessibility index" was formulated for each potential community resource, and comparisons were made between police and medical decision-makers. Compared to those who chose medical resources, persons who decided to use the police had significantly higher accessibility to the police and lower accessibility to physicians. This finding (Table 4) is more significant in view of the fact that the two groups did not differ in accessibility to any of the other facilities evaluated—clergymen, social agencies, psychiatrists, general hospitals, or psychiatric outpatient clinics. The greater accessibility to police by those using the police derives from their evaluating the police more favorably as a resource "to get help from with a mental problem." The police are rated lowest of all community resources by the medical patients and their relatives, but are ranked in the middle by the police patients and their relatives. Similarly, the police are seen as the "easiest and most convenient resource" by a majority of the police cases but by only one of the medical cases. Conversely, only one of the police decision-makers felt that physicians were the "easiest and most convenient resource" as contrasted with almost half of the medical decision-makers.

Consensus between patients and their key family members was high with regard to their relative preferences for different community resources. It should be noted that retrospective distortion may have biased somewhat the responses of the police and medical cases to questions

Table 4
Accessibility to police and physicians by decision-makers in police and medical cases

	ACCESSIBILITY INDEX FOR POLICE				ACCESSIBILITY INDEX FOR PHYSICIANS			
	High		Low		High		Low	
DECISION-MAKER	%	No.	%	No.	%	No.	%	No.
Police cases	65	(11)	35	(6)	29	(5)	71	(12)
Medical cases	11	(4)	89	(31)	66	(23)	34	(12)
chi square:	p<0.001				p<0.02			
police versus medical cases.								

dealing with their preferences for police and medical resources respectively. For example, those using the police may subsequently, because of their actions, accord higher ratings to the police than they would have if asked prior to their use of the police.

One police case exemplifies high access to police because of convenience. A middle-aged man and his wife moved to Baltimore from another state when his job was transferred. Under the increased demands of his new job the man became seriously depressed and implied to his wife that he might injure himself. She, being new to the city and without friends, did not know of any physician to call and therefore called the police when her husband began to play with a knife.

Despite differences in accessibility to police and physicians, both groups of decision-makers agreed in giving highest rankings to physician, clergyman, and psychiatrist as an "appropriate resource to treat problems like yours."

Family members calling for the police for help did so not because they lacked sophistication in defining the prospective patient's illness as mental, but rather with the foreknowledge that the police would help by certifying the sick person for hospitalization. This concrete and informed expectation was reported by 70 percent of those who called the police. A minority wanted the police to mediate family conflicts, for example, "I wanted the judge to tell my husband to leave me alone," or "I thought the judge would advise a divorce."

Utilization of Community Resources

In numbers of different community resources used, the medical cases averaged 4.2 and the police cases 3.3 (not a statistically significant difference). Table 5 shows the temporal sequence of community re-

Table 5
Temporal sequence of community resources utilized by police cases
(N = 17) prior to hospitalization

RESOURCE	TEMPORAL ORDER OF RESOURCES UTILIZED					
	1st	2nd	3rd	4th	5th–8th	
Medical doctor	4	3	3	1	0	11
Police	1	4	5	4	3	17
Psychiatric	2	5	1	2	0	10
General hospital, social agency, clergy, lawyer	10	4	3	0	1	18
	17	16	12	7	4	56

NOTE. Figures given are raw N. Ninety-four percent of cases utilized two or more separate resources and 41 percent four or more.

sources utilized by the seventeen police cases. Although nonpolice resources were consulted on thirty-nine separate occasions by these cases, they all ultimately were arrested and brought to the state mental hospital by the police. Part of the explanation of this comes from the network of referrals provided the cases as they move along various community resources.

A strong relationship exists between the very first resource seen by each case (police and medical) and the resource that initiates the hospitalization process either directly or indirectly via an unbroken chain of referrals to other facilities. If a patient is seen first by a physician, psychiatrist, or psychiatric clinic, 80 percent of the time he will enter the state hospital through the initiation of one of these resources (although not necessarily the same individual resource). On the other hand, if a patient is seen first by the police, a social agency, a general hospital, lawyer, or clergyman, 90 percent of the time he will end his help-seeking with one of these types of resources.

How this determinancy affects the police patients, who have low accessibility to physicians, can be appreciated from the fact that physicians are the initial resource used by 63 percent of the medical cases but by only 24 percent of the police cases. The physician, as the principal gatekeeper accounting for half of all initial community resources seen by our sample, is in a key position to make referrals that can determine the ultimate pathway taken by the individual en route to the state hospital. Of forty-eight referrals made by physicians, over 75 percent were to psychiatrists, mental health clinics, or mental hospitals. On the other hand, social agencies and clergymen, seen initially by 35 percent of the police cases, referred only 25 percent of all cases to psychiatric facilities.

The referral behavior of community resources is flexible and responsive to differences among the cases. For example, although physicians were visited eleven times by the police cases, none of these doctors made referrals to other physicians or psychiatric facilities. The doctors were not interviewed, but it is clear that the lack of motivation for treatment by the potential police cases was instrumental in their not being referred to specialized psychiatric resources.

Discussion

This study reveals that mental patients are brought into contact with the police because the patients have refused voluntary treatment and because other, more "appropriate," medical—psychiatric resources are not as accessible. The patient's family uses the police intelligently as a mental health resource; help and transportation to treatment are solicited, not control or imprisonment.

The typical police patient is not a violent, uncontrollable madman but is likely (1) to be either a paranoid schizophrenic or have a personality disorder (82 percent versus 40 percent for medical cases) and (2) to deny that he has a mental illness or needs professional help. This study confirms and elaborates upon a previous analysis of police patients from Baltimore done in 1957 (Maryland Association for Mental Health Report, 1961), which revealed that only 6 percent were suicidal and 75 percent were docile and manageable by persons other than the police.

The police case usually has low accessibility to the major community gatekeeper for treatment, the physician, and when he does visit a medical or psychiatric resource, his low interest in treatment makes it difficult for him to obtain needed services. One example of this process is a patient with a personality disorder who was unemployed, manipulative, and living at home with his mother. His mother visited a psychiatric clinic and asked for help (her son was moderately depressed and apathetic and destroyed some furniture) but was told that home visits were not made. Since the patient refused to come voluntarily for treatment, his mother called the police so that they would get him the help he needed. The police, then, made the necessary "home visit."

Bittner (1967) found that when requests for police aid came from physicians, lawyers, or employers, the police generally moved the patient to the hospital. It is assumed that these referrals indicate that other, more conventionally appropriate sources of help have been exhausted. Cumming (1962) reported fourteen of twenty-seven men reaching mental hospitals as having had contact with the police and indicated that the police enter the pathway to the hospital when "other attempts to ameliorate the situation fail." In the current study, nine cases were referred to the police by medical and psychiatric resources through recommendations given to the patients' families. These referrals were made after it was established that the patient would not volunteer for treatment since the resources involved (three social agencies, three physicians, one psychiatrist, one psychiatric clinic, one general hospital) would not offer services to a recalcitrant patient.

Additional evidence for the conclusion that the police are filling a gap in community mental health services comes from a study by Cumming et al. (1965) of phone calls coming to a police desk. Most of the calls for help with personal problems came after 5 P.M. and on weekends—hours when conventional sources of help are less accessible. Bittner's research (1967) shows that the police are unusually tolerant of deviant behavior, are supportive to individuals defined as "mentally ill" or eccentric, and are reluctant to interpose with arrests or commitments to hospitals, especially when other practical means are available

146 The Politics of the Emerging Professions

to manage the problem. The current study, focusing on the patient and his family, indicates that the enlightened handling of prospective patients by the police has had an impact on the public, which views the police as a reasonable "treatment" resource. Of interest is the finding that those family members deciding to use the police did not differ in social class from those using more conventional medical resources. Bittner has data that support the contention that police use is randomly distributed by social class (personal communication). Thus police interventions in cases of mental illness are not concentrated in the lower socioeconomic segments of the community, a fact that further attests to the sophisticated and intelligent use of the police when other resources fail to provide needed services. Until community mental health facilities develop more active evaluation and treatment programs for reluctant patients, for example, home treatment services and use of visiting nurses, the police will continue to serve a needed role in the care of the mentally ill.

Efforts are now underway to improve the effectiveness of the police as a mental health resource. Bard and Berkowitz (1967) report an ongoing program in New York City that is training police in family crisis intervention. The findings from the current research point to the great importance of familiarizing the police with knowledge of emotional disturbance and of equipping them with specialized techniques of intervention.

REFERENCES

Bard, M., and Berkowitz, B. Training police as specialists in family crisis intervention: A community psychology action program. *Community Mental Health Journal*, 1967, 3, 315–317.

Bittner, E. Police discretion in emergency apprehension of mentally ill persons. *Social Problems*, 1967, 14, 278–292.

Cumming, Elaine. Phase movement in the support and control of the psychiatric patient. *Journal of Health and Human Behavior*, 1962, 3, 235–241.

Cumming, Elaine, Edell, L., and Cumming, I. Policeman as philosopher, guide and friend. *Social Problems*, 1965, 12, 276–286.

Glasscote, R. M. Putting the mentally ill in jail continues to be common practice in much of U.S. *Psychiatric News*, May & June, 1966.

Hollingshead, A., and Redlich, F. C. *Social class and mental illness*. New York: John Wiley, 1958.

Liberman, R. Personal influence in the use of mental health resources. *Human Organization*, 1965, 24, 231–235.

Liberman, R. The role of physicians in the patient's path to the mental hospital. *Community Mental Health Journal*, 1967, 3, 325–330.

Maryland Association for Mental Health. *Finding the way to the mental hospital*. Baltimore: 1961.
Schwartz, Charlotte G. Perspectives on deviance: Wives' definitions of their husbands' mental illness. *Psychiatry*, 1957, *20*, 275–291.

VIOLENCE, LIKE CHARITY, BEGINS AT HOME

11

Ronald Sullivan

"All I've got for you is a little family trouble at Sixteen-Thirteen Madison." He'll tell you which floor and thank God it isn't the top, and so you'll climb, climb, climb, and all the while you'll be preparing to say, "Listen, what's the matter with you folks? Pipe down, can't you? Oh, shet ep, sister. Look— people are complaining; you're waking us folks in the building. O.K.—so you can't get along. O.K.—so you're drunk too. Now, look, I want you out of here. And quit socking your wife, and if I see you around her again before morning—before you're sober and ready to behave—I'll break your head wide open!"

That's the little speech, the succession of disciplinary directions that you'll be composing as you trudge upstairs; and then you hear the shuddering gasp, and somehow you're through the door before they've opened it for you, and he's standing there alone. The woman is on the floor with her skirts around her middle, and what beautiful red rosy tights she wears—all slick and damp—and the tights are extending themselves into a big evil patch on the floor. But beyond her he is there. He's very large; he looks colossal to you now. He doesn't have anything on except a pair of striped underwear shorts, and his eyes are rolling. He keeps watching you. He has a bloody bread knife in his hand, and you keep saying "Put it down, put it down—let go that knife," as he comes toward you a step at a time, and as the woman grunts and shifts on the floor in her blood, and still he keeps coming in, you've got to decide, and all in the instant. Do you shoot or do you try to use your stick? Do you try to take the knife away from him? . . . You don't like to be alone, nobody would like to be alone.

—MacKinlay Kantor,
"Signal Thirty-Two."

The threatened cop in Kantor's novel, like policemen everywhere, had every reason to feel alone. The odds were against him because it seems that violence, like charity, begins at home. According to the Federal Bureau of Investigation, one of every five policemen killed in the line of duty dies trying to break up a family fight. The President's Commission on Law Enforcement and the Administration of Criminal Justice re-

From *The New York Times Magazine*, November 24, 1968. © 1968 by the New York Times Company. Reprinted by permission. Ronald Sullivan is the *Times* New Jersey correspondent, based in Trenton, and a veteran police reporter.

ported last year that family disputes "are probably the single greatest cause of homicides" in the United States. And if policemen don't get killed in a family fight, they still stand a good chance of being bloodied. "There is a strong impression in police circles that intervention in these disputes causes more assaults on policemen than any other encounter," the commission reported in *The Challenge of Crime in a Free Society* (1968). In fact, the New York City Police Department estimates that 40 percent of its men injured in the line of duty were hurt while responding to family disturbances. Moreover, the department estimates that such calls take as much time as any other single kind of police action. "Yet the capacity of the police to deal effectively with such a highly personal matter as conjugal disharmony is, to say the least, limited . . . an activity for which few policemen—or people in any profession—are qualified by temperament or by training," the commission reported.

But that was before an experimental New York City police unit began intervening in family quarrels in upper West Harlem. Despite the high statistical probability of being knifed, shot at, gang-jumped, or pushed down a flight of tenement stairs, none of the eighteen volunteer patrolmen assigned to the Family Crisis Intervention Unit in the Thirtieth Precinct has sustained a single injury, much less a fatality, in the unit's first fifteen months of operation. Moreover, after intervening in more than one thousand individual family crises—an average of a little more than two a night—the unit has not been involved in a single charge of police brutality, and this is an area in which such accusations are commonplace.

But, perhaps just as important, none of the interventions resulted in either a homicide or a suicide. There are no conclusive records in the precinct to show how this deathless record compares with the outcome of family fights in the precinct in previous years. Nevertheless, [then] Police Commissioner Howard R. Leary, the United States Department of Justice, and the project's originator, Dr. Morton Bard, director of the Psychological Center at City College, are convinced that the new unit unquestionably has saved many lives.

There are no records connecting deaths with family fights because no police function is more misunderstood, more underrated, and more grudgingly performed than calls to break them up. Unlike other police activity, such as murder investigations or criminal surveillance, intervention in family fights is commonly regarded at all levels in the Police Department as a thankless job that poses the danger of grave personal risk and the distinct possibility of becoming embroiled in charges of police brutality, with very little, if any, promise of reward. A cop makes detective or becomes a sergeant by the big arrest or the daring rescue—not by breaking up a family fight. It is not surprising, then, that there are few references to the subject in police literature or at police training academies.

Now, however, it seems likely that the apparent success of the Family Crisis Intervention Unit will have an impact on the way policemen are motivated, trained, and ultimately rewarded by their departments. In fact, this year's report by the National Advisory Commission on Civil Disorders (1968) recommended New York's pilot program as a "model for other departments." The report said, "The commission believes the police cannot and should not resist becoming involved in community service matters. . . . Such work can gain the police the respect and support of the community."

Its importance was pointed up by the Governor's Select Commission on Civil Disorder in New Jersey. After investigating the causes of the Negro rioting in Newark in July, 1967, the commission reported that most complaints of police brutality originated from incidents that began as family-disturbance calls—and that these complaints had been increasing before the rioting broke out.

According to Dr. Bard, outmoded police organization is the silent factor underlying the growing tension between police and community, particularly in the urban ghettos. And the violence of family conflict in these areas is matched only by the indifference of society outside to its existence. Professor Bard emphasizes that only the police, of all social institutions, are present twenty-four hours a day, every day of the year, to answer the call when family violence threatens.

Thus, with the full support of Commissioner Leary, and $94,736 from the Federal Government, Dr. Bard's Psychological Center began a two-year experiment last year in training police to intervene in family fights. The pilot program, which is scheduled to end next April, does not aim to turn cops into psychologists or social workers. "That's just exactly what we're attempting to avoid," says Dr. Bard, who was a cop himself for a short time in the late nineteen-forties before he became a group worker with street gangs and ultimately a professor of psychology. "We have no intention of creating a family cop, or a family division, or making family crisis intervention an esoteric police specialty. All we're trying to do is give the ordinary policeman a new skill, one that will help him do better what he now does most—and that is help people in trouble." If, at the same time, he can become a primary mental health resource in the community, so much the better, of course.

The program also is part of a growing revolution involving the training of clinical psychologists and the development of community mental health programs in the cities. There simply never will be enough psychologists to treat poor persons in the slums, where most of the aggressive behavior and mental disorder is. So the idea at the center is to train psychologists to train other persons to do it.

At the same time, the university is given the chance to break out from its pedagogical shell by turning the surrounding community into a teeming psychological laboratory rather than a hostile environment. What better place is there than Harlem to study marital breakdown, aggression, sado–masochism, and the effects of violence on early childhood development? And who is better equipped to study it than the persons who face it every day, like Patrolman John E. Bodkin, a thirty-two-year-old, cigar-smoking, no-nonsense, seven-year veteran and member of the Family Crisis Intervention Unit?

"It was up on 145th Street," he said. "And the couple was from the South. We went in there and I could see right off that this guy was tight, very tight. He was a Negro fellow, about twenty-one or twenty-two years old, only up in New York six months. She had called the police because of a dispute—a minor thing. But there he was, a little guy, and he was really tense because when we walked in with our uniforms and our sticks, you could see that his earlier associations with police officers must have been very rough.

"You could see the fear in his eyes, the hostility in his face. His fists were clenched, and he was ready to do combat with us. God knows what he would have done if he'd had a gun or a knife. I moved toward the kitchen table and opened my blouse and I told him in a nice quiet way that I wanted to talk to him, but he's still tense and he's still looking at my stick. Well, the stick is under my arm so I hung it up on a nearby chair, purposely, to show there's no intent here. 'Look, I don't need it,' I'm trying to say to this guy. 'I don't need it because you're a nice guy in my eyes. You don't threaten me, so I'm not going to threaten you.' I've got to show this guy that I'm not a bully, a brute, a Nazi, or the Fascist he thinks all cops are.

"So he calms down a little. Then I took my hat off and I said, 'Do you mind if I smoke?' And he looks at me funny. And I say, 'I'm a cigar smoker and some people don't like the smell of a cigar in their house, so would you mind if I smoke?' And the guy says, 'Oh sure, sure,' and you could see he was shocked. I felt he saw a human side of us, that I had respect for him and his household.

"Then the guy sat down and he and his wife proceed to tell us what it was all about. When we explain to her why he's upset, she smiles. 'Yes, yes, yes.' You see, she thinks we're on her side. Then we tell him why he's mad and he smiles. 'Yes, yes, yes.' Now we're on his side. Well, they eventually shake our hands; they were happy and we never had another call from them."

Patrolman Bodkin and the seventeen other policemen in the family crisis unit operate in biracial pairs out of the ninety-six-year-old, four-story Thirtieth Precinct station house on the southwest corner of 152d Street and Amsterdam Avenue. The Thirtieth is one of New York's smaller and more insignificant precincts, running north from 141st to 165th Streets and east from Riverside Drive to Edgecombe Avenue. Most of the old apartment houses on Broadway have been taken over by Puerto Rican and Negro families. The remaining whites in the precinct, many of them apparently Jewish, are virtually barricaded in the big apartment houses overlooking the Hudson on Riverside Drive. Actually, the Thirtieth is just what Dr. Bard was looking for: a rat-infested neighborhood, but without the wretchedness of some of the other black precincts in Harlem, one free of big crime and big institutions and one that comes alive every week when the welfare checks roll in.

Like Bodkin, most of the cops in the family unit were already working in the Thirtieth before the program began. None of them was picked because he evidenced a bleeding heart for minority problems. All of them, and this includes the nine Negroes, were used to feeling hated, feared and envied in the ghetto. None of them has a college degree. They tend to be young, in their late twenties and early thirties, because it is very hard to teach old cops new tricks. What Dr. Bard, along with Dr. Bernard Berkowitz, a psychologist with twelve years as a policeman in his background, looked for in choosing from among forty-five volunteers were experienced cops who expressed enthusiasm for the experiment and frustration with their present inability to deal effectively with family crises, and who showed every indication of being sensitive to the changing role the police must assume in the cities.

The eighteen men, who were released from duty, spent nearly a month with professional psychologists at the center in mutual exploration of the best methods of successful intervention. The psychologists knew all about such things as aggression, trauma, neurosis, alcoholism and all the other behavioral patterns associated with family violence. And that is what they taught the men during the first three weeks of intensive psychological classroom work. But the center's pedagogy and its proclivity for reflective analysis generally failed the psychologists when they departed from the laboratory or the textbook for the explosive, instant-action world of police confrontation with family violence. "No one has a textbook for that. This is where we had to learn from each other," says Dr. Bard.

During the third week, the cops were subjected to three days of family-crisis psycho-skits staged by a group of professional actors. The short plays showed typical family crises and were written without conclusions; the endings were improvised by the patrolmen themselves, who intervened in pairs at the end. For example, in one play, a young Negro actress portrayed a wife who was cowering against the rear classroom wall, away from a tall, husky Negro, playing her wife-beating husband.

"He's going to hit me, he's going to hit me again," she screamed as the two cops burst on the scene and split, one of them going to the aid of the stricken woman, the other confronting the man.

"Whaddaya doing that for?" the patrolman snarled at the man as he pushed him toward a corner of the improvised stage. "That's no way to treat a woman, that's no way for a man to act. You're no man." With that, the Negro actor, even though he knew it was only a play, reacted angrily and moved toward the advancing patrolman, bellowing, "Who says I'm no man . . . ?"

At that point, the play was stopped and the cops and the actors analyzed their respective reactions. For one thing, the cop who confronted the husband was told this is how most cops get hurt—challenging a man's masculinity. Moreover, the cops were told that the wife may very well be a masochist who has spent the day provoking the man into attacking her. He gets an outlet for his aggression; she has the simple pleasure of getting beaten up. The idea, the policemen were told, is to give the combatants alternatives and the help they need to understand why they fight.

But an unsophisticated cop can go only so far, and this is where their fourth week of training came in. They took field trips to various social, health, and welfare agencies where experts explained the kinds of help available to poor families in trouble. Later, the men took part in human-relations workshops where they were prompted to examine, in group sensitivity discussions, their individual prejudices and preconceptions of disrupted family life in the ghetto.

After this, the unit began operating out of the Thirtieth station house in the precinct's special family car. Two members of the unit work each of the day's three eight-hour tours and are dispatched on all complaints involving family disturbances. They also continue their normal police duties—they give out parking tickets and speeding summonses; they patrol a given sector of the precinct; they are expected to respond to any emergency just like any other cop on the beat. At the start, they were subject to considerable jeering from other patrolmen, but their capacity to handle both missions effectively has turned the initial jibes at the station house into inquiries on how to deal with family crises.

Meantime, all of the eighteen men continue their training, taking part in six-man discussion groups led by professional psychologists. In addition, each man has a weekly private consultation with a third-year graduate student in clinical psychology. The consultation cuts both ways. The officer reports the way he reacted to a particular family crisis and is given advice on ways he might have responded differently. Some of the students have become intrigued with the research opportunities afforded by these exchanges. One has formulated a research proposal in which he will attempt to measure differences in aggressive threshold stimuli among children of families in which day-to-day violence is a part of the environment. These children will be matched with children raised in nonviolent homes.

Adriaan Halfhide, a twenty-seven-year-old Negro cop assigned to the family project, is convinced that 60 percent of the people in every block in the precinct are aware of the new unit. "We're more aware of them, too," he says. "We go into a family dispute and we can pick up certain signs, statements, gestures, looks and facial expressions that enable us to get a basic idea of what's going on. For example, I notice whether a man is gritting his teeth, whether the veins in his temple are throbbing. Before, I only looked for whether he had a weapon, or whether he was bigger than me. Later, when they just want someone to yell at, someone to use as a butt for their anger, I say, 'O.K., get mad at me.' Then everybody yells at me. But they're all together, yelling together, but at me, and that's groovy."

Halfhide and the other family cops have some fundamental ground rules. They always stay calm; they don't threaten and they don't take sides. They don't challenge a man's masculinity; they don't degrade a woman's femininity. They intentionally give people verbal escape routes to save face. And mother isn't always right—they know about Oedipus complexes. They notice that most family fights tend to break out on Sunday night after a festering weekend of drinking. They say the major causes of conflict are, predictably, money and sex. Families fight more in the summer because it's hot, and more in the winter because it's so cold outside they can't escape one another.

On the back seat of their patrol car the family cops keep two small wooden boxes with card files showing whom the unit has previously been sent to. The file is kept by street numbers so the men on duty can determine immediately whether any other team has called upon a family to which they are on their way. The cards show whether an earlier intervention involved any weapons so that the responding patrolmen can be on guard. The cards have thirty-five entries, including, besides usual vital statistics, "What happened IMMEDIATELY before your arrival? What do *you* think led up to the immediate crisis? (Changes in family patterns?) (Environmental changes, etc.?) Impressions of the family: How long has this family been together? Who is dominant? What is the appearance of the house? Appearance of the individuals? Other impressions? What happened after your arrival? (How did each disputant respond?) How was the dispute resolved? Mediation ( ). Referral ( ).

Aided ( ). Arrest ( ). Full details. *Summarize* the crisis situation and its resolution."

Every intervention is different, and each of the nine teams reacts differently. Nevertheless, there are some standard procedures. The patrolmen go in together, then split, with one of them going toward one of the antagonists, the second toward the other. Guns are rarely drawn. In fact, the cops often leave their nightsticks in the car. They don't shout, they don't push, and they don't threaten to lock up everyone in sight. All the while, the two men are scooping up any knives, scissors or other weapons, putting them where no one can get at them. Windows are checked in case the crisis involves a potential suicide. Children are accounted for.

Generally, the cops attempt to mollify both sides, taking the combatants into separate rooms so they can be questioned without one of them challenging the other's version of the crisis. The cops try to draw out the underlying facts, compare the differing versions and then, in a kind of group therapy, they attempt to explain to the family why it is fighting and recommend ways for it to stop. Normally, the family will be referred to a health or social agency. The cops carry printed slips with the addresses, offer to make the appointment—and in some cases drive the family down in the patrol car.

Many times, interventions do not involve violence. There is, for instance, a five-story walk-up on Amsterdam Avenue, a squalid rooming house taken over by prostitutes and narcotic addicts. But up on the top floor an old Negro couple—she in her late seventies, he in his eighties—were barely surviving in abandoned isolation in a tiny rear room. He was weak from advanced age and malnutrition and had fallen out of bed. She did not have the strength to lift him back. They had no children, no friends, no neighbors and no money. So she called the police, and the family unit was dispatched. Instead of just putting him back in bed, which is what a lot of cops would have done, the unit called the Visiting Nurse Service. The V.N.S. told them that they should call a physician. So the cops went out and got one. And the couple are now visited regularly by V.N.S. nurses who make sure the are getting along the best they can.

Violence, though, or the forestalling of it, is the rule—especially as weekends draw to a close and the relief checks are gone, some of them spent on gin. This particular night, Patrolman Bodkin and his partner, Frank Madewell, get the call on the police radio: "Man with a gun at One-Six-Three Street and Amsterdam." They weave fast against traffic and screech up at the address behind three other patrol cars. Upstairs, there are six cops in the third floor hall and a thin, hysterical woman in her nightgown shouting obscenities—alternately through a closed apartment door and *at* the cops for not breaking it down. "He's got my kids inside, and he's got a gun!" she screams.

From inside, the man roars, "You come in and I'll blow your——head off." With that, a burly sergeant pushes by the woman and bangs on the door. "Let's go! Open up, or we'll kick it down!" he shouts. "Come right ahead,——," the man bellows back.

Meantime, Madewell goes back to the car and checks the address in the card file. The couple has quite a file; he is marked as violent and possibly armed. Madewell goes back up and tells the sergeant, who jerks his thumb toward the closed door and replies: "O.K., you're the family cops. You go on in." And slides out of the line of fire.

"First, we used his first name," Madewell recalls. "We tried to con him. I said, 'I can't scream through the door, and besides it's cold as hell out here and all your wife wants is her clothes.' But he just tells me to do you-know-what and I'm sweating. 'You can at least give her her clothes,' I say to him. 'We won't say a word to you; we won't even look. C'mon, it's getting late and we can't stay here all night. Tell me what happened; you're a man, you can tell me. Did she try to put you down?' "

"God, I'm talking and talking to this guy, and the other cops are over by the stairs with their guns out. Finally—I can't say how long—I feel the lock give and the door open a crack and we go in and take him."

Later, detectives from the Thirtieth squad determined that the man had attempted to fire a .32-caliber revolver at the sergeant through the closed door, but that the firing pin failed each time to strike the shell hard enough to shoot the bullet. The man said he had stopped trying to shoot when Madewell called him by his first name and started to talk to him.

Or spend the early morning hours of a recent Saturday on duty with Albert Robertson, a forty-two-year-old family cop, a Negro with eleven years in the department, most of them in the Thirtieth. He and his partner, William Robison, a nonunit patrolman who has been pressed into family-car duty on this tour, prowl through the precinct's garbage-strewn streets.

The first radio call sends them to St. Nicholas Avenue, where they climb, climb, climb to the sixth floor. At an open door, the young, buxom Negro woman who called the police lets them in and jerks her thumb toward a big man asleep in the bedroom. "Robbie," she says to Patrolman Robertson, whom everyone on his beat seems to know, "he's nothin' but a bum who's been whippin' me for eight years. I want him arrested before he kills me. He beat me somethin' awful before he drank hisself to sleep."

"But, sweetheart," Robertson replies, "you know he'll be out tomorrow. And are you going to give him the bail money?" (It turns out later that she simply wanted to get rid of him for the weekend so she could go to Atlantic City.)

There's another call. And at 150th Street and Amsterdam a woman shouts down from a second-floor tenement window: "Robbie! Robbie! He's got a gun. He's messin' with us with his pistol."

So Robertson and Robison draw their guns this time and tell the woman to stand back. "Open the door!" yells Robbie. "For what?" the man inside growls. "That bitch is nuts." He finally opens up but he has no gun on him—and they have no search warrant.

Then it's back quickly to a big, run-down apartment house on St. Nicholas Avenue where a man and wife in a shabby basement apartment have been at each other all night. She says: "Look what he done to me; he kicked me in the belly. I want him locked up, officer." He says: "Hell, lock her up, too," and holds out his arm to show where his wife has cut him with a kitchen knife. "I'll go as long as she goes, too; otherwise, you got to fight me."

Carefully, with a look of weariness in his round, good-natured face, Robertson takes off his blouse and cap, lays his black notebook on the hall table, and sinks slowly into the only comfortable chair in the living room. "What's you folks been drinkin'?" he asks. "Scotch," the glowering, heavy-set man answers. "Sweetheart," Robertson says to the woman, "get me a small drink, will you?" Then he takes off his shoes and rubs his arches and wiggles his toes, and the man just sits and looks at him incredulously. The man gives Robertson the Scotch, but the drink has no ice, so Robertson asks the wife to bring him some.

"By this time," Robertson explains later, "they're so shook up with me sitting in *their* chair, sippin' *their* Scotch [he actually never drank it] that now we can find out what they're really fighting about. Before you know it, I'm part of the family."

She tells Robbie that they'd always drink and end up fighting. And it begins to come out, five years of it: He can't stand the dirty dishes, the food left for days on the stove, the messy apartment, and she knows he can't. She says she can't stand his all-night drinking, his playing around, and he knows it, too. So Robbie gives them a little advice— "Look at her side; look at his"—and tells them that next time they want to fight, call him up at the station house and they can fight with him and keep it in the family. He offers Robbie another drink. . . .

The car radio sends Robertson and his partner to Riverside Drive, where a young, attractive Negro woman is standing in the lobby of one of the better apartment houses facing the river. She says she had a fight with her husband and that he won't let her back in to get her baby or her clothes. She said he threatened to kill her, too. Robbie goes up and talks to him, and the man finally agrees to let her take the baby but not the clothes—"because I paid for them." But the cops persuade him to let her have them.

Suddenly as she's packing, he pushes by Robertson and grabs her, and as they escort her out, he lunges at her again. Then he rushes into the kitchen and comes back with a bread knife. "If she goes with the clothes, you're going to have to kill me tonight. Tonight I got to die," he says. Robertson ignores him. But as they turn to leave, the man moves toward them, waving the knife.

Robertson draws his revolver and tells the man: "Put that away and settle this in court tomorrow." The man keeps coming. Robertson cocks his revolver and says: "Buddy, it isn't a question of me shooting you, but where you're going to get shot." As the man hesitates, Robertson grabs the front door, shouts: "Merry Christmas, happy New Year and a good night to you," and slams the door in the man's face.

"You know what he was doing?" he says later. "He was looking for a little sympathy. And what better way to get it around here than get shot by a cop?"

Sometimes the intervention ultimately fails, as happened earlier this year when a woman, mumbling incoherently, her hands and legs covered with blood, staggered into the Thirtieth station house and threw a bloody paring knife on the desk. Two unit patrolmen, Tony Donovan and Joseph Mahoney, happened to be there and they led her gently to a side room.

"O.K., sweetheart," one of them asked her quietly, "where are you hurt? What happened?" They gave her a cigarette and lit it for her. And as she held it in her trembling hand, she moaned: "He kept nagging me. All day, kept after me. Couldn't stand it no more. Oh, God, go help him."

Six months earlier, the woman had called the police and the family unit had been sent to stop a fight between her and her husband. The unit determined then that both were alcoholics and tried to get them to go to Alcoholics Anonymous, but they refused. However, they did agree to separate, but he came back later. The drinking began again, and the inevitable happened. They began to fight. But instead of calling the cops this time, she had stabbed her husband, nearly killing him.

Or there's the night when Patrolmen John Edmonds, a quiet, forty-one-year-old Negro, and John Mulitz, a tall, thirty-five-year-old Pennsylvania Dutchman, get the call: "A man shot," and Mulitz, who's driving, turns on the flashing red light and uses the siren to get through traffic up Broadway to 163d Street. The address is not in the car's card file. The dying man, a middle-aged Puerto Rican, is on his back in the bedroom. Part of his intestine has bubbled through his abdomen where the steel-jacketed bullet came out. His wife mumbles incoherently to Edmonds: "We have ze argument. He goes into ze bedroom. . . ."

"Maybe if she called us earlier . . . ," Edmonds says.

Then it's another call and Mulitz and Edmonds pull up in front of a sagging tenement on 149th Street where a young, scrawny Negro, his right hand swathed in bandages, comes rushing out, screaming that one of his wife's sisters just threw acid on him. It seems that he and his wife had got drunk together earlier. They started to fight, and he put his hand through a bedroom mirror. When he tried to resume the fight after being treated at Harlem Hospital, one of his wife's three monumental sisters (they could have been a beef trust, Mulitz remarks later) heaved him out while another threw a panful of cleaning ammonia on him. In the scuffle, he stabbed his wife in the leg.

When Mulitz tells him that he must be arrested for this, the Negro takes out another knife hidden under his belt and snarls, "I ain't goin', and you can't make me." Mulitz orders him to drop the knife, but he continues to move up the front steps. Mulitz opens his holster and shouts, "Drop it!" but the man just looks at him.

Finally, Mulitz, who towers easily more than a foot over the man, crosses his arms and says, "Listen, you don't have to prove you're a man to me or to your wife and her sisters. I know you're a man; you already proved it to me. Now drop the knife like a good fellow." The man stops, wavers a few seconds, then bursts into tears—and drops the knife.

And one night, George Timmins, thirty-three, and his partner, Ernest Bryant, a thirty-three year-old Negro who cuts his hair Afro style and wears love beads off duty, pay their fifth visit to a Puerto Rican couple on 145th Street who are determined to destroy each other. This time, the husband has methodically dismantled the family bed and stacked the pieces neatly against the bedroom wall before leaving for his nighttime job. "She's no goin' to mess around in this bed while I gone," he says.

Normally, the man's wife would have tried to kill him for taking the bed apart. In the past sixteen years she has opened him up across the chest with a carving knife, shot him on three separate occasions, and once has thrown lye on his sexual organs. She is an obvious sadist. He, on the other hand, doesn't seem to mind much, and he proudly pulls up his workshirt to show the cops his battle scars. She only glares at him and turns to the cops. "You think he look bad now, ha," she says. "He keeps this up, he's really goin' to get hurt."

Federal officials such as Louis A. Mayo, Jr., the thirty-nine-year-old program manager of the family intervention project in the National Institute of Law Enforcement and Criminal Justice, a new agency within the Department of Justice, consider the experiment a success, even though its full results have yet to evaluated. "We are very encouraged," Mayo said recently. "For a very limited financial investment, there's been a handsome payoff on a cost benefit basis alone—and that doesn't include the personal agony that goes with a homicide."

"Look," says Mrs. Carole Rothman, a petite and attractive twenty-three-year-old graduate student in Dr. Bard's project, "I used to have the typical 'dumb cop' image. I simply couldn't believe a cop had the capacity to figure out the psychological nuances of family conflict. But you should see how fantastically sensitive they really are. They pick up on things that I would miss, and they challenge things I let go by. Now I've become intolerant of people who have cops stereotyped. I see cops as faces, not uniforms."

"If you ask the average psychologist, 'Who becomes a cop?'" says Dr. Bard, "you know what quick, glib answer you get off the top of his head? You get, 'A sadist, a latent criminal, a paranoid.' I have yet to have somebody answer, 'Somebody who wants to help.' I suspect very strongly that a significantly large percentage—not all—of the men who seek to become cops do so out of a wish to help. They're idealistically motivated.

"But the police establishment quickly disabuses any such notion. There's no mechanism for a guy to develop along these lines. He learns very quickly that the only way he can make it is to give up this helping aspiration. The system does not reward this kind of behavior and it does not encourage it because its guiding principles are repressive, restrictive, and in keeping with the horse-and-buggy days when conflicts were resolved in the middle of Main Street by the man with the quickest draw.

"Some of these guys make a compromise; they go into youth work or rescue service. A significantly large number quit. The ones who stay make more compromises and become the most cynical transmitters of the same values which they themselves deplored when they first came in. Now, a wholly different organizational structure of the police must prevail in which the system addresses itself to the problems that society really has, rather than those which society once had. The way it is now is neurotic.

"Let's face it. The very nature of the cop is to preserve the status quo. And the reason for the confrontation between the police and the intellectual is that, if there is anything the intellectual is for, he is for change."

A former New York City police official said, "It is a fact that until very recently a patrolman who got in a gun battle was immediately rewarded with a promotion to detective. And it is unfortunately a fact that the tradition of rewarding the man who winds up in a violent confrontation is still a very real part of the New York City Police Department and most other departments, too."

Dr. Howard E. Mitchell, director of the human resources program at the University of Pennsylvania, and an expert on police, contends that the day of holding a once-a-year Brotherhood Week at the station house, on the one hand, while beefing up the Tactical Patrol Force on the other, is over. "It's a different ball game now," he says. "The police are going to have to make a lot of changes, and it doesn't take any great intelligence to know that a person trained for riot control is not the one to send out to stop a family fight in a tense community."

In a sense that is pretty much what the Family Crisis Intervention Unit is all about. Or, as Capt. Vincent T. Agoglia, the commanding officer of the Thirtieth Precinct and a thirty-year veteran, remarked as he watched his men turn out the other morning, "You've got to have the people in the community on your side or else you can forget about police work. Look at the changes here in the way the community has reacted. We've got families now who come in here and ask for the family cops. Last year, they might have to come in here looking, instead, for the civilian complaint review board. It's not what the police *say*, but what they *do*, that counts."

REFERENCES

Report of the National Advisory Commission on Civil Disorders. Washington, D.C.: Government Printing Office, 1968.

The Challenge of Crime in a Free Society: A Report by the President's Commission on Law Enforcement and the Administration of Criminal Justice. Introduction by I. Silver. New York: E. P. Dutton, 1968.

SECTION
2
The New Breed of Professional

Not only are new training models required for educating new career-ists and non–mental health professionals, but new approaches toward undergraduate and professional education are also badly needed. Ledvinka focuses in on the problems of community training on the undergraduate level. He provides a conceptual scheme for planning an undergraduate program that emphasizes the differences between classroom and field experiences in terms of both methods and products.

Kelly, who is more concerned with professional education, obviously concurs, and, like Ledvinka, is searching for methods to involve the student meaningfully in local community process. Both emphasize the need for continuous interdisciplinary interaction and a longitudinal perspective on community development. Finally, both are committed to an ecological viewpoint that considers the interplay of mental health and social–political events.

The social work profession has also responded to the call for radical change in both the form and function of professional training. Rein insists that social workers should go beyond even radical casework that is individually focused and actually fight for the rights of all the people. He argues that his profession must go beyond the practice of community sociotherapy that emphasizes self-improvement and hence is a way of diverting radical forces from what he believes to be the true oppressors, namely, the middle-class run social welfare agencies. Rein would have social workers work *for* their clients rather than *on* their clients. But this in effect means that professionals can no longer maintain a neutral attitude toward the intense social and political issues that shape the lives of their clients.

However, as Wineman and James indicate, an educator has a tendency to avoid putting his action where his mouth is. The authors spell out a number of typical avoidance responses through which a social work school can continue to place students in a dehumanizing setting while simultaneously voicing great concern about the agency or institution. Wineman and James feel that no basic change in the profession is likely to come about until the educators stop supporting

163

just individual acts of advocacy and come out in direct support for an advocacy model that is based on a political theory of social change.

The final article in this section was written by a psychologist who was trained in a traditional manner but nevertheless immersed himself in the politics of a major city, but on the side of the mayor. In a sense, Dr. Klein became the mayor's advocate. It proved to be an unnerving and painful task for this professional psychologist. But one thing is clear: He was able to function in this capacity because he previously supported the mayor in his political campaign.

In looking back over this article, one gets the strong impression that the new careerists and the new breed of professionals may talk like clinicians, but they will act like politicians. And to the extent that they are politically ineffective, they may perish amidst a storm of social–political strife.

THE COMMUNITY AS A CLASSROOM
12
James Ledvinka

Higher education's growing concern with social issues has produced a number of new teaching methods. Among these new methods are programs designed to give students direct contact with community life and community institutions. The diversity of these programs is surprising to those who are familiar with orthodox classroom teaching only. Students serve as probation workers with juvenile offenders, tutors of public school pupils from low-income families, helpers in store-front drop-in centers of various kinds, sympathetic listeners on telephone crisis lines, observers of social life in small towns, participant–observers in mental hospitals and other institutions, consultants to rural community groups, informal community-relations trainers in police departments, unpaid staff in financially pressed Community Action Agencies, doorbell-ringers in voter registration drives, community organizers of ex–mental patients, nonprofessional legal advocates for convicts, and advocate-planners for unrepresented constituencies of planning agencies.

These programs of student involvement in the community bear some resemblance to the traditional internship model, but the spirit behind most of them is different in several respects. Student roles in community programs are usually not as narrowly defined as intern roles, and the supervision of students is usually not as close. In fact, some community programs are initiated and conducted by the students themselves, and most community programs are quite responsive to student direction and control. Also, not all community programs have the same close ties to a single agency or institution that internship programs have.

By freeing the student of the constraints that he would ordinarily encounter in an internship, community programs place him in a position of unusual responsibility and autonomy. In principle, that is intuitively appealing to many teachers. In fact, the whole idea of community programs is exciting to those who are tired of traditional classroom teaching. But there are pitfalls in mixing academics with the real world. Often the theory behind a community program is unrealistic, or the

This paper was expressly written for this volume. James Ledvinka is currently Assistant Professor, Department of Management, University of Georgia.

planning inadequate, or the execution incompetent. Programs that face those problems may die early in controversy or apathy. Or they may live on, a disappointment to the people who worked so hard bringing them into being.

Any successes beyond mere survival are probably due to luck, intuition, or natural acumen. They are clearly not due to collective wisdom, for collective wisdom in this area is by and large unrecorded. Most of the experiences of community programs are not preserved in the literature. And the program reports that do appear in the literature are narratives or informal case studies (for example, see Umbarger, Dalsimer, Morrison, & Breggin, 1962; Cytrynbaum & Mann, 1969; Lunneborg, 1970; and Ledvinka & Denner, 1972). Seldom does one find hard data on the conduct or outcomes of a community program.

What is especially needed is a framework to guide the program planner. Such a framework would identify the critical considerations in developing and executing community programs. The discussion below presents the beginnings of such a framework. It is based on the impressionistic, largely unpublished accounts of several community programs. Out of those accounts emerge three focal themes:

1. A program has an *environment*. It must relate itself to certain groups and organizations: the college of which it is a part, the students who participate in it, the community in which it takes place, the agency or institution in which it is housed, and the client or target population that it serves or observes. Each of these groups and organizations can be receptive or unreceptive to the program. Each can be supportive or resistant, benign or malevolent. Each has its own interests that can coincide or conflict with the program.

2. A program has a *mission*. The mission usually has an educational component and an intervention component. Different missions have different consequences for the fate of the program, and they also differ in their compatibility with the groups and organizations in the program's environment.

3. Programs undergo *transformation* as they are carried out. The transformation is in large measure due to misperceptions of the program's environment and to unanticipated consequences of the program's mission.

Environment

Environments differ from program to program. Nevertheless, the following are typical of the questions that one might ask concerning the environment's readiness for a community program:

The College

Would it tolerate the involvement of its students in the community's affairs?

Would it be susceptible to the sorts of influence from trustees, alumni, or the community that could damage the program?

Would it allow the instructor adequate freedom in the conduct of his instruction?

Would it provide adequate material resources to the program?

The Students

Would they want to work in a community setting?

Would they accept the political and value implications of the program?

Would they accept a nontraditional pedagogy?

Would they be able to assume the responsibilities and undertake the tasks that the program would ask of them?

Do they have the requisite mastery of the academic subject matter underlying the program?

The Community

Are there elements in it that are hostile toward the client or target population?

Would it tolerate the program as a social-change effort?

Could it provide the necessary material resources—meeting places, communications media, and the like?

Is it logistically suitable to the program—ease of access to the program site, distance from the college, availability of public transportation, and the like?

Do its economic conditions so disadvantage the client or target population that the program could not hope to succeed in its mission?

Would it provide adequate opportunity for collaboration with other human-service agencies?

The Agency or Institution

Would it be receptive to outside workers such as program students?

Would it tolerate the program's departures from traditional concepts of human service?

Is its own human service mission compatible with that of the program?

Would it provide access to the resources necessary for the operation of the program—clients, key personnel, records, equipment, and the like?

Is it respected and influential among the community's institutions?

Is it successful in its own service mission?

Is it free of the kinds of internal conflicts that could endanger the program?

The Client or Target Population

Would it tolerate the intrusion of program students?
Would its culture and values conflict with those that the students
would bring in?
Would it be receptive to the method of intervention that the program
would introduce?
Would its individual members be competent to undertake the roles
expected of them in the program?
Does it actually have the problems that the program would attempt
to solve?

Essentially, these questions concern either resources for the program or conflicts of interest with the program. The environment must
have resources: The college should provide freedom and encouragement
as well as the more tangible resources; the students must be capable;
the community should offer certain amenities; the agency or institution
should be strong and stable; and the client or target population should
have problems and the capacity to profit from the program's solution to
those problems. Moreover, the environment should have interests that
are congenial to the program: The college should be aloof from interests
hostile to the program; the students' values should make them receptive
to the program; the community should be tolerant of the clients and the
program; the agency should welcome the program and the outsiders it
brings; and the clients should accept the methods, motives, and personnel of the program.

The matter of interests is usually the more critical of the two. If interests are not compatible, then resources will not be provided. But conflicts of interest are common between program and environment, for
several reasons:

1. There is always an investment in the customary ways of doing
things. That is true for teachers, students, and helpers. But community
programs usually ask for a renunciation of the customary—an acceptance of new ways of teaching, learning, and helping. Accepting innovation is difficult and time-consuming for the person. Moreover, it usually
conflicts with beliefs and attitudes carefully cultivated by professional
groups, faculties, and fellow students.

2. Many community programs are ideologically sensitive. Some
ideological conflicts are obvious, such as the conflict between a program
with an ideological commitment and a college that sees itself as a bas-
tion of scholarly neutrality. But sometimes the conflicts originate in
unexpected places. For instance, a program could be opposed by the
subprofessionals who are asked to work alongside students in the program.

3. Programs can conflict with indigenous cultures. Both the com-

munity as a whole and the client group have indigenous cultures. But community programs are usually conceived by middle-class academicians who have little in common with the community or the clients. And community programs are carried out by students whose own life styles may be closer to counter-culture than to community culture. Those cultural differences present limitless opportunities for a program to meet hostility in the field.

4. Many community programs begin in the outspoken belief that established organizations perpetuate problems. But those organizations usually have considerable control over a program's survival.

5. Most community programs are uneconomical as instructional methods. That fact sets them against the cost-accounting criteria that colleges use to evaluate their activities.

Some conflicts can be resolved with little or no compromise of program missions. Potentially hostile groups and organizations can be consulted with before the program gets under way. Students can be briefed in an effort to sensitize them to indigenous cultures. They can even be asked to shed some of the paraphernalia of unconventionality if that would improve rapport with the community. But most conflicts of interest are more refractory.

Ultimately, the creation, implementation, and survival of a community program hinge on the resolution of conflicts with the environment. Each group and organization in the environment can exercise a "veto power" of sorts over the program by refusing to cooperate. In that way, the interests of the environment influence the form that the program takes.

However, there is also an implicit bargaining situation between the program planner and the environment. In return for cooperation by groups and organizations in the environment, the program can offer resources, prestige, or other commitments. For example, to gain agency support, it can agree to take on agency tasks that are extraneous to its mission. Or, to gain the university's permission, it can agree to restrain program activities that have touchy political implications. It is in those implicit bargaining situations that a program's resources are provided for.

Mission

A program's mission can be characterized in countless ways. The dimensions of education and intervention are chosen for their importance to the success and survival of the program. Those dimensions have value implications that bear on the interests of groups and organizations in the program's environment. They also affect the program's practicability in other ways that the planner is often unaware of when the program begins.

Education versus Intervention

Every community program that is part of a college's instructional effort is first and foremost an educational program. But most community programs have other objectives as well, as the list of programs at the beginning of this paper makes obvious. Most programs intervene in the lives of clients or the workings of organizations in an effort to bring about change. Thus, it must be decided how much to emphasize those intervention objectives as opposed to the program's educational objectives.

Intervention usually poses more problems than education does. Intervention ordinarily presents the greater threat to the program's survival. For it is intervention, not education, that often threatens the comfortable workings of an institution, or the clients' preferred methods of adapting to their environment, or the repose of the community, or the professed political and social neutrality of the college. Colleges are accustomed to justifying education, but not intervention, as part of their own mission. Community action is foreign to most colleges. They may be willing to treat the community as a book, something to be studied and analyzed. But they are less willing to treat it as a laboratory for experimentation with planned change. That is one reason why education is usually the primary mission and intervention the secondary one in a community program.

Moreover, intervention is sometimes seen as merely instrumental to educational goals. In other words, the intervention method is chosen not so much for its furtherance of the intervention objective as for its utility in promoting the education of program students. Implicitly, intervention goals are taken for granted or dismissed. Any involvement of students in social change is seen as good for "society" as well as for the students. Or, even if it is not good for "society," it is seen as acceptable so long as it does not inflict damage on the community or the client group.

It is easy to see, then, that the intervention methods in a program are usually not as well thought out as the educational methods are. The neglect of intervention is arrogant as well as naïve. It is arrogant in its disregard of clients, and that can endanger the survival of the entire program. Lower-status clients in particular are not inclined to suffer unthinking middle-class colonialism. Tutorial programs in low-income communities often encounter that problem. Many of those programs begin with a presumption of "cultural deprivation," which can put them in conflict with the racial or ethnic consciousness of their clients.

Neglect of intervention is naïve in its tacit assumption that the excitement and stimulation of community involvements are educational no matter what the nature of the involvement might be. Such an assumption amounts to saying that ineffective interventions are as educational as effective ones, that students learn no more from effecting the desired change than from failing to do so.

Any community program having an intervention mission must be based on a sound logic of intervention just as it must be based on a sound logic of education. That dictum seems so unassailable that it would hardly merit discussion if it were not so often violated in practice. Most community programs are developed by college teachers. And college teachers, being teachers, usually pay more attention to pedagogy than to planned social change. Moreover, there is little agreement among experts on what constitutes an effective social-change strategy. That lack of agreement can be confusing to the program planner who wishes to develop a sound logic of intervention. Consequently, intervention is often left to ideology or else given over to the tender mercies of agency administrators who are more concerned with what is efficient than with what is effective.

Intervention as a Mission

Every intervention attempts to bring about change in some *target* —a person, group, or organization. Also, every intervention has a *constituency*—someone it looks to for legitimization of its aims and methods. Thus a community program can be classified according to the target and the constituency of its intervention mission.

Targets can be categorized as *people* or *environments*. When the target is people, change efforts are directed at the individual rather than the individual's setting or environment. The two targets can be contrasted with the example of a program involving students and felons. When the target is people, students might help felons adapt to prison life. But when the target is environments, students would help improve prison life for felons. People are the province of the counselor and the teacher; environments are the province of the community organizer and the public administrator.

Likewise, constituencies can also be categorized as people or environments. When the constituency is people, the aims and the methods of the intervention are established by people, individuals representing no one but themselves. But when the constituency is environments, aims and methods are established by an agency or other organization.

The example of felons and prisons can make the distinction clear. When people (felons) are the target, a program with environments as a constituency would look to the prison administration for approval of its aims and methods. Its mission might be to prevent disorder or increase participation in prison programs by counseling felons. On the other hand, when people are both target and constituency, the program would look to the felons themselves for such approval. Its mission might be to organize groups of felons to discuss ways of winning parole or ways of avoiding prison discipline. The distinction is similar when environments (prison life) are the target. A program with people as a constituency might attempt to win concessions for the felons from the prison administration. On the other hand, a program with environments (the prison administration) as a constituency might attempt to reorganize the prison to cut costs or decrease recidivism rates.

The distinction between people and environments is not an absolute one. Schools, welfare agencies, mental hospitals, and planning boards are more in the character of "environments" than are community action agencies, legal service organizations, underground newspapers, and drug-user groups. For the latter organizations are more indigenous and more subject to client control. Generally, the more an agency or organization is responsive to people, the more it can be categorized as "people."

Taken together, the target and constituency of an intervention generate four categories of *student roles,* as shown in Figure 1. Students may serve as *facilitators, advocates, socializers,* or *consultants.*

Facilitators attempt to change people (clients), but the change is something the people themselves ask for. The student's implicit posture

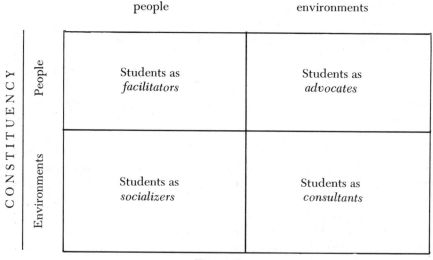

Figure 1

is, "Tell me how you want to change, and I shall help you bring about that change." An example is drug crisis-line programs. In these programs, a telephone number is publicized as a place to call for help with drug problems. Students who man the telephone in these programs receive calls for various sorts of help: information on physicians and drug antidotes, advice on how to give up drugs, and sympathy during bad trips. Changing people, then, does not necessarily mean changing their personalities or changing anything else enduring about them. It can mean giving them advice and information. Indeed, facilitators can act as information resources, teachers, trainers, counselors, or therapists. They serve people in much the same way that consultants serve organizations.

Advocates attempt, on the client's behalf, to change the behavior of the people and organizations with which the client must deal. If the crisis-line students were to leave the telephones and intercede in the caller's behalf with landlords, police, spouses, and the like, then those students would become advocates. Though people remain their constituency, environments become their target. The students would be attempting to change the client's situation rather than to change the client himself.

Socializers attempt to change people in a direction desired by some organization having authority or influence over people. A student tutor is usually a socializer: He works with the school's definition of the child's problem. He may tutor the child in the subjects for which grades are unsatisfactory, or he may attempt to relieve the child's "cultural deprivation" by providing some sort of cultural enrichment. In the rare cases when the tutor is a facilitator, he works with the child's own definitions of his problem. He might help the child learn how to take tests, or how to control teachers, or how to avoid school discipline.

Finally, consultants attempt to change an organization in ways that the organization requests. Just as the facilitator does not necessarily attempt to change anything enduring about the person, so the consultant does not necessarily attempt to change anything enduring about the organization. Like the facilitator, the consultant may simply give his target information, serving an intelligence function of sorts. For example, students can give planning boards information about the sentiments of critical groups in the community. The consultant differs from the advocate in that he attempts to change an organization on its own terms, terms that may conflict with the interests of the people who are affected by that organization.

Education as a Mission

Traditionally, education has been said to comprise three *domains*, the cognitive, the affective, and the psychomotor (Bloom, Engelhart,

Furst, Hill, & Kratwohl, 1956). Those domains correspond to thought, feeling, and action, respectively. Community programs, as educational enterprises, can be directed at educating the student in any of the three domains. Also, community programs either may or may not have a *collateral learning agenda*, an outside body of knowledge or a discipline, that the student is supposed to learn besides learning how to work effectively in the program. Thus, every community program's educational mission can be classified according to its domain and according to its use of a collateral learning agenda.

Most discussions of educational domains contrast the cognitive domain with the affective and psychomotor domains. Traditionally, formal education has emphasized the cognitive. A community program that emphasizes cognitive learning attempts to give the student an intellectual understanding of the phenomena he observes in the program. On the other hand, a community program that emphasizes affective or psychomotor learning attempts to give the student an ability to handle the phenomena in nonintellectual ways. It attempts to help him understand his feelings about what he encounters, or else it attempts to help him act effectively in the program.

A collateral agenda is present in a community program whenever any material to be learned or applied is laid out in advance. Collateral agendas may be embodied in lectures and readings, as in community programs that are merely laboratory adjuncts to a regular college course. Or they may be embodied in the student's prior learning experiences, as in most internships. To the extent that collateral material is laid out in a community program—or to the extent that the program instructor or supervisor imposes his own biases or preferred strategies on the students—a collateral agenda is present.

Taken together, domain and collateral agenda generate four categories of *pedagogy*, as shown in Figure 2: *deduction, induction, relevancy*, and *competency*.

The educational objective of deduction is mastery of the collateral material. The student's experiences in the program are used to illustrate that material. Often the objective of this pedagogy is said to be "demonstrating the usefulness of the material for understanding the real world."

Many instructors of community programs have misgivings about strictly cognitive learning. And many reject the predetermined cognitive agendas that go into most college courses. Both stances imply a bias against deduction. Yet it is difficult to find a community program that does away with deduction altogether, for that would be tantamount to rejecting all the accumulated scholarly and professional wisdom that relates to the program, and few colleges will tolerate such a program.

An inductive pedagogy does away with advance specification of

DOMAIN

		cognitive	affective or psychomotor
COLLATERAL LEARNING AGENDA	Present	*Deduction*	*Relevancy*
	Absent	*Induction*	*Competency*

Figure 2

what is to be learned. The student's experiences in the program are not used to illustrate any collateral material. Instead, they are the data out of which the student may develop his own material. Explanatory concepts and theories emerge from those data; they are not imposed on the data beforehand. Whereas the emphasis in deduction is on testing hypotheses, the emphasis in induction is on discovering them. Thus the student must actively confront his observations and construct an explanation for them. The education objective is "discovering what has to be learned."

Induction is appealing to those instructors who believe that the student must overcome his passive reliance on academic authority and develop his own understanding of the phenomena he observes. It is also appealing to those who are dissatisfied with existing explanations, instructors, and professionals who sense profound weaknesses in current professional wisdom and current professional education. But, as was already noted, colleges are unwilling to do away with such things, and professional agencies are usually just as unwilling. Perversely enough, the instructor too is usually ambivalent about inductive pedagogy. Having been educated by means of a deductive pedagogy himself, he is all too familiar with the authoritarian education he would reject.

Relevancy employs collateral agendas only as a guide to action. Readings, lectures, and the like, are provided to the student for whatever use they may be in helping him carry out his activities in the program. But the student, if he is graded, is graded on how well he performs those activities, not on how well he absorbs the collateral material. Whereas the objective of deduction is to demonstrate the usefulness of the material for understanding the real world, the objective of relevancy is to demonstrate the usefulness of the material for *effecting change.*

Relevancy is seldom the principal pedagogy in a program, but it is often used as a secondary pedagogical device. In tutorial programs, for example, students are often given handbooks on tutoring techniques. And in programs with students serving on legislative staffs, students are often lectured on the legislative process, and reference materials are placed on reserve at the college library. The student is expected to assimilate those collateral materials only insofar as they are useful to him.

When competency is the pedagogy, the student is forced to use his own experiences as the material out of which he develops an ability to function effectively in the program. The objective is "developing the ability to deal with the real world," or "learning to handle one's own feelings about the real world." While induction is concerned with discovering concepts and theories, relevancy is concerned with discovering methods of action or methods of managing feelings.

Competency, like relevancy, is seldom the principal pedagogy in a program. When competency is incorporated as a secondary pedagogy, it is usually carried out through group discussion. For example, in the various mental hospital programs, small groups of students meet weekly with an instructor or supervisor. One purpose of these meetings is for students to discuss the problems they have been encountering in the program. The student confronts his ambivalence toward mental patients as well as his inability to work effectively with them. In searching for a resolution to these problems, he can draw upon the collective experiences of the group as well as the insights of the instructor or supervisor.

Thus, many community programs can profit from the application of two or more pedagogies. The principal difficulty is that academicians are, as a rule, both unaccustomed to thinking beyond deductive pedagogies and unimaginative in planning the flexible pedagogical strategies that their programs demand. For example, a crisis-line program may begin with a deduction pedagogy, using collateral learning materials in the areas of counseling and psychotherapy. But these materials may be found wanting as a guide to action. This would necessitate the development of new materials, using competency or induction as a pedagogical strategy. Many instructors and many instructional programs seem unable to provide for this kind of shifting pedagogical emphasis.

Missions and Environments

There are other choices facing a program planner besides choices of mission. He must decide whether to seek official sanction for the program from the college or agency, and he must decide how closely to supervise the activities of program students. These choices determine the degree of control over program activities. Often they amount to choices between a program that is responsive to creativity on the part of students and a program that is acceptable to the college or agency. The program planner must also decide the manner in which students are to be involved in the program. Students can be involved as a group—which could be threatening to the agency, the community, and the clients. On the other hand, they can operate as individuals having little or no contact with one another, as in most internship programs. Finally, the program planner must decide the degree to which students are to be active participants as opposed to passive observers. These choices are important. Nevertheless, the primary choices are choices of mission, and other choices usually tend to rest on mission choices.

One part of mission design is the matching of missions to groups and organizations in the program's environment. Consider a typical program environment: The college is not exceptionally innovative or reformist; the agency is a typical human-service organization; and the clientele is of low social status in the community. First of all, in such an environment the advocacy role tends to conflict with the interests of the college and the agency. It also tends to militate against the prevailing community sentiment. The consultant role can avoid those problems, but by definition it is directed at changing the agency, a difficult task. And the facilitator role will attract support only if it is directed at something that everyone agrees is absolutely of crisis proportions, such as drug use in the community. That leaves the socializer role. This is the most acceptable role, for it is harmlessly aimed at changing the individual in ways that the agency and community prefer and that the college can live with.

However, a dilemma emerges when one considers the clients. They usually tend to reject the socializer role, for it imposes an alien set of values on them. On the other hand, the advocacy role is often the most appealing to clients, for it furthers their cause by attempting to change the organizations that affect their lives. There are clients who will acquiesce in socialization, just as there are organizations that will underwrite advocacy programs, but nowadays neither is very easy to find.

The choice open to the program planner, then, is sometimes between a program that cannot win material resources from organizations and a program that cannot gain the cooperation of clients. The same may be said of other social interventions besides programs of student involvement in the community. Most interventions can have but a single constituency. If logic does not dictate such a conclusion, then politics does.

There is less difficulty in matching education missions with the environment. Only the college has an abiding interest in pedagogy. Nevertheless, colleges often seem to share pedagogical preferences with agencies and communities. All prefer the safer pedagogies—cognitive pedagogies and pedagogies with collateral learning agendas. Cognitive pedagogies help assure that the student be more concerned with thought than action. And collateral learning agendas help guide the student into acceptable forms of action. By dispensing with innovation, agendas keep the program from getting out of hand. Thus, in educational missions as in intervention missions, the most bold and exciting community programs are the ones least likely to enjoy the support of established institutions.

Transformation

There are at least three causes of unwanted transformations in a community program:

1. The program's environment may be misperceived. Students may not tolerate alien pedagogies. Clients may not accept alien intervention strategies. And the college, agency, and community may not allow reform.
2. The program's mission may be inadequately thought out. For instance, its pedagogy may fail to prepare students to undertake the intervention roles intended for them.
3. The program may have unanticipated impacts on its environment. Unexpected "incidents" can occur whenever students carry out unfamiliar tasks in an unfamiliar setting. Or else the program may succeed. Success can be a problem in that established institutions sometimes tolerate a program only because they are convinced that it will fail to bring about the social change it attempts.

When any of those things happen, the program must usually be transformed if it is to survive. And it seems safe to generalize that most such transformations tend to restore tradition and blunt innovation. When environments are misperceived, they are usually misperceived wishfully as tolerating more innovation and reform than they actually do. When the program's mission is inadequately thought out, the most common reaction is to tighten the logic behind the mission by reverting to old, reliable methods. And, when the program has unanticipated impacts, the most common reaction is to give it more predictability and less caprice. Error begets caution.

However, there are models that avoid these unwanted transformations. One model worth discussion here is to begin the program on a scale so small that established institutions do not have to be approached for support. This model is popular. Oftentimes a program begins with a single instructor and a carload of his students going into the community once a week for as long as the activity remains enjoyable to them. Clearly, such a model will revolutionize neither higher education nor human services. Nevertheless, it has some advantages as a way of starting a program on a trial basis.

One advantage of the out-of-car program is that it can be freely altered without clearance from the college or an agency. Another advantage is the pure, manageable simplicity of the program. A small-scale program avoids the bureaucratization and routinization that can hopelessly burden down a larger program and make it a joyless experience for the person running it. A final advantage of the out-of-car model is that it gives a chance for mistakes to be made without the program being destroyed in the process, errors that are minor nuisances in a small program are often catastrophic in a larger one.

Once the errors are made and the program is adjusted to the satisfaction of all concerned, expansion can be undertaken on sounder ground. At that point, the program will probably have something of value to offer the college and the agency in return for official sanction and material resources. And, if the college and the agency are still reluctant to cooperate, the program might possibly turn itself into an independent agency in its own right, possibly along the lines envisioned by Anne Roe (1970) in her discussion of Community Resource Centers. Independent programs can be funded by foundations or government agencies, and outside funding of a program makes collaboration with it a more attractive prospect to community agencies. Moreover, outside funding allows the program greater autonomy than it would have if it were to owe its day-to-day material survival to a community agency.

None of that would provide for all the resources a program needs, however. The university and the community must be tolerant, if not generous. Students and clients must be competent to a degree. No amount of planning and no amount of outside financing can assure these requisites. And no amount of outside help can overcome the problem of a community that is stagnant and impoverished or an agency that is powerless and inflexible.

Moreover, there is an additional problem in that the spirit of reform and innovation often gets lost as a program becomes institutionalized. But there are examples to the contrary. The Outreach program at the

University of Michigan is a large program that has become institution-alized, but it appears to have retained much of the spirit of reform that characterized its modest beginnings in 1965 (Cytrynbaum & Mann, 1969). Programs similar to Outreach have begun on campuses as diverse as Yale and Eastern Michigan University. Moreover, on a number of other campuses there are programs somewhat less reformist that quietly flourish, bringing a measure of effective innovation to teaching and per-haps a measure of change to communities. These programs are success-ful to the extent that they pay heed to the realities that this discussion has attempted to capture.

REFERENCES

Bloom, B. S., Engelhart, M. D., Furst, E. J., Hill, W. J., and Kratwohl, D. R. *Taxonomy of educational objectives.* New York: Longmans, Green, 1956.

Cytrynbaum, S., and Mann, R. Community as campus: Project Outreach. In P. Runkel, R. Harrison, and M. Runkel (Eds.), *The changing college class-room.* San Francisco: Jossey-Bass, 1969. Pp. 266–289.

Ledvinka, J., and Denner, B. The limits of success. *Mental Hygiene,* 1972, 56, 30–35.

Lunneborg, P. W. Undergraduate psychology field work: The unwashed take over. *American Psychologist,* 1970, 25, 1062–1064.

Roe, A. Community resource centers. *American Psychologist,* 1970, 25, 1033–1040.

Umbarger, C. C., Dalsimer, J. S., Morrison, A. P., and Breggin, P. R. *College students in a mental hospital.* New York: Grune & Stratton, 1962.

ANTIDOTES FOR ARROGANCE: TRAINING FOR COMMUNITY PSYCHOLOGY

13

James G. Kelly

The thesis of this article is that if psychologists can broaden their definitions of therapeutic activities, expand their definitions for the criteria of competent helpers, become participants in their local communities, and alter their time perspective, then they can help to build a psychology *of* the community.

A redefinition of the psychologist's job is advocated, and a new set of criteria for the hallmarks for this profession is proposed. Being a community psychologist is more than being a good psychologist, for community psychology is a sufficiently different activity. To achieve valid training or able professional role models for this field, accommodations to the heritages, assumptions, and styles of previous training are sharpened and redefined. Developing competences for work in the community is a different task and requires new political alliances and new criteria for personal and joint accountability between the community and the psychologist.[1]

The spirit of the community psychologist is the spirit of a naturalist who dotes on his environment; of the journalist, who bird-dogs his story; and of the conservationist, who glows when he finds a new way to describe man's interdependence with his environment. The recommended way to prevent professional extinction is participation in the local community; the preferred antidote for arrogance is an ecological view of man.

Psychologists sneer and smart over the arrogances and disdain of radicals, militants, or the citizen with conservative reflexes. The most arrogant guys around are often we professionals who *analyze, position, re-*

Revised and edited version of the Presidential Address, Division of Community Psychology (Division 27), presented at the 77th Annual Convention of the American Psychological Association, Washington, D.C., September 3, 1969. Reprinted from *American Psychologist*, 1970, 25, 524–531. Copyright © 1970 by the American Psychological Association, and reproduced by permission. James Kelly is currently with the Department of Psychology, University of Michigan, Ann Arbor, Michigan.

[1] The final report of the Task Force on Community Mental Health suggests additional emphases for the psychologist working in community mental health (see Glidewell & Brown, 1969).

flect, *study*, *commission*, *postpone*, *garble*, *intrude*, and *play with*, but rarely play out, the crosscurrents of community events. It is our quiet and sometimes folksy and affable arrogance that can interfere with colleagues' and students' opportunities to adopt tentative explorations and offbeat enterprises that are an integral part of psychology. For many of the younger generation, too often, psychologists have been models for community change that represents, at best, tokenism; sometimes in moments of haste, we have generated the seeds for alienation.

Elsewhere, the present author has stated how concepts from biological ecology can be applied to designing social interventions (Kelly, 1966, 1968; Mills & Kelly, in press; Trickett, Kelly, & Todd, in press). If all of the stimulating ideas from biology are distilled into a single theme, it is a fondness, a commitment, a love, if you will, of the very community where you live and work; an involvement that engulfs your attention and draws your curiosity to make an adventure out of knowing all there is to know of its heritage, its conflicts, its people, its political forces, and its efforts to launch campaigns for social goods, as well as its failures when the status is quo. Few of us have been trained to cathect to a locale. I am confident that few psychologists have been taught to worry about our communities, and still fewer of us have given our time to see the promotion of a civic cause fulfilled.

How did psychology get into such a fix? One of the key events can be attributed not to the heritage of psychology, but to the reluctance of psychologists to chart a course of action that is around our roles, beneath our status, and beyond our scientific canons. Perhaps we psychologists have been too hung up with ourselves and have been able to see our world only through the mirrors of ourselves. How many articles or books on community psychology discuss the community? Klein's (1968) recent work is alone in this respect. How many conferences at professional meetings talk about the development or evolution of communities? Few, if any.

We certainly seem to be in a fix! Are we addicted? These charges may seem severe, undisciplined, and untestable. Perhaps they are! I would also like to take this opportunity to express some ideas on how we might right the fix and get ourselves spruced up for a campaign that can be, in William James' (1911) terms, a moral equivalent for war.

What follows is a recitation of some concrete ways in which psychology as a science and profession can create a point of view for training ourselves and our students as community psychologists. Then, psychologists can ask APA and our colleagues to come and see the crop; to do something other than yell at the APA Central Office for the fertilizer! The following are seven ideas for pulling ahead of social crises, for being professional *and* revolutionary without rhetoric and without arms.[2]

Each of these seven principles is offered as a way in which training for community psychology can be created and nurtured. The focus on training is not an emphasis on how to tinker with the curriculum, but refers to the socialization of a new profession. The initial premise is that, since community psychology is different from other forms of psychology, then its socialization will need to be different. For the training of the community psychologist demands a critical period in which he learns the styles of work that are going to be relevant for his own future adaptation. If the differences in requirements are real, training programs will need to be designed to reflect these varied conditions.

In all of these comments, references to university-based training will be emphasized, particularly those relationships between the university, the community, and the training program. The following principles, however, also could apply with appropriate modification to field training centers and their relationships to the community.

Field Assessment and the Selection of Community Psychologists

I cannot decide whether my interest in community psychology is in spite of my training in psychology or in addition to my training in psychology. As I look back on my development, the most critical events seem to be the planned and unplanned experiences of working and dealing with the broadest range of persons. Some important occasions were related to the opportunities I had as a graduate student at the University of Texas in the late 1950s. Most of them, however, were not; they involved the people I worked with, the people I worked for, and the stress I dealt with as I tried to make and find my way. Persons I have known to be turned on about the excitement of community work also seem to be accidentally a part of psychology. I certainly do not know of any doctoral training programs in psychology that begin with the goal to train persons who are effective change agents and then proceed to select and train persons for that very purpose.

What I think we need as a start are ways to locate potential com-

[2] An important source for several of the following ideas is the report, "Ecological Concepts and Mental Health Programs."

Acknowledgment is expressed to George Coelho, Project Officer of the National Institute of Mental Health, for the contract to conduct this study. Appreciation is given to him and to the author's colleagues for their collaboration in this work (see Kelly, Goldsmith, Coelho, Randolph, Shapiro, & Seder, 1967).

munity psychologists as early as the high school and provide a series of activities that can prepare them to be responsive to the tough tasks of community work. Rather than rely only on the Graduate Record Examination, Miller Analogies Test, testimonials from eminent psychologists, and matriculation at Ivy League schools, the new training program should expend its resources to create field tasks of moderate intensity and difficulty. Such assessment procedures would not be designed just to meet the requirements of a pass–fail situation, but would suggest the various combinations of skills that the applicant has developed up to a particular time. Such an assessment would be so designed to provide alternative ideas for obtaining training that can adapt to his needs. Under these conditions, universities could join together, create a national academy, pool resources, and encourage the student to enter the university that is most congruent with his developmental level. The new student would have the option to continue his training at other universities of his choice at a future point in his career.

Such a training program could provide the additional benefits of relating the university to additional resources, like undergraduate and high school instruction, and encouraging students to enter their graduate career when (1) their interest, (2) their competence, and (3) their field performance suggest, and *not* just when they have accumulated the necessary credit hours or meet the resident requirements. The field assessments, where the student tries to solve a community problem, can also include provisions for advisory committees, with representatives of the applicants, as well as community leaders and faculty, all helping to design the assessment procedures. Mechanisms could be worked out so that the criteria for performance can shift to accommodate changes in communities, generational shifts of interest, and the development of new knowledge by the faculty. What happens after selection?

Continuous Interdisciplinary Interaction

One of our hangups that must be resolved is our inability to work effectively with members of other professions. I am not preaching tolerance for all disciplines, nor am I suggesting that we create a multidisciplinary project that collects representatives from other disciplines, *nor* do I mean sending psychology graduate students across campus to pick up a course in anthropology or sociology *after* they complete all other requirements. I am affirming that the entering students should be given the chance to become involved with multidisciplines, both faculty and students, as they work toward the solution of a problem that lies outside the territorial boundaries of their discipline. Under these conditions, the student has the opportunity to work toward the resolution of complex problems in the presence of faculty and students outside his discipline, and he has the chance to learn the process of collaborating with other professions *by doing it.*

New settings can be created to assist the student in solidifying the collaborative skills that he is just learning. For example, the faculty member tutoring the student will be expected to have been through such an experience, or committed to go through it for the first time with the student. It also is assumed that the group of students going through such training will have a chance to view their own group process and reflect and achieve clarity about their own participation in that process. The premise is that listening and engaging others can be learned directly from the practice of working in natural field conditions. If the student uses such experiences, he will have acquired an internal resource that helps him generalize to new settings, and he has taken an essential step in learning how to be a change agent. The hypothesis is suggested that if the student can work effectively with other disciplines, he will be able to reach out and work with citizens, independent of their beliefs, even when they conflict with his own. He has learned how to make the resolution of personal conflicts and confrontations be generative for himself and others.

One of the important contexts for encouraging such work at the departmental level is the support from the university administration and the federal agencies; both must support more than the spirit of working across disciplinary boundaries. Working out all the right conditions for a collaborative enterprise at the local level is limiting if the federal agencies preach good deeds but are not able to make these deeds count and actively nourish interdisciplinary training. It may be completely naive to think that federal agencies can leave their catacombs, but universities must do a better job by encouraging, cajoling, and gigging federal officials to function as interagency ombudsmen.

One of the important by-products of the successful interdisciplinary process is that it devises a training ground for a generalist, a generalist who is not a dilettante or world traveler, but a person who has achieved a working perspective via direct and sustained experience in a local community. I also think the ability to collaborate implies a seasoned toughness of spirit, a point that reemphasizes the importance of the field selection for students entering the program. Here, the student first learns how to work on a problem with a group of nonpsychologists. Graduates of such a program with this type of socialization are expected to have a greater chance to be effective colleagues, even when the substance of community psychology changes and the problems shift.

The Longitudinal Perspective

The development of persons, like the evolution of communities, requires a view without restrictions on time. One of the most difficult tasks facing community psychology is to learn how to tune into a community and assess how transitory or how deep-rooted the issues of the day are. This task is critical for the survival of the community psychologist. *If he misjudges gossamer for grit, he is dead before he starts.* Mapping out the antecedent factors that have contributed to the current balance of political events is an exciting activity that forces the community psychologist to draw on professions and involves processes that may be unfamiliar to him. If such an effort is made as a cross-sectional analysis, the risk of making programmatic error rises sharply. A value for the longitudinal perspective is that it reduces the community psychologist from appraising effects of environmental conditions from being "good" or "bad." It allows him to hang loose and relate the processes that have appeared to be disruptive to processes that can contribute to community development at a future point in time. The longitudinal perspective also helps to make explicit ideas that are useful in dealing with complex events and cautions against the packaging of monolithic formulations of the change process that are so pervasive and contagious. The longitudinal perspective also can give immense satisfaction in working with persons over time.

How does the university go about achieving this? To my mind, the criteria for training would be shifted from defining units of courses to creating segments of training. In sum, the student would participate in training until that particular activity is completed—when the particular segment is achieved. If a student is learning consultation skills, he may be working with a client system for a period of several years, depending on the particular characteristics of the client system. To view graduate training in an unstructured fashion requires efforts by both faculty and students to be accountable to each other and to be open and confrontable. Unless the curriculum can be replaced by the personal accountabilities between faculty and students, a program without credit hours and without courses could be anarchic or at least anomic. To start, the faculty must be prepared to get with an open-ended process. Such a longitudinal program also requires an unusual amount of documentation and archival recording of critical periods. Such an activity is expensive and involves supporting staff. Certainly, the typical departmental secretary is not enough of a framework for such a training program. Fulfillment of this principle requires new resources for the university, resources that are urgently needed if the community psychologist is to reorder his way and restructure his home environment.

Mixing Theory and Practice

The challenge of community psychology to me means that the psychologist puts aside all of his polarities and his hyphenated role conceptions and plunges right into a practice to create ideas that are pragmatic. This is what Reiff (1968) has been telling us for years. The essence of the task of the psychologist is to conduct himself so that his behavior expresses the integration that he has made of the development of his theoretical and his practical ideas. This does not mean assigning students to the classroom under one faculty member and then assigning them for a practicum under another faculty member, with the result that the student is left to cope with two supervisors and their idiosyncracies. The ecological perspective affirms that acquiring competence for community psychology involves direct personal experience in building practice and theory, so that the two feed on one another and assist the community psychologist to become a generalist who is relevant, who can become an advocate, and who has a survival potential that lasts beyond several years. The guess is that the training program that creates such a mix assists the psychologist to be adaptive to changing environmental conditions.

As the student works toward the integration of these ideas for himself in the presence of other students and faculty, all learn in still another way to be accountable to each other for actualizing these values. The attainment of this integration for me implies something, if you will, that is precious, namely, that the conversations, confrontations, dialogues, and "rappings" are reciprocal. The faculty's participation is enhanced when they are able to say clearly and concisely how their efforts worked and did not work. The students' contributions are real when they can ask the searching questions. Such aspirations may seem like having counsel from a favorite uncle, niece, or nephew. This may not be so farfetched, for the frequency and quality of interaction approaches the definition of a community. It is these types of informal interactions that are the sources for personal and professional integration.

But this type of interaction asks a lot of both students and faculty —it means the professor drops his Socratic ways, his citations, and his defensiveness about being professional, and even says quite frankly that he does not understand a particular problem any better than anyone else. The student can no longer hide behind padded bibliographies, simulated silences, and he is not allowed to "cop out" and be uninvolved in his own graduate career. Shedding such role-sets can make a whale of a difference to faculty and students independent of substantive interests. Such freedom from professional sclerosis can generate a whole new profession!

These thoughts are suggested not as a way of creating a club, or a new commune, but as settings to help develop disciplined and integrated professionals that the field demands. The criteria for seeing whether the theory and practice do mix *is* that the theoretical products are valid if they explain what is happening today; the practices are relevant if they help the community psychologist anticipate the effects of interventions for some future time. Working for such criteria affords a climate for students and colleagues to create a viable society. This is definitely a nice bonus.

Taking Advantage of Community Events

Another hangup that we professionals have is our tendency to structure our lives and fill our curriculum as if our pieces of knowledge were bits of honey in a beehive. We so preempt our lives with our definitions of professional practice that we allow little room for picking up a piece of the action, and we give ourselves few chances to move with the changing conditions. The community psychologist needs free hours for both faculty and students. Community events, whether they are crises or public holidays, represent our laboratory and require that we be in attendance to observe and participate and earn a right to contribute. It is on such occasions that persons who may be intensely involved and yet alienated from their communities can be noticed and persuaded to become new resources for the community. When the community psychologist is free with his time, he is free to replenish his energy that is so quickly spent when he involves himself in situations with persons who are strangers. The intellectual and affective resources involved when dealing with emergency events can be an exhausting experience—an experience that you must be up for. I personally have been impressed with the effectiveness of persons who perform in stress situation. When I have checked, one of the critical ingredients of their success is their lack of fatigue rather than particularly novel or provocative words they have spoken.

Freeing the curriculum of structural requirements and replacing it with alternative ways to seed learning without a calendar is an essential hallmark when embarking on the training of the community psychologist. To try to model the training along the traditions of the university and the heritage of training in professional psychology is worse than shortsighted. It is fraudulent! The adaptive tasks of the community psychologist are not to accommodate to the university; his tasks are to follow the life course of the community and to adapt to the community's environments. Advocating care for the locale means giving it the first option. Representing the university happens when the community psychologist acts; the academic side of the role is the presence of the community psychologist in the center of things. Accountability for this role must be shared, and it demands resources within the community and the university for this new joint accountability. It is likely that such resources will have to be identified and created; we have no clear roles for these functions in our society.

This is a difficult principle to see born, let alone keep alive, for it means that the university administration must see its faculty on detached service and not expect the faculty member to perform functions previously identified as marks of a university professor. I am not advocating a new elite, for the community psychologist should replace these deleted functions by involving colleagues in his work, by defining the validity of work via relating it to others. Such dialogues may require more tact, more tolerance, more clarity of purpose, and more humility than we would like. But what better training ground for the community psychologist than rapping with colleagues. Besides, we might learn something!

There is another facet of taking advantage of community events, namely, that it requires a sense of personal identity that is constantly tested. Being on the battlefield means that the psychologist does not call "foul" or does not go home mad when things get rough. In fact, his validity as a professional is reinforced when he remains involved, when he has a sense of how the battles are affecting him, what they are costing him, how his performance stacks up, and when he needs help. This sense of personal integrity cannot just be hoped for, and we cannot refer back to child-rearing practices for an understanding of it. This personal integrity must be learned via the socialization of mastering community events, including those occasions when the community psychologist looks like a loser. It is this *kind* of laboratory where coping with unplanned events can generate the future development of the community psychologist and a psychology *of* the community.

Identification of Community Resources

The recitation of these ideas may sound like the community psychologist is either a guru, a saint, a mayor, a ward healer, or a new kook. What has been intended is that, as the effective community psychologist works, an initial premise is that he makes for himself a program of community development that depends on encouraging others to work with him. He turns over to others work that for him is a major investment. Being able to collaborate is a very high priority as he searches for persons who can replace his own activities. This coping style is a very infrequent part of the socialization of the psychologist, but a behavior that is vital for the psychologist who is going to be an effective community resource. I noted that when psychologists try to function in the community in the same way that they try to function in their departments or agencies, and play out the same political battles that are relevant there, they often fall flat. A particular city or town may operate like a university, but the operating guideline for the community psychologist is that *every* setting, organization, and subgrouping of society has a culture that is ecologically distinct and requires different channels for expressing social influence. A hedge against his own limited political idiosyncrasies is his effort to locate and develop resources out of the local culture.

If community psychologists are going to be open and resilient and draw on the resources of others, then they too will need help. The organization that sponsors the community psychology training must become involved with the surrounding environment, must be alert to identify and accommodate persons with talent, and must have a commitment for being involved in the exciting *and* the boring, the repetitive, *and* the ephemeral events that are the media for community change. We professionals too often sneak away from such daily chores. How often do we in psychology not only ask persons to change to fit our aspirations, but then add the additional burden that they march to our drum while they do it? Finding ways and having commitments to work with persons with varying ideologies is a tough, exhausting, but actualizing experience. It is an interaction, nevertheless, that is mandatory for the development of an effective community program.

For me, the social revolutions in our society mark the end of the professional as *the* policy-maker! When I keep saying this to myself, I realize how incomplete, how fragile, and how invalid some of my own training has been. I begin to think how I can begin to create conditions so that the committed, the involved, and the curious student and citizen can find settings to create his own competence and enlarge his world view. One thing I am convinced of is that our frame of reference must shift, and our training programs should be redesigned so that the settings for the personal development of the community psychologist are viable, coherent, and of the highest quality. One way to create a richer and more valid enterprise is by teaching the community psychologist to identify with *all* the people in his community and to become involved in the creation of *new* community resources.

Updating the Community Psychologist

If the community psychologist works toward implementing such principles, how is he himself going to generate new ideas and mobilize energy for adapting to change? Of all the people, he will most frequently need to revive his concepts, shift his perceptions, rotate his ideologies, and learn how to manage new environments. How can this be achieved? One idea is for the academy of training facilities, who were participating in the selection of new students, to work together again in creating a facility for the continuing education of the community psychologist.

I have been struck by the historical accounts of the role that the Marine Biological Laboratories at Woods Hole, Massachusetts, has played in the development in biology (Conklin, 1968a, 1968b). For many years, Woods Hole served as a social setting with a mixture of functions. It was a place where biologists could come to work; it was a place where the leadership attracted the stimulating and provocative minds. It was a place where faculty came with their students and, under very informal and casual conditions, worked, talked, and shared their ideas and hopes that so frequently do not appear in the final publication of scientific reports. Biologists with whom I have spoken are unanimous in their praise for this institution and for the major influence that the setting has had in the development of their own work.

The picture of Woods Hole, as sketched by those who have been associated with it, can take on the properties of a romantic South Sea island. Putting aside such reveries, the creation of an analogue to Woods Hole for the training of community psychologists seems to me to be an idea worth pursuing on its own merit. An idea that, if implemented, could play a critical role in the updating of the faculty and the generation of students who can become the eminent and accomplished innovators.

When I begin to consider the means by which a Woods Hole laboratory can be created for the training of community psychology, some features occur to me that are different from those of a research laboratory located in a scenic marshland along the Massachusetts coastline. Such a facility would not be in one place, but would be scattered in different parts of the country and would be located in geographical areas where there are varying political conditions, different opportunities for the delivery of community services, and where each of the laboratories would have contrasting styles of working with citizens. Such facilities could provide a mode for regenerating community psychologists rather than create totally new communities.

As I think about how social change occurs in the practice of professions, I am struck with the apparent need we have to identify with *new* bureaucratic structures. Social innovations seem to be symbolized only through the creation of new buildings, new departments, and new professions, with intact identifiable social structures. What also occurs to me is that the innovative life history of such social organizations is over almost at the time of the birth of the new institution. What we have been unable to do is to devise alternative social settings that relate to the workings of society, and then to consider how to use ad hoc and temporary groupings of persons to nurture the development process. Glidewell's (1968) ideas regarding the relevance of temporary societies as media for self-development are an intriguing set of ideas because they force community psychologists to focus on the form and style that is congruent and relevant for the change activity, rather than to expect that any new structure *or* formal social organizations will replenish us and our society. I am proposing that a loose collection of laboratories situated in strategic sites can achieve for community psychology what Woods Hole did for an earlier generation of biologists.

Conclusion

All of the aforementioned ideas are options we have. They are ideas that I think can make our commitments clear, our interventions long-lasting, and our knowledge adaptive. I hope that these seven points offer a set of conditions that spell out channels and opportunities for community psychology to make its way. The task of community psychology is to educate ourselves and our communities to the fact that social change does not *only* occur as a result of reactions to specific crises or demonstrable technologies, but can be a product of social processes— processes that have their origin in the design of social settings arranged for innovation *and* for change.

REFERENCES

Conklin, E. G. Early days at Woods Hole. *American Scientist,* 1968, *56,* 112–120. (a)
Conklin, E. G. M. B. L. stories. *American Scientist,* 1968, *56,* 121–129. (b)
Glidewell, J. C. The professional practitioner and his community. Chairman's Address, Mental Health Section, presented at the meeting of the American Public Health Association, Detroit, November 1968.
Glidewell, J. C., and Brown, M. *Priorities for psychologists in community mental health.* Report of the Task Force on Community Mental Health, Division 27, 1969.
Graziano, A. M. Clinical innovation and the mental health power structure: A social case history. *American Psychologist,* 1969, *24,* 10–18.
James, W. From the moral equivalent for war. In, *Memories and studies.* London: Longmans, Green & Co., 1911. (Also in, *The philosophy of William James.* New York: The Modern Library, 264.)

Kelly, J. G. Ecological constraints on mental health services. *American Psychologist*, 1966, *21*, 535–539.

Kelly, J. G. Towards a theory of preventive intervention. In J. W. Carter, Jr. (Ed.), *Research contributions from psychology to community mental health*. New York: Behavioral Publications, 1968.

Kelly, J. G., Goldsmith, R., Coelho, G., Randolph, P., Shapiro, D., and Seder, R. *Ecological concepts and mental health programs*. (Final Report: Contract No. 67-1488) Chevy Chase, Md.: National Institute of Mental Health, 1967.

Klein, D. C. *Community dynamics and mental health*. New York: Wiley, 1968.

Mills, R. C., and Kelly, J. G. Ecology and cultural adaptation: A case study and critique. In S. Golann & C. Eisdorfer (Eds.), *Handbook of community psychology and mental health*. New York: Appleton-Century-Crofts, in press.

Reiff, R. Social intervention and the problem of psychological analysis. *American Psychologist*, 1968, *23*, 524–531.

Trickett, E. J., Kelly, J. G., and Todd, D. M. The social environment of the high school: Guidelines for individual change and organizational redevelopment. In S. Golann & C. Eisdorfer (Eds.), *Handbook of community psychology and mental health*. New York: Appleton-Century-Crofts, in press.

SOCIAL WORK IN SEARCH OF A
RADICAL PROFESSION
14
Martin Rein

There is a great deal of interest today in the radicalization of professions. A restless search for relevance to public policy is being undertaken in social work, psychiatry, psychology, city planning, sociology, and political science, to name a few fields. One form that the radicalization is taking is to question afresh the role of the professional association in the area of public policy. In the last few years, this reassessment has been most striking. At the 1968 National Conference on Social Welfare, for example, black activists pressed the conference to change its preamble, which defines the conference as a forum for discussion that "does not take an official position on controversial issues." The city planning profession has split recently into what Gans calls

> the progressive and conservative wings: with the former calling for social planning to reduce economic and racial inequality, and the latter defending traditional physical planning and the legitimacy of middle class values.[1]

Sociologists seem especially vigorous in calling for a radical sociology. Gouldner's review of Parsons' book *American Sociology* captured the discontent seen at the 1968 Conference of the American Sociological Association. He quotes one angry sociologist who asserted:

> The profession of sociology is an outgrowth of 19th century European traditionalism and conservatism wedded to 20th century American corporation liberalism. . . . The professional eyes of the so-

The author expresses his appreciation to Mrs. Sylvia Scribner, Albert Einstein College of Medicine, New York, N.Y., for her help in clarifying the argument developed in the paper. Discussions with Philip Lichtenberg, a colleague at Bryn Mawr College, were an important source of stimulation. Reprinted with permission of the National Association of Social Workers, from *Social Work*, April 1970, *15*(2), 13–28. Martin Rein, Ph.D., is Professor, Graduate Department of Social Work and Social Research, Bryn Mawr College, Bryn Mawr, Pennsylvania.
[1] Herbert Gans, "Social Planning: Regional and Urban Planning," *International Encyclopedia of the Social Sciences*, Vol. 12 (New York: Macmillan & Free Press, 1968), p. 135.

ciologists are on the down people, and the professional palm of the sociologists is stretched toward the up people.[2]

Gouldner and Seeley define a radical social science as one critical of the emerging forms of the welfare state, which they view as a new social control system seeking "conformity as the price of welfare." Reform should not be limited to "melioristic efforts within the system," they hold, but should "develop alternatives to the *status quo*." [3]

The press for radicalization has taken another form as well. It is directed not only at extending the ròle of the professional as citizen and member of a professional organization, but at changing the very essence of his professional activity. In this sense we are witnessing today a search for radical professionalism rather than a quest for the professional who acts as a radical. Preassessment of the professional role is taking two major forms. The first is a reexamination of the profession's sources of legitimacy, a process that has been accompanied by a growing disenchantment with its avowed role as gatekeeper of tested knowledge. Some social workers are now trying to derive their legitimacy—their right to intervene—from the clients to be served, rather than from the technology they have accumulated. It is not uncommon to find in the new professional literature a call for social workers

. . . [to] join with . . . clients in a search for and reaffirmation of their dignity. . . . Let us become mercenaries in their service—let us, in a word, become their advocates. . . . Let our clients use us . . . to argue their cause, to maneuver, to obtain their rights and their justice, to move the immovable bureaucrats.[4]

[2] Alvin Gouldner, book review of Talcott Parsons (Ed.), *American Sociology* (New York: Basic Books, 1968), *Science* (October 11, 1968), p. 247.
[3] Letter by Alvin Gouldner and Jack Seeley to Frank Riessman, New York University, September 10, 1968. A conference on "Revitalizing Social Science" was held at New York University on October 14, 1968, to discuss the letter. This conference may be considered as a first meeting of representatives of the radical caucuses of the various social science associations. There is interest in creating a policy-oriented magazine and an organization. Unity on the left may be hard to maintain, as it always has been, but a start appears to have been made.
[4] Henry Miller, "Value Dilemmas in Social Casework," *Social Work*, January 1968, *13*(1) p. 33. Social workers are also dismayed by the criticism that casework "*systematically* excludes many of the persons most in need of attention [and even] when properly applied to persons disposed to use it," is ineffective. *See* Scott Briar, "The Casework Predicament," *Social Work*, p. 6, same issue. To meet these charges, the field has shifted its emphasis from the application of tested knowledge and accepted standards of "sound" practice to experimentation. Demands for innovation, experimentation, and accountability to service-users all illustrate a willingness to challenge established standards of practice.

This principle of accountability to the consumer departs from traditional professionalism, which has always been colleague-oriented rather than client-oriented, a distinction captured by Everett Hughes, who defined a professional as someone respected by his colleagues and a quack as someone respected by his clients.

The second broad approach to radicalizing professional activity has been to advocate intervention in larger systems, such as the community, rather than in the life of the individual. Today community intervention is an idea in good currency among the helping professions. Witness the growth of community psychiatry, community psychology, and community organization in social work. One need only read such journals as *Psychiatry and Social Science, American Psychologist,* or *Social Work* to recognize this shift in the professions to social action with neighborhood groups. This shift will be discussed in further detail later and the author will argue that, by itself, community intervention represents an inadequate index of radical activity.

These two trends suggest a basis on which to elicit the creed of social work as a profession. But before proceeding, the obstacles to formulating a professional relief system will be discussed. It is hoped that a review of these impediments will serve as an introduction to a discussion of the development of a radical social work creed.

Obstacles to a Professional Creed

Throughout social work literature, one finds references to the fact that social work is a value-laden profession. Hence it might seem an easy task to summarize the values that comprise its belief system and then explore the relevance of this creed to today's urban problems. But the literature deals with values only globally; the discourse is confined to a high level of abstraction. For example, there is the widely held proposition that each individual has dignity and worth. Surely this is an important statement, but, unless its implications and consequences are drawn for professional practice, it is not a useful frame for action.[5]

What is more, social work literature contains the implicit assump-

---

[5] Consider the recent debate on whether war-injured Vietnamese children should be brought to the United States for medical treatment. The National Association of Social Workers' Commission on International Social Welfare asserted that such a plan disregards a basic child welfare principle that "children have the right to grow up in their own families in their own cultures." Such a conclusion, Kelman explains, has political consequences, for it supports the United States "government's desire not to call attention to civilian casualties of the war in Vietnam." Moreover, the preservation of life is a more important value, Kelman asserts, than respect for cultural diversity. Rose B. Kelman, "Vietnam: A Current Issue in Child Welfare," *Social Work,* October 1968, *13*(4), p. 20.

tion that there is a consensus on professional values and one must join in this consensus as a precondition for professional practice. All values are presented as though they were mutually reinforcing. The possibility of a conflict in values is never suggested, although, in actuality, opposite sets of values are often embraced simultaneously. Timms, a prominent British social worker, notes:

> Caseworkers have asserted a faith in the potentialities of the human being to change himself and his society whilst, on the other hand, espousing a group of psychological theories which appear to place severe limitations on the capacity of individuals to change.[6]

One obstacle, then, is to recognize that the values in a professional creed are problematic rather than self-evident and that they frequently conflict.

Another obstacle arises from the difficulty of defining the profession. What, after all, is social work? An exhaustive study of social work education in the early 1950s concluded that "social work and social workers should be looked upon as evolving concepts that are as yet too fluid for precise definition."[7] By the late 1960s this fluidity had hardly become solidified. Indeed, to the extent that social work is involved in a fundamental reassessment of its major organizing principles, it is even more fluid today than it has been in the past. Because social workers serve as policy planners, reformers, social critics, and clinicians, it is difficult to identify the single professional creed that binds together these diverse activities.

A further problem in identifying the professional creed arises from the inability to separate clearly the procedural and substantive aspects of professional activity. Social work, like other professions, was influenced by the pragmatism of John Dewey. Dewey stressed the continuity of experience and the importance of process. In accord with this formulation, means and ends became blurred, professional technology became defined in terms of process, and social workers came to emphasize method and neglect purpose. Hence it is exceedingly difficult to find out what social workers believe and what they are trying to accomplish. There is nothing more challenging to a social agency than to ask what its objective is. The emphasis on process rather than outcome tends to obscure the role of ideology. What social workers believe must be inferred from what they say and do.

---

[6] Noel Timms, *Social Casework, Principles and Practices* (London: Routledge & Kegan Paul, 1964), p. 61.
[7] Florence V. Hollis and Alice L. Taylor, *Social Work Education in the United States* (New York: Columbia University Press, 1951), p. 54.

The last obstacle to be discussed is the disparity between rhetoric and reality, between what professionals say and do. A failure to implement ideals runs through the history of social work. The field developed out of a deterrent ideology, which sought alternatives to sending poor persons to the workhouse and would permit them to stay in the community while at the same time keep welfare rolls low. A common practice underlying the celebrated Elberfield system in Germany, the work of Thomas Chalmers, and the later activities of the Charity Organization Society was the use of strict investigation and close supervision of paupers as a way of making life on the dole uncomfortable and intolerable. So harsh were the ideals of political economy on which the social work ideology of the nineteenth century was based that it is not surprising to discover that humanitarianism and common sense inhibited their full expression. Reality and rhetoric diverge today as well. For example, social workers may believe that a precondition of good casework is full employment, a decent income, adequate social services, and a sound physical environment. But if this rhetoric were insisted upon, there would be no casework for the poor.

From a review of these obstacles, it seems reasonable to conclude that the search for a single, common professional creed is illusory. There are many creeds and many belief systems. The question now becomes: What are the critical components of the multiple belief systems? The author thinks these may be found in an examination of the different orientations in social work to behavioral goals and change processes.

Standards of Behavior

Norms and standards can be examined from several perspectives—standards that judge client, professional, or organizational behavior. In this analysis, the primary focus will be on the standards or norms of acceptable social behavior to which social work clients are held accountable. From this focus, the author is examining the social purposes of social work practice. What then are these norms? As Titmuss has astutely observed:

> The attitudes that society adopts to its deviants, and especially its poor and politically inarticulate deviants, reflect its ultimate values. . . . We must learn to understand the moral presuppositions underlying our action.[8]

One of the principal moral presuppositions underlying social work practice in this country has been acceptance of society's linkage of work

[8] Richard Titmuss, Foreword, in Noel Timms and H. F. Philips, *The Problem of the Problem Family* (London: Family Service Units, 1962), p. vi.

and income. With the exception of keeping women and the aged out of the labor force during the Depression, social workers have supported those policies designed to get the able-bodied poor to work. Industrial society is organized around the preservation of the middle-class ethic that rewards the industrious. But are there criteria by which to judge men other than market-productivity standards? To respect the dignity of man and to assert that each man has inherent value must clearly repudiate these dominant norms.

Since the issue of conformity to established standards is so crucial a component of a professional creed, it requires further discussion. For example, school performance is judged by the individual's ability to meet competitive standards (based on mastery of a body of information) and socialization for achievement. The ideal of helping people reach whatever level of performance they are capable of, that is, self-actualization without reference to minimum standards, is a radical ideal that challenges accepted social standards. Teachers and social workers know that educational attainment largely determines life chances and they strive to do what they can to equip their pupils and clients to compete. Hence they are naturally attracted to those most likely to succeed, those whose achievements will reward the social workers' and teachers' efforts. It is, after all, not perversity but realism that leads professionals to make this assessment. The school cannot care equally for the education of every child, whatever his skill, unless society values all men for whatever contributions they can make. And this, our performance-market-productivity-oriented society is unwilling to ensure.

Social workers must choose whether to help individuals meet prevailing standards or whether to challenge the standards themselves. If they choose to challenge values, they cannot do so by creating new ones. As professionals they must show that established norms conflict with other still more fundamental values in the society or that they are inconsistent or irrelevant to the specific task at hand.

In most situations, there is an overwhelming urge to bypass the issue altogether, with the argument that happiness and self-fulfillment can only be achieved when individuals conform to the standards of the society. Thus, helping people conform to the work ethic in our society assures their contentment because the conforming man is the happy man. This dubious proposition is lucidly challenged in *The People Specialists*, a book about the human relations movement in industry. Personnel men share much in common with social workers. The personnel movement has two conflicting roots—one in scientific management, which was concerned with the study of men at work to determine how their material output could be best increased, the other in social welfare, which was concerned with improving the workers' levels of living. Which aim were the personnel workers to accept: "to make workers more productive or to make them happier?" Personnel theory, like social work theory, pro-ceeded under the assumption that to do one is to do the other. But as the author shows, "there is no clear evidence to support any direct rela-tionship between high morale and high productivity." Indeed, there is some contradictory evidence:

In most corporations maturity is not a prized quality. On the contrary, the infantile qualities of passivity, dependence, submissive-ness seem to be the hallmarks of "good employees." [9]

This is not an abstract philosophical debate. Most social work prac-tice, whether in industry, prisons, probation, public welfare, or mental health, must accept the conflict between the individual's needs and the imposed and often arbitrary standards of society. When such conflicts arise, social workers must decide whether they support or challenge these established standards. Of course, some may try to define themselves as neutral arbitrators between contending parties. A radical ideal holds that the social worker must choose sides and is obliged to protect the in-dividual against the system.

Industrial social work, which never fully blossomed in the United States, had to make such a choice. The difference between the French and Indian schemes illustrates the general dilemma. The French hired social workers on the assumption that happy workers were productive because they came to work regularly and were not distracted by mari-tal, health, or other problems. In India it was assumed that the firm had more power than the individual and there was a natural tendency for power to corrupt. Hence the individual needed to be protected against this more powerful system. The social worker's role was to even out the odds.

Intervention Strategies

Theories of change can be divided into two broad categories.[10] There are those that accept social conditions as a constraint and con-clude that change must start within the individual. They are based on the premise that if the individual himself would only change, he would be able to move toward altering the external resources in the social en-vironment. By contrast, other theories treat external conditions as the targets of change, rather than as constraints. Their argument is that man cannot change until the world he lives in is transformed. His mate-

[9] Stanley M. Herman, *The People Specialists* (New York: Knopf, 1968).
[10] For this distinction the author has relied heavily on James S. Coleman, "Conflict-ing Theories of Social Change." (Mimeographed by the author, 1967).

rial circumstances must change first because man's emotional responses are adaptations to the external circumstances in which he lives. This distinction should be made as concretely as possible because what is implied are two alternative courses of action. As an example, the dichotomy just drawn will be applied to the area of manpower policy for disadvantaged groups. One approach emphasizes the necessity of direct efforts to modify the attitudes of the disadvantaged before introducing them into job situations. This is based on the principle of preparing people in advance for a change in their environment. The other approach brings the subemployed into a job situation first, thus changing their occupational environment as a precondition for individual change. Social services are then looked upon as supports to help the individual handle the demands of his new environment. This shift from preparation to support is important in understanding the role of social services and social work in manpower training programs.

One further approach must be mentioned. It is the position that change in the character of the individual can be brought about by the process of social action. As man organizes to change his world, he changes himself. This change theory is more subtle than the others. It appeals to the conservative–traditional camp as well, where it is more popularly known as a self-help ideology, by which individuals take action on their own behalf. There is radical and revolutionary support for it as well. In a thoughtful report on "Race Relations and Social Change," Coleman explains the revolutionary argument for participation, as revealed in the writings of Sorel, Sartre, and Mao Tse-Tung:

> Participation in revolutionary action transforms the previously apathetic masses, by giving them a goal and the hope of achieving the goal. The revolutionary action itself and the rewards of success it brings to hard work create men who are no longer bound by traditional customs, inhibited by ascribed authority patterns, and made apathetic by lack of hope. This psychological transformation, according to these authors, is a necessary prerequisite to the social and economic transformation. Applied to the case of Negroes in the United States, it would state that the real benefit of the civil rights movement is the psychological change it has produced and is producing in those Negroes active in it. A more radical application would be that only by engaging in a real revolution will Negroes be psychologically transformed in such a way that they can achieve their goals.[11]

But what if the external conditions do not succumb to action programs? This approach is not altogether explicit about this awkward

[11] James S. Coleman, "Race Relations and Social Change" (Baltimore: Johns Hopkins University, July 1967), p. 17. (Mimeographed.)

question and how it might be resolved. One interpretation holds that even in failure, personality change can be achieved. The self-help position could argue that personal dignity is won by the process of striving to better one's conditions. Character is forged by the activity, rather than the outcome. The more radical position would appear to suggest that change can be brought about by the total submission of the individual in the collectivity. Although his material circumstances may not be altered, his social–psychological environment has nevertheless been dramatically altered. Although social change approaches are often considered inherently radical, they are not. The purposes of social intervention theories, whether revolutionary or conservative, can either be directed at freeing men to build new standards or encouraging them to accept standards of proscribed behavior. It is for this reason that an intervention strategy, separated from the *purposes* of intervention, does not provide the basis for a creed.

Carried to its logical conclusion, this distinction between changing individuals and changing social conditions tends to break down. A theory that asserts that the starting point for change is the individual is incomplete if it leaves out the political and hence environmental processes that have led to the creation of an organized effort to induce change in the individual. Moreover, the availability of an authentic helping person is in itself a change in the external environment if other human beings are accepted as environmental resources. Similarly, only considering a change in social conditions leaves out the intervening processes by which an altered world produces individual change. Why are some groups and individuals able to exploit changes in the external environment and others are not? Thus, when applied to specific situations, the distinction becomes less convincing, and most reasonable men prefer a more differentiated argument that specifies the conditions under which one or another theory of change is more appropriate. But in the absence of a scientific theory of change, passion and ideology have a rich soil in which to blossom. It is for this reason that in this paper these theories are treated as elements of an ideology.

It should be emphasized again that the important generalization that arises from these observations is that both individual and social change theories can be used either to accept or repudiate established standards of behavior. Strategies of change can be used for different goals and, therefore, both goal and process become inseparable components of an ideology.

By dichotomizing the two dimensions of standards and theories of intervention in a two-by-two table, it is possible to identify four major professional creeds. They are (1) traditional casework, (2) community sociotherapy, (3) radical casework, and (4) radical social policy. (See Figure 1.)

THEORIES OF CHANGE

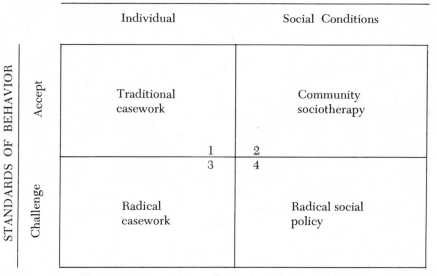

Figure 1. A typology of social work ideologies

Traditional Casework

The literature of social casework abounds with references to helping the marginal, deviant, and mentally ill meet standards and, thereby, achieve self-actualization and fullfillment. That conformity is viewed as the road to self-fullfillment is evident.

As Davis pointed out, advice about life problems is given in terms of moral ideals rather than actual practice. It is assumed that "one can best secure mental health, best satisfy one's needs, by conforming." [12] The social worker is thus trapped into what Hughes has called the "fallacy of one hundred percentism"—the refusal to admit the possibility of less than complete acceptance of moral, legal, respectable norms for behavior.[13] It is not surprising then to find that Hamilton, perhaps the leading modern casework theoretician, describes the function of diagnostic casework as "adaptation to reality." [14] As Keith-Lucas pointed

[12] Kingsley Davis, "Mental Hygiene and the Class Structure," in Herman D. Stein and Richard Cloward (Eds.), *Social Perspectives on Behavior* (Glencoe, Ill.: Free Press, 1958), p. 334.

[13] Everett Hughes, unpublished lecture, Brandeis University, 1961.

[14] Hamilton is sensitive to the awkward moral problem that arises when casework practice emphasizes adjustment. Therefore, she tries to distinguish between adjustment and acquiescence, emphasizing that casework helps "the client to identify what is real." But there is no systematic treatment of what reality is or how acquiescence could be achieved without adjusting to one's situation. *See* Gordon Hamilton,

out, diagnostic casework "can be used to justify the caseworker's desire to urge or dwell on the moral standards of the community though identifying these with the client's 'reality.' " [15] Biestek makes the implications explicit:

> The important fact to a caseworker is that these standards are realities in the client's life. . . . The client's personal adjustment must include a sound, realistic social adjustment, because as an individual he lives in a definite social community. . . . The function of the case-worker is to help the client accept and adjust to these standards.[16]

Thus, by falling prey to the fallacy of one hundred percentism, many caseworkers hold their clients to a higher standard of morality than the one to which the community itself adheres.

Throughout the literature of social work, a discerning reader can note that many social workers believe the task of social work is

> to reconcile the poor to their station in life . . . to plaster up the sores of an unjust society . . . to get the grit out of the administrative machinery—to persuade recalcitrant old ladies to go into institutions, to empty urgently needed hospital beds, to chivvy rent arrears from difficult tenants.[17]

These are, after all, the various realities to which the clients of social work must adjust—the realities of the economy, racial injustice, and bureaucracy.[18] In an effort to discredit this interpretation of the social

---

Theory and Practice of Social Case Work (2d., rev.; New York: Columbia University Press, 1951), p. 237.

[15] Alan Keith-Lucas, *Decisions About People in Need: A Study of Administrative Responsiveness in Public Assistance* (Chapel Hill: University of North Carolina Press, 1957), p. 143.

[16] Felix J. Biestek, "The Principles of Client Self-Determination," *Social Casework*, November 1951, 32(9), p. 374.

[17] D. V. Donnison in a book review of Barbara Wootton, *Social Science and Social Pathology* (New York: Humanities Press, 1959), *The Almoner*, July, August, and September 1959, 12(4, 5, and 6), p. 172, notes that "the social workers who have to resist these pressures often work in isolated and exposed positions."

[18] For a similar criticism, see C. Wright Mills's famous study, "The Professional Ideology of Social Pathologists," *American Journal of Sociology*, September 1949, 35(2), pp. 179–180. Pathologists are sociologists who write textbooks about social problems. Mills believed that "these writers typically assume the norms which they use and often tacitly sanction them. There are few attempts to explain deviations from norms in the terms of norms themselves, and no rigorous facing of the implications of the fact that social transformations would involve shifts *in them.* . . . If the 'norms' were examined, the investigator would perhaps be carried to see total structures of norms and to relate these to distributions of power."

worker's function, Titmuss has pointed out that two questionable assumptions underlie the insistence on adaptation to reality.

The first is that reality is something which the caseworker knows, but the client does not; the second is that if adaptation is genuinely to take place, reality must genuinely be accepted by the caseworker. The ultimate logic of this is to make the caseworker a prisoner of the collective *status quo;* consequently, she will have little or nothing to contribute to the shaping of the social policy; she will not, in fact, desire to do so.[19]

But this discussion of traditional social work is theoretical, being based only on what social workers say. Obviously, the literature may be subject to other interpretations. Only scattered empirical evidence is available on the attitudes and behavior of social workers, but these seem to support the author's exposition. The author has found no study directly concerned with the issue of getting clients to meet standards of behavior; studies deal with agency rules or, more generally, with personal values.

In 1967 Rossi et al. analyzed welfare workers in fifteen cities who worked primarily with Negro clients. They reported that their sample

came out about evenly split on making decisions largely based on agency rules or largely on the circumstances of the client. However, the breakdown by race showed the whites considerably more rigid, with fifty-four percent (as compared with forty percent of the Negroes) saying they usually obey the agency rules.[20]

Billingsley, in his study of professional child welfare workers in Boston, obtained data on the choices social workers make when their assessment of the needs of their clients conflicts with agency procedures. He discovered that "in spite of the social worker's intellectual and emotional commitment to meeting the needs of his clients," more than three-quarters complied with agency rules even when these conflicted with "the workers' own estimation of the needs of the client." [21]

McLeod and Meyer at the University of Michigan conducted a study in which they compared the values of professionals, nonprofessionals, and social work students on a number of issues. One of these dealt with belief in change versus tradition, that is, "the willingness to

[19] Richard Titmuss, *Commitment to Welfare* (London: Allen & Unwin, 1968), p. 42.
[20] Peter Rossi et al., *Between White and Black: The Faces of American Institutions in the Ghetto* (Baltimore: Johns Hopkins Press, 1968), p. 144.
[21] Andrew Billingsley, "Bureaucratic and Professional Orientation Patterns in Social Casework," *Social Service Review*, December 1964, 38(4), pp. 402–403.

accept change as contrasted with the orientation that is committed to the traditional ways of the past." Their findings are suggestive. They found that the nontrained were oriented to the status quo (71 percent), but what was of special interest was the shift in values between those who were in training and those who were fully trained. Most students supported innovation while in training (54 percent), while most trained workers were committed to the status quo (52 percent).[22]

These findings are suggestive only, and it is hazardous to make firm generalizations based on them. They do appear however to indicate that the dominant value commitment and behavior of professional social workers support in theory and practice a posture of getting others to meet standards of acceptable behavior. They reveal the extent to which social workers personally comply with bureaucratic norms even when these conflict with clients' needs.

Radical Casework

Not all social workers are prisoners of the collective status quo when they work with individuals. Many overtly and covertly resist these pressures. Resistance to established norms can, as has been already suggested, take several forms. It can challenge the standards, either by appealing to other standards with which they conflict or by showing that the standards themselves are inconsistent and lead to contradictory and unintended consequences. A latent functional analysis, when properly done, is, after all, a form of muckraking or social criticism. Gouldner's critique of practices in adoption offers an illuminating example.

Adoption agencies require or recommend that adoptive parents be of the same religion as the mother of the adopted child. What proof is there that this practice is desirable or effective either for the child or for the parents? In this instance, it seems probable that the policy derives not from evidence of its effectiveness at all but from the pressure of various interest groups.

It may well be most injurious to a child to be adopted by parents of a religious persuasion similar to that of his biological mother, if members of this denomination regard illegitimacy with moral revulsion. . . . Yet, here, as in many other instances, agencies' practices are shaped by community pressures and legal requirements and do not rest on evidence of their effectiveness for the clients.[23]

[22] Donna L. McLeod and Henry J. Meyer, "A Study of the Values of Social Workers," in Edwin J. Thomas (Ed.), *Behavioral Science for Social Workers* (New York: Free Press, 1967), Table 30-2, p. 409.
[23] Alvin Gouldner, "The Secrets of Organizations," *The Social Welfare Forum, 1963* (New York: Columbia University Press, 1963), p. 167.

Gouldner presents the hurtful consequences of certain adoption procedures in such a way that his statement becomes a useful instrument of social criticism. Critiques of this kind offer one framework from which a radical casework practice might emerge.

More typically, social workers try to activate those values that they accept as morally right and society accepts but fails to act on. They then organize their research and action to serve as moral witnesses, documenting the failure of society to implement the ideals it has already asserted in law or policy.

Another approach is suggested in the writing of Lichtenberg. In a discussion of the prerequisites necessary for the cure of the psychotic, he asserts:

> If we compare the organizing principles relevant to a therapeutic community with those embodied in the present-day organization of the society, we discover that the principles underlying the therapeutic community are superior. . . . Equality, cooperation, openness and frankness between persons at all levels of authority, two-way flow of communication with whatever hierarchies exist, control of the governed not only over themselves but over those who govern, preoccupation with one's true feelings rather than with masking one's attitudes, confrontation with poor communication so that it does not escalate difficulties, sexual freedom, . . . all of which have been found to be essentially ingredients of [the] therapeutic community.[24]

It is the structure of the community that is faulty, since it lacks what the psychotic requires for his cure. Lichtenberg clearly insists that the world must be changed if the emotionally disabled are to be cured. Of course, Freud's work, which had an enormous influence on social work pratice, is a brilliant example of a systematic critique of and challenge to society's standards of sexuality and its principles of individual responsibility.

Casework practice, then, can challenge the standards of society by showing that they are irrelevant or have hurtful consequences, that valid and relevant standards are not implemented, or that the standards men live by are faulty.

But the discerning reader might well ask: Is radical casework an empty cell, logically plausible but nonexistent in reality? The author resists accepting this formulation, for he is convinced that radical casework does exist. One form that it takes is when the caseworker acts as an insurgent within the bureaucracy in which he is employed, seeking to change its policies and purposes in line with the value assumptions he

[24] Philip Lichtenberg, "And the Cure of Psychosis Is for Us All," pp. 12–13. Unpublished manuscript, Bryn Mawr, Pa., 1968.

208 The Politics of the Emerging Professions

cherishes. Caseworkers can act as rebels within a bureaucracy, humanizing its established procedures and policies. One cannot read the literature in social casework today without finding some examples of radical casework. In the writings of Briar, Miller, and Piliavin, one finds caseworkers repudiating the traditional norms of helping clients adapt to reality. They are at the frontier, trying to find ways to make a radical casework live.[25]

Community Sociotherapy

Community sociotherapy has to do with the belief system that holds that such processes as organizing groups for self-help, protest, access to community facilities, or even revolution can create a transformation of the individual personality. Participation in social action is viewed as a sociotherapeutic tool. HARYOU–ACT, the Community Action Program in Harlem, put the argument as follows:

If it is possible to establish a core program of social action, it would be reasonable to expect that the energies required, and which must be mobilized for constructive and desirable social change, would not then be available for anti-social and self-destructive patterns of behavior.[26]

The report claims, for example, that crime in Montgomery, Alabama, declined during the period of the civil rights protest.

This energy displacement theory was in an earlier period used to justify the notion that recreation reduced crime. It is a theory that explains how activism can be transformed into compliance. Other theories are also at hand, including claims for the positive effects on personal health of power, integration, cohesiveness, community competence, identity, and so forth. All of these have in common the proposition that, as man tries to change his social condition, *he* changes in the process.

The attempt by sociologists to get social workers to use social action and self-help as strategies for promoting individual conformity has a long history. Part of the history that spans the twentieth century yet has a consistency in ideology that would almost suggest a linear theory in its evolution will now be reviewed. The first example is drawn from Znaniecki and Thomas's study of the Polish peasant written in 1918. The authors explain:

[25] See, for example, Briar, *op. cit.*, pp. 5–11; Miller, *op. cit.*, pp. 27–33; and Irving Piliavin, "Restructuring the Provision of Social Services," *Social Work*, January 1968, *13*(1), pp. 34–41.
[26] *Youth in the Ghetto: A Study of the Consequences of Powerlessness* (New York: Harlem Youth Opportunities Unlimited, 1964).

It is a mistake to suppose that a "community center" established by American social agencies can in its present form even approximately fulfill the social function of a Polish parish. It is an institution imposed from the outside instead of being freely developed by the initiative and cooperation of the people themselves. . . . Its managers usually know little or nothing of the traditions, attitudes, and native language of the people with whom they have to deal . . . [Although] the "case method" that consists in dealing directly and separately with individuals and families . . . may bring efficient temporary help to the individual, it does not continue the social progress of the community nor does it possess much preventive influence in struggling against social disorganization. Both of these processes can be attained only by organizing and encouraging social self-help on a cooperative basis.[27]

The argument is clear. Organizing and encouraging self-help will reduce social disorganization. The failure to help the Polish immigrant conform to American standards, according to the authors' criticism, is based on two factors—imposition by alien institutions, which today is called "welfare colonialism," and the individual case approach.

In the 1930s, the prescription for action took an organized form in the Chicago Area Project under the leadership of Clifford Shaw and Henry McKay, when a social action program was launched to reduce crime and delinquency. It is perhaps of interest that Saul Alinsky was a student of sociology at the University of Chicago at the same time and, according to Morris Janowitz: "Some of his notions of community action and organization are strikingly parallel to those developed in this project."[28] Perhaps so, but it seems that the distinguishing feature of this and the later programs the Chicago project inspired is the absence of a political ideology and the commitment to sociotherapeutic aims. In the 1940s, New York University supported a project directed by Rudolph Wittenberg that was designed to promote personality change through social action in East Harlem. In the 1950s, New York City's Youth Board Gang Project turned to community organization as a strategy to help create an integrated community that could reduce crime and delinquency. In the 1960s, community organization as sociotherapy can be found in Mobilization For Youth's program, which was originally conceived as a delinquency prevention program and was financed by

[27] Florian Znaniecki and W. I. Thomas, *The Polish Peasant in Europe and America,* Vol. II (Boston: Gorham Press, 1918), pp. 15–26.
[28] Many of the observations in this section are based on an interview with Morris Janowitz. He later developed his insights in "A Note on Sociology and Social Work" (Chicago: University of Chicago, undated), p. 3. (Mimeographed.)

the National Institute of Mental Health and the President's Committee on Delinquency and Youth Crime.[29]

The critique of social work in these examples was not directed at the purposes of intervention, but at its effectiveness. Sociotherapy was not a new ideology, but a new technology for getting marginal groups to meet standards. Znaniecki and Thomas's criticism is not the established orthodoxy accepted by community psychiatry and community psychology. Dumont, a psychiatrist at NIMH, commenting on the role of mental health programs in Model Cities, asserts that "community organization is itself a major mental health service, an end in itself." [30] Scribner, while stressing the varied interests of "social action" psychologists, makes evident their common commitment to "social action without . . . political movements as forces of change." While the purposes of change are varied, they all center on different aspects of the problem of compliance—"correcting deviant behavior which interferes with individual progress, . . . controlling mass hysteria . . . or changing child-rearing practices. . . ." [31]

The concern for compliance through social action now seems to be taking a new turn. It is calling for an indirect strategy of involving the middle classes to control the lower classes, in whom it is assumed the roots of nonconformity to established standards grow. Glazer describes the Negro bourgeois as "the missing man in the present crisis." According to this thesis, black power, black capital, and black participation must mean the involvement of the Negro middle class rather than the Negro poor and disaffiliated groups.[32] Long develops the argument. He explains:

> The key question is whether there exists or can rapidly be produced sufficient middle class cadres to govern the black governed city. . . . The greatest fear clearly is that the middle class Negroes cannot dominate the lower class culture of Ghetto life.[33]

A change in social conditions is being called for to enable the middle-class Negro leadership to police its own poor more effectively. Apart-

---

[29] For a further analysis of community organization as sociotherapy, see Peter Marris and Martin Rein, Dilemmas of Social Reform (New York: Atherton Press, 1967), p. 167.
[30] Mathew P. Dumont, "A Model Community Mental Health Program for a Model Cities Area" (Washington, D.C.: Center for Community Planning, U.S. Department of Health, Education, and Welfare, August 1967), p. 3. (Mimeographed.)
[31] Sylvia Scribner, "What is Community Psychology Made Of?" American Psychological Association, Division of Community Psychology, Newsletter, January 1968, 11(1), p. 5.
[32] Nathan Glazer, "The Problem with American Cities," New Society, March 21, 1968, p. 3.
[33] Norton Long, "Politics and Ghetto Perpetuation," in Roland L. Warren (Ed.), Politics and the Ghettos (New York: Atherton Press, 1969).

heid in South Africa is justified on much the same grounds: By walling off the Negroes from white society, Negro leaders must police their own lower class. Social stability is more effective when imposed by indigenous institutions than by welfare colonialism.[34]

Radical Social Policy

The link between social action and sociotherapy has been stressed in this paper because the author believes it is not widely understood and because it is the dominant pattern of the social environmentalist position today. But there is also evidence of a social action program that challenges the established standards of behavior and also tries to replace existing institutions rather than merely transferring organizational slots from white to Negro leaders.

Perhaps the best-known example of radical social action by a social worker and a city planner who teach at a school of social work is the work of Cloward and Piven in the welfare rights movement. Wilbur Cohen, Elizabeth Wickenden, and Winifred Bell dominated the intellectual leadership in welfare policy. They were committed to incrementalism as a strategy of change and liberalism as a social philosophy. Cloward and Piven substituted a more radical approach to social policy. Their *immediate* aim was not to improve the social conditions of the welfare poor; they were not trying to strengthen the welfare system, but rather to replace it. They believed that this apparent conflict of aims between improving conditions, which inhibits the urgency to introduce more fundamental change, and disrupting the performance of an intolerable system could be avoided in the case of welfare because an improved welfare system would be politically unacceptable. Amelioration would lead to metamorphosis.[35]

While these are important tactical issues, they should not obscure the essence of their radical creed, which is the commitment to redistribution, reducing inequalities, and altering social conditions—political, economic, and social—as a precondition for individual change. Cloward and Piven are not primarily concerned with the problems of compliance, of getting individuals to meet standards or promoting social stability. Rather, their emphasis is on altering institutions, redefining norms and purposes, and reassessing the standards by which professional performance is judged.

The ideals of a radical profession must be able to find expression in specific forms. Social workers already perform a great variety of profes-

[34] For a discussion of the conservative argument for Black Power, see Martin Rein, "Social Stability and Black Ghettoes," in *ibid.*
[35] See, for example, Richard A. Cloward and Frances Fox Piven, "A Strategy to End Poverty," *The Nation*, May 2, 1966, 202(18).

sional roles as reformers and organizers, policy analysts, planners, researchers, consultants who are inside the bureaucracy, critics who are outside the established system, and "insider—outsiders," a role that enables them to be relevant, but critical. Like all creeds, the radical creed may contain inconsistencies and contradictions. When rigidly applied, it can become dogma and theology. The function of a belief system is not to provide answers but to offer goals and objectives toward which one's professional activities can be oriented.

Of the four professional creeds discussed in this paper, the author has given more attention to traditional casework and community sociotherapeutic ideologies because they are better developed and experience has sharpened the understanding of them. It is not altogether surprising that the more radical doctrines have failed to win wide support and hence remain at the margin of the profession. But the margin in one era may become the center of another.

Professional Creed and Urban Problems

Which of the professional creeds seems most appropriate to urban needs? America faces many urban crises—the crises of race, class, managerial competence, and financing services. While the problems overlap and reinforce each other, they must also be distinguished from each other.

The problem of race cannot be solved without a redistribution of authority, resources, and power. The problem of poverty requires a redistribution of income and resources. The issues of race and class need to be sorted out, and the trade-off between redistributing income and power (those aspects of the one goal that would be acceptable to proponents of the other goal) has to be clarified. The movement for school decentralization in New York City has by and large not demanded more resources for the ghetto, but only a different decision-making system.

What can be said about the relationship between professional doctrine and urban–racial problems? Which creeds are most relevant to this problem? In the search for a better solution to the problem of race, the liberal ideology, from which the spectrum of professional creeds previously examined are derived, has been assaulted. That the cherished beliefs about integration have been challenged is evident, but the insistence on separatism opens new issues. That the distribution of power among the social services is ethnically determined is a disquieting reality that has been long forgotten. Irish control of police, Italian control of sanitation, Jewish control of education, and perhaps Negro control over the new social services in community action agencies illustrate the neglected relation between service control and ethnicity. A redistribution of power may alter these established patterns. It has been relatively easy in ideological terms to accept a redistribution of power at the neighborhood level. A nineteenth-century leader of the settlement house movement asserted:

> Poverty, pauperism and other social evils could not be cured by alms, or by a redistribution of wealth, but only by creating [a] genuine neighborhood reestablished as a feature of civic life.[36]

Many still believe that creed today; for them the neighborhood remains a tool for sociotherapy.

But the great racial crisis will emerge as Negroes and other ethnic groups insist on a redistribution of power not by "turf," but by function. The struggle for power over education in New York City has already opened up the question of who controls the social services. For many Negroes, control of the social services offers a much better leverage for the redistribution of power than does control over economic institutions. The accountability system in the social services has always been vulnerable. The demonstrated weaknesses of elite accountability, democratic accountability, and professional accountability are already evident. We may be witnessing a new demand for ethnic and racial accountability.

The traditional and community sociotherapeutic belief systems, on which professional social work ideology rests, will not be able to cope easily with ideological issues that the crisis of race has already presented. A more adequate creed will have to be developed if the profession wishes to be relevant to the issues of race.

Poverty cannot be dealt with simply in terms of overcoming apathy through more intelligent service or through social action programs, however dedicated. What is needed is a national redistribution of resources that deliberately redresses the imbalance of opportunities between rich and poor communities, between Negro and white communities. Sociotherapeutic approaches, whether individual or social, run the risk of deceiving themselves and others if they function without a complementary national reform.

A dispassionate analysis of current social policy would confirm the conclusion that social work programs have been used as a substitute for more searching policies to redistribute income, power, and resources. There is a perverse tendency in American social reform to repudiate social work and then to embrace the very ideals that have been rejected. The Economic Opportunity Act stressed institutional change initiated

---

[36] Quoted in Roy Lubove, *The Professional Altruist: The Emergence of Social Work as a Career* (Cambridge, Mass.: Harvard University Press, 1965), p. 15.

214 The Politics of the Emerging Professions

by the poor. Shriver harshly reprimanded the social work community at the 1965 National Conference on Social Welfare for social work's preoccupation with individualized methods and failure to reach the poor.[37] Yet as Kahn observed:

The heart of the community action program is in the field of individual remediation help, retraining, counseling and aid. . . . A social-change strategy, thus, continues to require case and individual elements, and political realities may even render individual services primary despite ideological commitment.[38]

Community sociotherapy and traditional casework appear to have a stubborn vitality. The more they are rejected, the more thay seem to survive, flourish, and expand. In the author's judgment, the viability of the professional doctrine that emphasizes therapeutic solutions has produced a great dilemma in American society insofar as the solution of poverty is concerned because it seems that social policies have been based on it. Accordingly, we have tried to stimulate the economic participation of the poor through training to support the work ethic, employability and counseling programs, and citizen participation, but have failed to develop an economic policy to achieve social objectives. In short, social policies have been generated to meet economic aims, but economic policies have not been used to meet social ends. Thus America lacks a policy of using up its available labor force or redistributing income among poor individuals and resources among low-income communities. Social work doctrine has inhibited the profession from openly repudiating the claim that casework can reduce dependency and social work can contribute to the reduction of poverty.

Conclusions

Social work, *by itself,* has almost nothing to contribute to the reduction of the interrelated problems of unemployment, poverty, and dependency. Therefore, if you interpret social work as radical social policy committed to altering political and economic institutions that affect well-being (on the assumption that social welfare activities to compensate individuals for the diseconomies generated by the political and economic system have been insufficient), then it ceases to be social work.

[37] Sargent Shriver, "Poverty in the United States—What Next?" *The Social Welfare Forum, 1965* (New York: Columbia University Press, 1965), pp. 55–66.
[38] Alfred J. Kahn, "From Delinquency Treatment to Community Development," in Paul Lazarsfeld et al. (Eds.), *The Uses of Sociology* (New York: Basic Books, 1967), p. 497.

Individual social workers may, of course, function as reformers in the areas of employment, income redistribution, and political power, but these activities are marginal to their professional tasks. In this sense, they are professionals who are radical rather than members of a radical profession. In recognition of this dilemma, some social workers have urged that the present profession be forsaken and a new one built that is committed to the problems of inequality of wealth, power, authority, and so forth, and to strategies of redistribution. These major unresolved problems of public policy also touch the limits of the contribution of social science to social purpose. Hence it is especially crucial that the problem not become subordinated to methodology. But in this broader area of social reform, social work will need to compete with new programs that have been developed at such universities as Harvard, the Massachusetts Institute of Technology, the University of Michigan, the State University of New York at Buffalo, and the University of California at Berkeley and have been variously called public policy, public affairs, social policy, and urban policy. Can social work recruit able students, attract competent faculty, and win institutional resources and support to embark on this new venture and compete with these new centers of training? It clearly has not done so in the past. Whether past history is a prelude to the future must remain an open question.

What can social work do short of full repudiation of its present mission? It can contribute greatly to improving the quality of urban life, humanizing institutions, and altering the priority of social values. It can perhaps implement these objectives by defining its present mission more broadly, and it must do so in terms of the way it interprets its clients' needs. A radical casework approach would mean not merely obtaining for clients social services to which they are entitled or helping them adjust to their environment, but also trying to deal with the relevant people and institutions in the clients' environment that are contributing to their difficulties. That is to say, social workers must get the school to adjust to the needs of poor children as well as getting poor children to adjust to the demands and routines of the schools. They must force landlords to maintain their clients' housing as well as help poor families to find somewhere to live. They must get public welfare agencies to change their procedures to make it easier to use welfare as a resource for help, as well as help clients fulfill the requirements of the welfare bureaucracy. In short, then, a radical casework approach would mean not merely obtaining for the clients the services to which they are entitled or helping them adapt to the expectations of their environment, but it would also encourage the individuals to alter their external circumstances as well as seek directly to change the framework of expectation and the level of provision that are contributing to these difficulties. Social workers need to emphasize skill in practicing casework in a hostile rather than a benign environment—casework that is directed not so much at encouraging conformity (adjustment to reality) but to marshaling the resources of clients to challenge "reality."

As social work moves away from altering the environment on behalf of a given client to altering the environment in general without reference to a specific client, it moves to social reform and to the boundaries of its main concern. Action at the boundary is crucial and should be encouraged, but it should not lead, as it has done, to the neglect of its center. If we try to redefine the present margin so that it becomes the new center of social work activity, then we accept the position that social work must move toward a radical social policy approach. However, a radical casework approach may prove, in the end, to be the more enduring strategy to pursue.

THE ADVOCACY CHALLENGE
TO SCHOOLS OF SOCIAL WORK
15

David Wineman
Adrienne James

There are prisons with and without walls. A prison is here defined as a social arrangement in which a captor–captive relationship exists. Public assistance, probation, and parole agencies are prisons without walls. All forms of incarceration—jails and mental hospitals—are virtual prisons. And the American public school system chronically oscillates between potential and actual prisonhood.

Captor–captive states are inherently inimical to the human condition because they jeopardize the humanity of both captor and captive. Yet they appear to be inevitable in most complex societies. The degree of civilization of a society is demonstrated by how it treats its various classifications of captives, by the extent to which it displays a consciousness of its destructiveness, and by its readiness to undertake countermeasures against dehumanization.[1]

Reprinted with permission of the National Association of Social Workers, from *Social Work*, 1969, *14*, 23–32. David Wineman, MSW, is Professor and Chairman of the Human Behavior Sequence, School of Social Work, Wayne State University, Detroit, Michigan. Adrienne James, MSW, is Executive Director of Operation Friendship and a part-time instructor at Wayne State University.

[1] Treatment is the inverse of dehumanization. It is significant in this respect that a body of law is beginning to develop in which the right of the mentally ill to treatment is upheld. Cardinal to the court decisions that have begun to lay the foundation for this evolving juridical principle is the concept that when government (society) deprives a person of his right to liberty, that person is entitled through constitutional protections to prompt treatment so that his chance to regain the freedom of community life is maximized. See, for example, the three landmark decisions written by Chief Judge David Bazelon for the U.S. Circuit Court of Appeals (D.C.) dealing with the criminally insane, the sexual psychopath, and the senile aged in *Rouse* vs. *Cameron*, 373 F2 451, *Millard* vs. *Cameron*, 373 F2 468, and *Lake* vs. *Cameron*, 364 F2 657. The Rouse decision is especially noteworthy since it clearly reflects the court's opinion that in some cases an order of conditional or unconditional release may be the appropriate remedy in the absence of treatment. In an especially striking decision, one claimant has been granted damages of $300,000 from the state for negligence of state doctors in providing psychiatric and ordinary medical care in a state hospital. The opinion notes: "We believe we understand the immense difficulties faced by the State in financing, staffing, and administering as vast a complex as Mattawan State Hospital, as well as the other state hospitals. However, society denominates these institutions as hospitals and they should be so conducted.

The social work profession is currently experiencing its main moral outrage and drive toward advocacy with respect to one of these client captivity statuses: the public assistance recipient. The other client statuses or states of captivity through which one may be equally attacked and buried in a subhygienic world have for the most part failed to excite recent writers on client advocacy. The statuses of schoolchild, mental hospital patient, probationer, parolee, and detention home, training school, or prison inmate have been virtually ignored.[2]

There is a kind of "bandwagon vision" operating that makes the poor and the black visible mainly in the status of public assistance client but not in these other statuses.[3] The stark horror of these more shadowy statuses of captivity should be spotlighted. There is a need to broaden the advocacy will of social work to attack the breakdown of democratic decency in whichever client statuses it occurs.

In the complex struggle for change that is visualized in building an advocacy norm into the profession, the school of social work is in an embarrassingly undefined position. A large number of social work students are spread among courts, public welfare, correctional agencies and institutions, mental hospitals, and schools. On campus, schools float out theory, technology, and ideals that represent the knowledge–value mix of the social work profession.[4] Theory may be weak, and sometimes

---

If they are to be no more than pens into which we are to sweep that which is offensive to 'normal society' then let us be honest and denominate them as such. . . ." *Whitree* vs. *State*, 290 NYS 2d 486, in *The Mental Health Court Digest*, September 1968, *12*(3), pp. 3–4.

[2] Perhaps the clearest exhortation for broad client advocacy comes from Scott Briar, who uses the poor in his examples but also stresses that the principles of advocacy are "no less applicable to other groups in the society." A survey of *Social Work, Social Casework, Social Service Review, Journal of Education for Social Work, Social Work Education Reporter,* and *New Perspectives: The Berkeley Journal of Social Welfare* since 1965 reveals that captor–captive settings other than public assistance are seldom dealt with as specific advocacy targets. Exceptions to this are Specht, who uses a probation example; Brager, who cites school systems and housing authorities as possible targets for advocacy interventions; and Miller, whose focus on the involuntary status of certain clients includes the settings described in this paper. See Scott Briar, "The Social Worker's Responsibility for the Civil Rights of Clients," *New Perspectives: The Berkeley Journal of Social Welfare,* Spring 1967, *1*(1), pp. 89–92; Harry Specht, "Casework Practice and Social Policy Formulation," *Social Work,* January 1968, *13*(1), pp. 42–52; George A. Brager, "Advocacy and Political Behavior," *Social Work,* April 1968, *13*(2), pp. 5–15; and Henry Miller, "Value Dilemmas in Social Casework," *Social Work,* January 1968, *13*(1), pp. 27–33.

[3] Hollingshead and Redlich, for example, show that among neurotic patients, "Custodial care [as a type of treatment] is limited largely to Class V [lowest]"; and "There is clearly a strong inverse relationship between class status and whether a psychotic patient is in the state hospitals." August B. Hollingshead and Fredrick C. Redlich, *Social Class and Mental Illness* (New York: Wiley, 1958), pp. 267, 282.

[4] The words theory and technology refer to the theory and technology base of psychoanalytic ego psychology. The settings in question, it is being argued, are incom-

techniques melt in front of the worker's eyes. A more eclectic program with a unified theory of social and human behavior is needed. But even if all these problems were solved immediately, it would not make much difference, because any model of theory, technology, and ideals, regardless of what it is or might become, will be useless the minute the student tries to apply it in the face of the contamination of the field work settings.[5]

A critical index of the integrity of the school of social work will increasingly be found in its willingness to engage in a reexamination of the relationship between its teaching and the action imperatives of its field work agencies. In facing this challenge, the school finds its place in the crisis of higher education today: the confrontation between knowledge and social injustice.

Forms of Dehumanization

The following kinds of things, which frequently occur in captor–captive settings, are destructive to the total functioning of the person and preclude any rational application of the theory, technology, and ideals of the social work profession.[6] With respect to all of the following, social work students (and others) either are direct witnesses or are so close that de jure–tight cases could be made from their testimony.[7] There are other types of dehumanization, but those cited are meant to be representative of the most severe forms.

---

patible with the therapeutic ideology drawn from this model. The inference (if it were to be made) that there would be a higher compatibility with drastically different approaches—for example, the sociobehavioral—is distinctly dubious. Examination of the sociobehavioral approach, or any rationally based extrapolation of a variety of current change models, will reveal that none of them could coexist with the capricious and arbitrary handling of human functioning endemic in these settings.

[5] Obviously, the focus on dehumanization and comments on the inutility of knowledge in captor–captive settings do not imply that there is no body of knowledge that, if followed, will permit the development of humane and useful settings. In the children's field, for instance, the works of Fritz Redl and Bruno Bettelheim alone present a detailed theoretical exposition of such humanely based and therapeutically focused residential care. John Brown's efforts in Canada, so vividly portrayed in the movie Warrendale, are provocative in this regard. Gisela Konopka has also written productively for this field, and a further contribution is A. E. Trieschman, L. K. Brendtro, and J. K. Whittaker, The Other 23 Hours (New York: Aldine Press, 1967).

[6] Many of the areas mentioned—especially those identified as civil liberties or constitutional issues—have been investigated by the Metropolitan Detroit Branch of the American Civil Liberties Union of Michigan, primarily through its Committee on Civil Liberties of Children and Youth. Mimeographed material on these issues is available from the committee, 234 State Street, Detroit, Mich. 48226.

[7] In those areas in which the possibility of a constitutional or other legal violation may occur, cooperation of the legal profession is essential and represents a resource

1. *Physical brutalization.* This occurs in the form of beatings, food deprivation, enforced immobility (for example, standing for hours without being allowed to move), sensory deprivation (for example, the use of quiet rooms for hours with little light or other signs of reality), spontaneous use of group sadism "to teach a kid a lesson," to mention but a few. When they occur in state agencies, these may violate the constitutional right to freedom from cruel and unusual punishment.

2. *Psychic humiliation.* This includes a variety of tactics for stripping a person of all semblance of human dignity. Examples are shaming, exploiting weaknesses, needling and teasing, refusing to permit a person to tell his side of a conflict, arbitrary use of authority, surveillance activities in public assistance and corrections, and the use of invidious terms like "animal," "bastard," and "nigger" directed by persons in authority to patients, inmates, clients, and public school students.

3. *Sexual traumatization.* This occurs in settings where more powerful and institutionally sophisticated residents force the homosexual equivalent of rape on the weaker and less sophisticated.

4. *Condoned use of feared indigenous leaders for behavioral management.* A usually tacit but sometimes open deal is made between those in authority and such leaders, who are then permitted wider leeway than normal, given certain privileges, and the like, in exchange for the exercise of brutal control measures on weaker group members.[8]

5. *Chronic exposure to programless boredom.* Certain settings simply provide nothing for people to do. They sit and deteriorate mentally or engage in physical conflicts with each other in outbursts of tension and/or "symptom blowups" because of a systematic drainage of activity structures.

6. *"Unclean" grouping.* This includes enforced living together of clinically incompatible mixtures of human beings who cannot avoid symptom and trait clashes that worsen their problems. Too wide a range of sophistication, toughness, psychosis, delinquency, developmental levels, socioeconomic classes, and cultural styles is clearly contraindicated by any professionally based theory but may occur under certain conditions of policy stupidity, downright decadence, shortage of institutional space and personnel, and/or neglect.

7. *Symptom-squeezing forms of punishment.* Punishment of dis-

---

that social workers have encouragingly utilized in public assistance but not with other captor–captive client statuses. See, for example, Charles F. Grosser and Edward V. Sparer, "Legal Services for the Poor: Social Work and Social Justice," *Social Work*, January 1966, *11*(1), pp. 81–87; and Betty Mandell, "The Crime of Poverty," *Social Work*, January 1966, *11*(1), pp. 11–15.

[8] This phenomenon is described vividly in Howard W. Polsky, *Cottage Six* (New York: Russell Sage, 1962).

turbed children and adults is contraindicated because of their ego impairment. In many residential settings for disturbed people, however, there is wholesale violation of this principle. Moreover, in the eagerness of the authorities to get some kind of pleasure/pain hold on the person, a special attack on his functioning is mounted by selection of certain punishment experiences that squeeze already existing symptom-loaded areas.

Thus, for example, restriction of home visiting privileges is apt to do just that. These are people who have broken down in the family system in a society in which the family unit is viewed as the basic protective and status-giving experience. Yet this pathology-infected area becomes the very one used to control the person's behavior in the institution. This is not to imply that home visiting should be uncontrolled—the criteria that control it should give priority to individual needs, not the behavioral control requirements of the institution. Another example of symptom-squeezing is the use of dark isolation rooms, regardless of whether the person has a severe phobia about being alone and in the dark.[9] Restriction of food with severely regressed people and the use of suspension from school with poor learners are cases in point —so are physical punishment of youths already fixed on a delinquent identity stressing toughness and any punishment at all of an individual whose ego functioning is heavily masochistically oriented.

8. *Enforced work routines in the guise of vocational training.* While it is possible that an educationally well-designed work training program may be integrated with housekeeping and maintenance chores, this is rare in most public institutions. Usually it is designed more to take the place of programming, which is ignored, or to save on administrative costs. When there is no central theory that relates it to the patient's or inmate's problem, it is simply not defensible and arguably constitutes a violation of the right to be free from involuntary servitude.

9. *Violations of privacy.* These range all the way from having to live in extremely overcrowded quarters in institutions to unauthorized searches of person and property. The latter occur in institutions and schools, in the operation of welfare and probation and parole agencies, and in the form of unauthorized home visits in which the client, probationer, or parolee must admit the worker or suffer some penalty. These assaults on personal dignity may represent violations of constitutionally guaranteed rights.

What is new about this list? Nothing. There is a tradition—a cul-

---

[9] Isolation need not be antitherapeutic. See, for example, William C. Morse and David Wineman, "The Therapeutic Use of Social Isolation in a Camp for Ego-Disturbed Boys," *Journal of Social Issues*, January 1957, *13*(1), pp. 32–39.

ture of abuse—in these captor–captive settings that is protected by a complex web of human weakness and deceit, including the most treacherous form, self-deceit.[10]

Conventional Faculty Reactions

Students go into these settings every year—like so many ants marching out of the hill—all with their shiny new theory and methods gear in their little knapsacks, ready to "help." (None of them was ever born that naïve, but that is the pretend game they and their faculty play.) They are systematically taught to abandon reality.

From out of the wasteland of the field work settings students come back with angry perplexity: "Do you know what the attendants are doing at——?" "I saw a principal knock a kid across the office!" "This counselor cut this kid down, wouldn't listen to him. How can I get anywhere if I can't protect the kid from that?" "Did you ever see the Hole at——?"[11] "This boy at——is terrified of the older boys' sexual attacks. Nobody will talk about it there." "Dr. X threatens the patients with shock if they act up." "This student has been suspended for six weeks with no plan." "The kids at the youth home have to stand for hours 'on the line.'"[12]

When students express these concerns, the faculty more or less falls back on avoidance responses, which can only be characterized as a system of defense against change:

1. *Avoidance through instant clichés* is represented by the following examples: (a) That is work among the heathen—"You have to *work*

[10] The captor–captive phenomenon described in this paper is presented in a highly conceptualized form by Goffman in his focus on the dehumanization of prisons and mental hospitals. Erving Goffman, *Asylums* (Garden City, N.Y.: Doubleday, 1961). In the writings of Szasz the same theme is certainly implicit, but his main thrust is to reveal and indict what he considers the subversion of the psychiatric profession as the means by which the state creates a condition of captivity of the mentally ill. See especially Thomas S. Szasz, *Law, Liberty and Psychiatry* (New York: Macmillan, 1963).

[11] The "hole" refers to isolation facilities in detention homes, state training schools, and prisons. It is typically a dimly lit, locked cubicle about 9 ft. × 9 ft. × 12 ft., sometimes with a small window either dirt-encrusted or deliberately glazed to screen out light, a slot in the door through which food is passed, a grade toilet and washbowl, and a concrete slab practically at floor height on which a mattress without linen and a blanket may be provided. There is no clock on the wall, and the person being isolated typically is not permitted to have any activity materials, including reading matter.

[12] "On the line" refers to the punishment practice by which a person is required to stand in one spot without moving for a stipulated length of time, for example, thirty minutes to an hour. If he moves, time is added.

with these people, to help them because 'they know not what they do.' We have tools, and they need to learn from us." (b) The child still knows you are his friend—"You can still help the kid even if you can't stop some of these things from happening. It's important to him that you're there and *understand*." (c) Search for the silver lining—"Are you sure it's that bad? Isn't there anything the client gets that's useful?" (d) Study it—"Do a process record of one of those, and let's have a look at it," *or* "Why don't you make that your term paper topic?" (e) The staff is human, too—"The girl does have to know that staff have feelings (although I don't think the attendant should have hit her). Maybe you can work on that with her." (f) The administrator is getting ulcers from it, too—"I'm sure the administrator would do something if he could. I've known him for a long time. But he's got the legislature to deal with. He suffers, I'm sure. He's got a pretty good record. . . ."

2. *Avoidance through the emotional control demand system of the professional model.* How many students have been challenged with: "Are you sure you're not overidentifying with your client? You're pretty angry, you know." There is something wrong with the fear of affect in the casework and group work model. The importance of feeling is stressed, but students are taught never to show it to the client. Students are taught that their subjective lives are dangerous to the client's interests. It is necessary to be clear about this: It is true that worker needs and client needs should not be confused. But the way in which this has been incorporated in teaching and supervision has resulted in enculturating generations of caseworkers and group workers with fear of feelings for the client, not only those they may show *to* him but those they may show to their supervisor *about* him. That "sin" of overidentification with the client is avidly sought and rated low on evaluations. But identification with the agency, with the profession, is *good* and gets high ratings. (Has anyone ever heard of a student or worker about whom it was noted in an evaluation that he overidentified with the agency or the profession? That is a sin beyond imagination!)

There is something seriously amiss in the eager embrace of identification with the agency as the hallmark for the emerging professional identity, while warning of the precariousness of such identification with the client. The objection to this does not mean that self-discipline in relating to clients should not be taught or that theory, technique, and ideals should be abandoned. But agencies and professions are tools, instrumentalities toward an end: helping the client. To inject agency identification into the professional ego by dint of reward/punishment techniques inherent in evaluation and admission to elite membership among the "anointed" is really a betrayal of the fundamental values of the profession.

3. *Obsession with big-system change magic* is the newest avoidance tool that has come along as part of the enthusiasm about social movements and institutional reform. This should be supported, but not at the cost of the total expenditure of social work advocacy will and energy. The phenomenologically real system for caseworkers and group workers is what they experience in their dealings with the human beings they are committed to serve. The system is ubiquitous, but it comes in different sizes, shapes, and organizational patterns. Social work should continue to experiment with different-size targets for mediating and changing the system in its constraints on human functioning and human happiness. These should, however, be maneuverable targets, lest the advocate become like everyone else who has been shown the big-system world and its fierce determinism, powerless before the god of macro-organization.

Teaching by Doing

What should schools of social work do, then, when the "ants" come marching back with their embarrassing questions? *Schools must back their students in unflinching criticism and attempts at changing the settings they are in when those settings hurt the people they (and the schools) serve.*

Imagine the student—caseworker, group-worker, or community organization practitioner—who is witness to an act of client dehumanization. If he wants to enter the lists of advocacy in behalf of a client, only one condition is both necessary and sufficient for initiating such action: that his school will regard his action with enthusiasm and support.[13] This can occur if the traditional partnership between school and agency and their complementarity on the teaching continuum, which gives them power over the student, is somehow restructured so that the student's normal fear of reprisal is liquidated sufficiently for him to take the moral and tactical actions implied in the advocacy concept.

Of these two partners in the student's educational destiny, it may be validly asserted that the school is the more powerful. In the final analysis, when the agency complains about a student, it is still the school that determines his ongoing status as student. This power differential, while both complex and not absolute, is still extremely critical in the overall

[13] It seems unnecessary to point out that NASW should also support its member (and nonmember) advocates, and the authors note that Briar's paper, *op. cit.*, which was accepted in October 1966 as a working paper of the NASW Commission on Social Casework, has been approved by the Cabinet of the Division of Practice and Knowledge and referred to the Ad Hoc Committee on Advocacy.

strategy and tactics of evolving a training model that "builds in" student advocacy. For it is the superior power of the school that opens the door to deliberate and planned protection of the student advocate, and this protection will itself involve the school in direct confrontation with agency systems.

This asserted power differential in favor of the school has always existed and been used. Thus, the school has not always bowed to agency perceptions of student incompetence. Schools have refused to accept such judgments and subsequently arranged another placement or negotiated retention in the original agency. That there may have been far fewer instances of such an outcome than acceptance of the agency's recommendation does not vitiate the argument with respect to the school's possession of the "final vote" on the student.

Limitations on School Power

Yet, for reasons that are quite clear, schools have been chary in using this power. First, the schools have not felt free to reject the agency's judgment about a student; they fear they will lose the agency's goodwill and participatory zeal in student training, which may extend to loss of placements. Second, they face a certain embarrassment and loss of status in graduating students whom agencies regard as inferior candidates. These strings on the use of school power are illustrative of the complexity and relativity of its freedom to differ with cooperating agencies.

However, it must also be remembered that these limitations have been most urgently operative outside the issue of advocacy. The typical case of the student whom the agency considered untrainable involved his presumed lack of potential as a clinical change agent and focused on what were considered defects that dulled or obviated such potential.[14]

If, however, a student should present evidence to the school that a given agency behaves toward the client in ways that violate the requirements of the professional action model, this certainly would constitute a totally new paradigm of agency–student–school conflict. There is a vast

---

[14] In referring to clinical social work training and the criteria employed by agency field instructors in making judgments about student potential, the authors are not in any way attributing to this a negative or antiadvocacy taint. The whole judgment-making process about who will or will not be a good clinical worker is drawn from a totally different set of data, with different motives and for different reasons than those that would apply if a student took an advocacy position and then was attacked by a field agency and labeled undesirable.

difference between a student who is a passive target of a field instructor's criticism of his suitability for social work and a student who is an active critic of an agency's social work morality—especially in the context of a school's sympathy and support of such sensitivity.

In the face of such novelty the two strains on the school enumerated could be inverted:

1. *Loss of placements.* Should the school keep such placements in the name of good education without at least trying to change them?

2. *Loss of status.* Should the school feel embarrassed about graduating students who point to such defects?

Yet, some may say, schools will still lose placements and still be maligned for graduating "crackpots." And do students know enough to criticize the agency? Is that not a contradiction in terms (a student who faults his teacher)?

It should be kept in mind that what is being dealt with is not a complex knowledge problem. It does not take intensive training, or perhaps any training at all, to recognize gross dehumanization. The student's sense of decency may be enough. Further, students vary widely in degree of social work knowledge, standing in the formal training process (that is, newly arrived to almost graduated), previous practical experience, presocial work education, individual intellectual endowment, and value dispositions. While some advocacy issues are more borderline than others and some do require technical training, many do not. Primarily, the considerations here are basic human values that must be guaranteed before treatment can be launched.[15] Many students, espe-

---

[15] Of course, the student may react to a treatment method with which he disagrees or that he misunderstands as dehumanization. So may a fully fledged professional. Professional colleagues may have sharp differences about the "right" approach such that one terms the other's therapeutic plan as ruinous to a client's interests. Such conflicts cannot reasonably be approached through an advocacy procedure. Dehumanization is simply something that in commonsense terms is qualitatively distinct from conflict arising out of competing theoretical orientations. There is usually no theory base in the situation in which dehumanization occurs except perhaps the belief that people can be forced to change by pain and humiliation. Lay rather than professional thinking dominates, often accompanied by open ridicule of the more sophisticated or professional rationale. Creature needs of the dehumanizers tend to be served, not the needs of the client. Frequently, disregard for and contempt of the client are openly present. Further, there is an entirely separate and important conceptual issue relating to the compatibility between the treatment and advocacy functions of the social work role. The authors believe that many clinicians tend to be hung up on this but that there are guidelines for positive balancing of these two functions that could be described in a more theoretical and technically relevant analysis of this issue. This is needed for both teaching and practice of clinical social work, especially in the client-service ecologies discussed in this paper.

cially in today's academic environment, are keenly aware of these issues and have been for a long time. In fact, their instructors' apparent apathy, uncertainty, and evasiveness have caused many students to wonder about the integrity of the profession.

As to loss of placements and status, one does not know without testing the model under discussion how things will turn out. Obviously one can visualize (or hypothesize) other than negative outcomes.

Certainly ability to maintain placements is a serious and critical issue.[16] Still, given an aggressive stance on the part of the school, an agency (or an administrative department of the state that controls certain placements) cannot with impunity just terminate placements. Schools have options they can use under such conditions. There are legal, political, and public relations moves that could restrain such agency or bureaucracy responses. Obviously, this is important.

Schools *should* fear losing placements, not because they will not have places to send students and thus will thwart their own enterprise, but because the client will be the loser. So schools that support student advocacy may have to resort to complex strategies and tactics in order to keep placements for the sake of the client. In so doing they will at the same time be fighting the very issue of dehumanization.

In this way the double function of schools becomes clear vis-à-vis teaching and advocacy: (1) they support the trainee in protest against defection from the values of the profession in which they are training him, and (2) they fight the issue of dehumanization and in this respect realize a completely separate function in becoming themselves active agents of system change. So, paradoxically enough, the school that supports its student advocates as a matter of policy and action tries to keep "inferior" placements, but in the act of keeping them calls attention to them and engages in change attempts.

The question might be asked that if students with school backing begin to launch protests against such practices, will agencies not come to regard them as spies and schools as spy-breeding organizations, a kind of CIA? This pejorative argument can be quickly voided when schools make known to agencies in advance their explicit policy of backing students in stands against client dehumanization. Espionage does

---

[16] A question that will occur to some is whether the student's job future is jeopardized by his "advocacy history." If he becomes somehow labeled as a "troublemaker," even in an advocacy-protected school, does he not possibly face some difficulty in being hired? This eventuality cannot be discounted. The strongest credential for a job in social work, however, is the MSW degree, and the disproportion between social work manpower and jobs is certainly in the student's favor. Furthermore, a record of advocacy may be considered a plus in some agencies.

not proceed by public announcement. The act of announcing to the professional community that schools are concerned with client dehumanization and that they will support and participate with their students in doing something about it effectively vitiates the spy argument. At the same time, such an act is a form of preconfrontation by the school itself of client mistreatment by agencies.

Implementation Model

So far a principle has been argued. In what form should it be implemented? Imagine that a school has put itself on record as being in support of student advocacy against client dehumanization and has so notified students and agencies.[17] Beginning experimentation appears to have three essential ingredients: informality, simplicity, and protection of the client's right to self-determination.

"Implementation form" refers to just that and not to content, that is, how and with what theory, strategy, and tactics a given advocacy action would be carried out. Simplicity, informality, and protection of client self-determination are conceived of as basic ingredients for setting a climate for advocacy experimentation by schools. Content would be supplied by analysis of given incidents of dehumanization and selection of strategy and tactics from a number of options described in the pertinent literature. While none of these deals directly with school-based, student-supported advocacy, they could be reviewed for their adaptability to this.[18]

---

[17] The faculty of Wayne State University School of Social Work unanimously adopted and distributed to students, field instructors, and agency directors on April 8, 1968, an official position statement supporting client advocacy as a viable option for its students and on June 17, 1968, adopted an implementation model that had been proposed by a committee of faculty, students, and agency representatives. "Advocacy of Action Against Client Dehumanization" and "Memorandum," and "Advocacy Implementation Model" (Detroit: School of Social Work, Wayne State University, April 8, 1968, and June 17, 1968, respectively). (Mimeographed.)

[18] In addition to articles previously cited, see, for example, George A. Brager, "Institutional Change: Parameters of the Possible," *Social Work*, January 1967, *12*(1), pp. 59–69; Wilbur J. Cohen, "What Every Social Worker Should Know About Political Action," *Social Work*, July 1966, *11*(3), pp. 3–11; Charles F. Grosser, "Community Development Programs Serving the Urban Poor," *Social Work*, July 1965, *10*(3), pp. 15–21; Irving Piliavin, "Restructuring the Provision of Social Services," *Social Work*, January 1968, *13*(1), pp. 34–41; Martin Rein and Frank Riessman, "A Strategy for Antipoverty Community Action Programs," *Social Work*, April 1966, *11*(2), pp. 3–12; Paul Terrell, "The Social Worker as Radical: Roles of Advocacy," *New Perspectives: The Berkeley Journal of Social Welfare*, Spring 1967, *1*(1), pp. 83–88; and Daniel Thursz, "Social Action As a Professional Responsibility," *Social Work*, July 1966, *11*(3), pp. 12–21.

Informality. In an advocacy-committed school, the freest and most spontaneous use of faculty resources is visualized as the desideratum for the student witnessing client dehumanization and wondering what he can do. Setting up a procedure that requires him to meet with a standing committee, with the executive office of the school, or to submit to any screening device must be avoided simply because it becomes too cumbersome in the climate of a felt need for active intervention. Collegial rapport and esprit between student and faculty are indispensable.

Thus, when a student becomes aware of and/or observes policies and practices that dehumanize clients and when he has decided to advocate in behalf of such clients, he should be encouraged to go directly to a faculty member or members of his choice. This structure would enable the student to view the faculty as a resource pool and would free him to select among them in terms of their expertise and interest in specific areas. Thus, the student should not be required to select his own advisor or field instructor as consultant, although he may do so if he chooses. This student–faculty cadre is then free, without other faculty review and consent, to develop an action plan based on analysis of the circumstances.

Simplicity. The fewer the number of steps and tasks required, the more feasible the procedural model becomes. Yet, terse, succinct documentation cannot be dispensed with. The student should be required to describe in writing the policy or practice that dehumanizes the client. Records of each case should be kept and periodic reports to the total faculty should be planned (for purposes of information only).

Protecting client self-determination. No advocacy action should be undertaken without client consultation and consent whenever such action will result in identification of the client either by name or implication. With some clients this will prove a stumbling block either because of the predicament they are in or because (as would be the case with some mentally ill clients and some children) they simply are unable to conceptualize the problem.

The predicament they are in might be illustrated by the following example: Suppose the student has for a client a child who is in a youth home and has been brutalized. The student wishes to carry out a protest action, but the child is fearful that he will be mistreated more if this happens. Such a step will then have to be forgone, although there may be some permissible leeway for trying to work it through with him, especially if meaningful protection that he can comprehend can be thrown around him. On the other hand, when the advocacy action is directed at a policy per se or a procedure that is applied to a group, client consent may not be at stake.

Toward a New Professional Identity

The thesis of school-based client advocacy is not limited to a heroic adventure of students and their teachers. Involved is not only a redirection of the energy and power of the school to change agencies but equally to change the professional identity of the social work practitioner it graduates. The reaction patterns described earlier of the typical faculty to students' anguished questions about the indecencies of captor–captive settings point to one set of factors explaining why so few professionals have gained distinction in the battle for agency reform. Their ingenuous strivings in this direction as students have been extinguished by the avoidance behavior of their teachers.

But the student who emerges from an advocacy-centered school will have had the antithetical experience to the above: He will have seen his school "put its action where its mouth is." He will have been witness to real struggles and will have experienced some of these together with his teachers. Instead of having been exhorted by inactive teachers to carry the activist torch in his professional future, he will have been a participant with his teachers in carrying that torch as a student. Not the least of such torch-bearing, while moral in its nature or source, will have been shared technical thinking about advocacy and examination of both failure and success by student and faculty.

Such an academic environment and its constituent experiences provide the germ plasm for a new breed whose preprofessional moral distaste for human injustice will have been honed and hardened to the level of professionally informed instinct. Such professionals will find it unavoidably natural to stand and fight for client rights as a first priority, instead of fleeing to the "suburbs of the professional environment"—the agencies with better standards—postcommitment refugees who could not wait to get out [19]; or, lacking the energy required for such mobility, to remain self-committed captives, bitter, cynical, and passively helpless in agencies that dehumanize.

Thus, if social work's dream of the client-advocating professional is a real dream, the profession, along with the schools, ought to welcome the challenge of the shift to advocacy of social work faculties and to back this one tiny but tough step toward bringing that dream closer to reality.

[19] "One of the favorite ploys of social work supervisors and educators is to advise students that when conditions become intolerable in agencies and they can no longer support their administrator, they should resign and go elsewhere. *This is too easy,* for it leaves those whom social workers are supposed to help to the tender mercies of the inhumanity they themselves cannot stomach. A better answer might be not only to refuse to quit but also refuse to engage in unethical acts." Russell E. Smith, "In Defense of Public Welfare," *Social Work,* October 1966, *11*(4), p. 97.

PSYCHOLOGIST AT CITY HALL
—A PROBLEM OF IDENTITY

16

Stanley D. Klein

In recent times, citizens have become increasingly aware of the social problems within society. Along with this awareness has come the wish on the part of individuals and groups to actively "do something" about these problems. The call for involvement on the part of psychologists is heard within professional meetings and on the pages of professional journals. In fact, the theme of the 1969 Convention of the American Psychological Association was "Psychology and the Problems of Society."

Psychology as a body of scientific knowledge about behavior and professional psychologists as individuals would appear to have some part to play in solving social problems.

How applicable is psychological knowledge? The answer may seem obvious: Since psychologists know about human behavior and the solving of problems, they are ideally suited to confront today's social problems.

This article describes my personal experiences as a representative of the Mayor of Boston. More specifically, it reviews the identity conflicts I experienced as I tried to utilize my knowledge and experience as a psychologist in a new role and in new situations.

Professionally I identify myself as a clinical psychologist, dividing my time between undergraduate teaching and private psychotherapeutic practice with children and young adults. As a private citizen living in Boston, I have been active in local politics.

In the spring of 1968, I was appointed to the staff of Mayor Kevin H. White of Boston as a special assistant, charged with the responsibility of "taking care of the hippie situation." This appointment evolved from discussions between city officials and myself about the expected influx of young people to Boston in the coming summer. It is important to note that these discussions occurred primarily because I was known per-

Paper presented at the annual meeting of the American Psychological Association, Washington, D. C., September 4, 1969. Reprinted from the *American Psychologist*, February 1970 25 (2). Copyright 1970 by the American Psychological Association, and reproduced by permission. Stanley D. Klein is at the Department of Psychology, University of Massachusetts, Boston, Massachusetts.

sonally and politically at City Hall, rather than because of any judgment by city officials of my professional competence as a psychologist. That is, I had been a working colleague of a number of individuals who were now key city officials because I had served in an administrative capacity in Mayor White's election campaign in 1967. The fact that I was a responsible and loyal political worker was both a key factor in my appointment and a source of some of the subsequent identity conflicts on the job.

City officials felt that a psychologist familiar with young people and their problems would be helpful in dealing with "hippies." I implicitly agreed and felt that my experience as a teacher and a therapist would be applicable because I expected to serve principally as a liaison person between the Mayor's Office and the various individuals and groups involved in the hippie situation. I expected to be a listener and a communicator, both familiar roles. Furthermore, I expected that my psychologist's behavioral style (which, of course, is part of my own personality style) would be relevant to the situations.

In the months that followed, hundreds of young people, all labeled hippies by the mass media, came to Boston. The complexities of problems for the city administration exceeded the springtime expectations. It was necessary for many departments within the executive branch of city government, such as Parks and Recreation, Law, Housing Inspection, Health and Hospitals, Youth Opportunities, and Police, to become directly involved. In addition, private agencies and citizens' groups involved themselves. As a result, as the representative of the Mayor's Office, I had to face a wide range of situations, some of which had not been anticipated. Some, such as coping with runaway adolescents, challenged my psychological knowledge about such behavior. Others, such as coping with the grievances of irate citizens' groups, challenged my political skills. Finally, some crises, such as observing a midnight demonstration on the Boston Common, and visiting demonstrators in jail a few hours later, challenged my physical stamina.

As the summer progressed, I realized that my role was much more that of politician than psychologist. I had expected my psychological knowledge to be particularly helpful; however, I discovered that my knowledge and my style were of limited value. As a representative of the Mayor, it was necessary for my orientation to shift from helper or teacher to negotiator, judge, detective, manipulator, and sometimes defender of "hippies," or police, or politicians. While my professional training was helpful to me in some ways in this political role, most of the decisions that I made were based primarily upon political, rather than psychological, considerations. To my disappointment, I found that my psychological knowledge was, at best, secondary to my understanding of the politics of the situations.

My role at City Hall proved to be different from my previous professional roles as teacher, researcher, or therapist in four ways.

First, in these traditional psychologist's roles, one's primary responsibility is to the welfare of the client, who usually invites the psychologist to provide a specific service in an area in which the psychologist is an expert. In my role at City Hall, my clientele seemed to include "hippies," private citizens, police officers, and many others, individually and collectively, but my primary responsibility was to the welfare of my boss —the Mayor.

Second, in the protective confines of my office or classroom, my clientele come to me and I am in charge. What I say represents my point of view, and my clientele and I are the only ones who observe my behavior. In contrast, as a representative of City Hall, I went wherever the "action was." I had to present and defend policies that did not always represent my point of view. Furthermore, I was always subject to public as well as private scrutiny.

Third, my function as a teacher and a therapist is relatively clear to me, my students, and the people who consult me for psychotherapy. However, on my city job, not only did I experience some confusion about my role, but I was perceived in a variety of conflicting ways: To conservative police officials, I was a hippie or hippie advocate; to some hippies, I was a plainclothes police officer; to radicals, I was a "fascist pig"; to the press, I was a "psychologist advising the Mayor," or "doing research on hippies."

Fourth, as a teacher or therapist, my goal is to facilitate change within individuals. The direction of the change is usually mutually agreeable. As a representative of the Mayor's Office, I could direct external environmental change, and sometimes the direction of the change might be totally disagreeable to some of my constituency.

These four role differences are not mutually exclusive, nor do they exhaust the possible ways of conceptualizing my particular experiences. The conceptual framework itself evolved after the summer of 1968. Nonetheless, it has proven personally functional because it has decreased my identity conflict as I have continued to work in 1969 as a member of Mayor White's staff—as a politician with the credentials of a professional psychologist.

Utilizing the role differences as points of departure and keeping in mind the issue of the value of psychological knowledge, I will describe some of my specific experiences during the summer of 1968.

Welfare of Client (Mayor)

To be primarily concerned with the political welfare of the Mayor, rather than the personal welfare of an individual client or the social welfare of a community group, was difficult and distasteful, and the most important role change. This reorientation away from the recipients of service pervaded all the other role changes.

My "street work" illustrates this issue. Some social workers and most police officers have experience working with their "clients" on the street. My role, as I toured the Boston Common and the surrounding areas where the young people were "making the scene," included the friendly, helpful, observer-type roles of these two professions. However, the implications of my activities for my actual client remained my primary concern.

My experience in relating to young people and my therapist's tolerance of unusual behavior made it relatively easy to maintain personal contact with the hippies. While I knew the language and customs of the group, I also knew that I did not have to adopt them in order to be an acceptable person. Most importantly, I knew how to listen and how to try to understand. At the same time, I represented the Establishment and had the responsibility of assessing the situation; that is, I had to judge the level of tension of the situation and, if necessary, notify law enforcement officials of any potential trouble. Here, my clinical training was helpful in enabling me to judge the reliability of some of my "informants." However, this detectivelike role was strange to me, and I had to gain my experience "on the job."

In the street-work setting, confidentiality of communication—a sacred commandment for me as a psychotherapist—was a complex issue. Here, I experienced conflict concerning the use of information that was given in trust, particularly when it involved illegal activities. Once, at a time of high tension on the Common, two youths gave me concealed weapons (knives) that they had allegedly found. Frequently, I observed the sale and use of illegal drugs and acquired knowledge of the whereabouts of runaways. Violence, drugs, runaways, and similar problems are perplexing to me clinically. However, in this context, they represented unlawful behavior, potential danger for large numbers of people, and a bad scene politically.

Public Self and Self-Determination

As a psychologist, I have enjoyed relative autonomy in my professional career. Supervisors and department chairmen notwithstanding, I am accustomed to deciding what I teach, what I research, or how I therapize. In addition, I usually perform these functions in safe, relatively private places. In contrast, going wherever "the action was" was part of my political job.

A number of times during the summer, I was confronted by large unruly groups in meetings as well as in organized public demonstrations against the Establishment. In the confines of my office, I am prepared to be harassed by an individual or a family who feels it is not getting what it wants. Furthermore, in individual or group psychotherapy, and in teaching to some extent, interpersonal struggle, tension, and similar phenomena are part of the process and occur in the context of the transaction between people who have some kind of relationship with one another. Possibly, máss meetings and public demonstrations also evolve according to particular processes. Generally, my knowledge of individual and group dynamics did not seem applicable in these confrontation situations. Although at times I could demonstrate my understanding of "their side," the value of such empathy seemed short-lived. For the most part, I felt that all I could do was to "maintain my cool" and try to figure a safe way out politically and physically for myself and others.

Often, my job was to communicate administration policy. Sometimes, in the process of policy formation, my personal recommendations did not prevail. Subsequently, I had to present and defend the policies. Thus, before large groups and occasionally in response to queries from the press, I had to restrain my "academic freedom" and "therapeutic honesty."

Clarity of Role

It is comforting to know one's own role, and it is usually helpful if others understand it. As has been suggested previously, I was often unclear about my role. In addition, I seemed to be perceived differently by different groups with whom I had contact. Furthermore, my role in relation to different groups changed over the course of the summer.

In the early part of the summer, I attended many meetings of separate groups of businessmen, police officials, hippies, "hippie helpers," and others. Here, particularly in the beginning of the summer, I was acceptable to myself and to the groups as an information gatherer and observer. Later on, as individuals and groups began to demand action from me, it was difficult to know how and when and to what kinds of demands to be responsive. I found that it was essential to know the background of the various groups' relationships with the city government in order to assess their demands. Such knowledge could only come from discussions with other city officials, not from my particular background or knowledge.

Some of these separate groups were in conflict with each other. I had information about each group that the other groups wished they had. For example, I knew about planned demonstrations as well as police operational procedures. Here again, I tried to retain my professional commitment to confidentiality of communication. Political considerations often threatened this commitment.

At administrative policy meetings, my role and function were again perplexing. Some of my colleagues at City Hall perceived me as the psychologist "hippie expert." According to this percept, I was expected to deliver certain statistical information on numbers (how many hippies are there?), psychopathology (how many of them are crazy?), and other matters. As a scientist, I had insufficient data. As a clinician, I had decided that it would be both ethically inappropriate and socially destructive for me to discuss the psychopathology of individual young people. I had gathered some information and was expected to report on it. The problem was how to communicate in an understandable and helpful manner, while clarifying my role for others and for myself.

I found that some psychological knowledge could be communicated in a useful manner at policy meetings. For example, I successfully argued against confrontation by suggesting that many youths unconsciously (and some consciously) were desirous of a destructive encounter with the police. Therefore, the Establishment would be "giving them what they wanted," while thinking it would be resisting their wishes.

Psychological knowledge was pertinent to policy formation in two other ways. First, sterotyping was popular among all groups. Over time, I was able to describe and differentiate different groups within the so-called "hippie" group stereotype. This enabled the administration to develop policies that accounted for these differences. In my work with the youth, I tried to undo stereotypes about "politicians" and "cops." Second, I advised against the use of affect-laden words in public statements. Thus, we tried to substitute "closing hour" for "curfew" and "youth" for "hippies."

Within policy discussions, I altered some of my own stereotypes. For example, I learned that public policy decision making often involves far more than the content of the situation. Also, I vividly experienced that there are more than two sides to many questions. In addition, I gained an appreciation of the power struggles that take place between different city agencies—struggles that may be unrelated to the social problem itself. Retrospectively, my work with families and groups should have prepared me to expect such power struggles as well as to appreciate the many sides of a question. However, I was unable to make this transfer of learning until after I had experienced it.

Change Agent

Facilitating change, be it in individuals, groups, or systems, is an important function of applied psychology. With my particular background as therapist and teacher, I knew something about the facilitation of internal change. For the most part, I had to abandon my theoretical orientation, which tends to emphasize internal change as a prerequisite for external change. Instead, my energies were directed toward the manipulation of external factors with the diffuse goal of a "cool scene."

In the interests of this goal, I organized and led a weekly meeting of representatives of all groups involved—"straight" citizens, hippies, hippie helpers, police, city officials, and others. It was at these meetings that my psychological background was of particular value. I knew that communication between individuals could occur in a group setting. I also knew that such meetings were potentially constructive or destructive to individuals and/or groups, and would require careful leadership.

In early June, I met separately with the different groups involved with the youth. This provided me with an opportunity to understand points of view and to note key individuals within each group. Next, I invited representatives of each of these groups to meet together. At the first meeting, small discussion groups were formed with representatives of each faction in each small group. Later, these small groups reported to the entire group. This format worked successfully as an initial encounter, as individuals had an opportunity to talk with each other as individuals. Apparently, it made it possible for individuals with different points of view to meet with one another as human beings and to share their ideas. The meeting format was then changed to a large group meeting, which I chaired. The invitations to attend were broadened. As a result, about forty people attended weekly meetings through July and August. The meetings were a principal vehicle for communication among the various groups and factions within groups.

Although these meetings were incorrectly labeled "group therapy" by some participants, my experience as a group therapist was helpful in this setting. I was able to keep the meetings focused on problem solving, while allowing intensive expression of affect. These meetings were exciting, frightening, informative, and sometimes comical. Often, threats and counterthreats, accompanied by illustrative profanity, were tenuously balanced by understanding, firmness, and consistency. As a trained group psychotherapist, I was prepared to accept hostility. Often I invited such hostility toward myself as the Mayor's representative in order to channel it away from other protagonists. In addition, I was prepared to respond to "hidden agendas," unconscious communiqués, and nonverbal messages, while not becoming trapped by verbal content. For example, in the midst of a heated argument between youth and police, I interrupted the discussion to point out the pleasant, friendly greeting exchanged between a police officer and a young person who had just arrived. I was thereby able to illustrate that such relationships are possible.

Once again, because I also had the role of communicator of city policy, political considerations intruded on my group leadership style. I had powers that were quite different from the powers of the group therapist. I could influence decisions that could affect the lives of the participants outside of the group setting, especially because what they said during the group sessions might well be used against them by me or by others. In addition, I was not unbiased. Rather, I had to be prepared to present a relatively united position of city officials and to avoid an open conflict between officials of the Mayor's Office and other city agencies. Any such conflicts had to be settled elsewhere.

As a scientist, I lack specific criteria to evaluate the impact of these meetings as a factor in change, internal or external. Much tension continued; there were troublesome events. But the feedback from participants indicated that the meetings were helpful to them and to their groups.

Conclusion

In the previous example of the group meetings, my psychological background was particularly relevant. In the other examples, my psychological knowledge was helpful sometimes. In retrospect, it had been naïve of me to think that my professional background had adequately prepared me for the particular situations in which I found myself.

My personal identity problem was determined in part by my inability to define my area of competence ahead of time. Erroneously, I had generalized my experience on some matters pertaining to youth to a broad community setting. By the time I realized the need for setting limits on myself, I had committed myself to certain responsibilities beyond my own limits and could not retreat without putting myself or the Mayor in an embarrassing position. In time, I resolved my identity problem in a way that was somewhat unsatisfactory to me as a psychologist. I identified myself as a politician serving the city, and, specifically, the Mayor.

My experience suggests that the psychologist has some knowledge that may be helpful in the social action arena. However, the psychologist should be extremely cautious in accepting the willingness of society, including some psychologists, to perpetuate two fantasies: first, that the psychologist "knows everything" about people; and second, following from this omniscient position, that the psychologist can be especially helpful in social–political situations.

I have described my activities as an assistant to the Mayor of Boston within a framework of role differences between my usual role as a psychologist and my role at City Hall. However, I am concerned that the focus of this article was such that the key factor in my entry into the political system might be overlooked. As I noted at the beginning of the article, I was a trusted political worker, known personally to key city officials. I am not suggesting that such partisan political activity is the only way into the system. Instead, I wish to conclude by emphasizing that person-to-person trust and understanding, although it may not be sufficient, is necessary if the psychologist or any other human science specialist is to be invited to have the opportunity to "do his thing" within the social action arena.

PART

3

The Politics of Community Control and Its Repercussions

The changing concepts of mental illness, the new mental health workers, and the new breed of professionals have had a significant effect on community politics. Perhaps in rural areas, or in stable, homogenous small towns, the third revolution in mental health can be a bloodless one. But, as the papers in Part 3 clearly show, in larger cities where people are already in conflict, community forms of intervention can actually *intensify* the conflict.

In order to fully appreciate the dynamics of community control, one must first understand the dilemma psychiatry has found itself in by creating communities called "catchment areas," which are very often geographical units that ignore the boundaries of human communities. Secondly, one must distinguish between a *gemeinshaft* community in which people are held together by common bonds like the extended family and a *gesellschaft* community in which people come together in formal institutions often quite removed from their family ties and obligations. Panzetta argues that community-oriented professionals tend to act as if the catchment area contained a *gemeinschaft* community whereas in reality most catchment areas are pieces of a larger *gesellschaft*. Thus, the professionals are forever looking for a community that does not exist. Panzetta would have us avoid the issue of community and citizen control and instead emphasize organizational sensitivity to the life-styles of the people being served. Brody, also, is disillusioned with the way public programs have attempted to include local people. He points out the ambiguity in the Model Cities concept of "widespread citizen participation" and the OEO notion of "maximum participation of the poor." Brody raises doubts about the sincerity of the professional who talks about fostering local control without providing any mechanisms to accomplish this goal. He asks, if the Federal Government is so interested in local citizen participation, why are they so often ignorant of state and local programs? Unlike Panzetta, Brody believes in the importance of community control, but he recognizes that this must be given a *political* form in specific situations, or else it remains empty rhetoric.

The papers by Roman and by Schiff are concerned with the early attempts of two mental health centers situated in urban black communities to involve local citizens directly with the policy of the center. Roman, who lived through the harrowing experience of the incidents that took place at Lincoln Hospital in New York City, still maintains that community control is a means of developing local resources and eventually making state and public institutions accountable to the people.

On the other hand, Schiff, who directed a Center in a similar neighborhood in Chicago but with fewer repercussions, reviews the Lincoln Hospital situation and rejects the notion of community control. In fact, Schiff argues that the majority of neighborhood residents are not interested in control but in performance. He finds that those individuals most vehement about control are those professionals and nonprofessionals interested in increasing their own power. In contrast, people in grassroots organizations are much more concerned with making certain that agencies and institutions carry out their responsibilities in accordance with the highest professional standards. Schiff strongly recommends that a mental health center be responsive to an advisory board made up of local people and professionals representing the institutions carrying out the mental health program.

Freed and his associates, working in a mental health center in another Chicago black community, are particularly interested in the political forces that shape the history of their center. Their first paper concerns the problem of factional control and traces the early stages of the program during which professionals found it necessary to subcontract to local black militant groups. The second paper focuses on the history of a drug program. It brings us up to date and clearly reveals that the decision to subcontract services and to create an advisory board did not solve the problems of community control and participation. It did, however, permit the community program to deliver essential services. Part of the difficulty as the authors see it, is that this program had to cope with a multi-ethnic population. Given this situation, it may not be possible to bring all the people together. Nevertheless, Freed and his colleagues are dedicated to a concept of community development that implies that professionals should support strong community groups, though they do recognize the dangers in such action.

In addition, the program described by Freed and his colleagues has had to continually face the problem, also explored by Panzetta, that groups strengthened through community organization can eventually turn against those people who originally supported them. Hence, they argue for a delicate balance between politically feasible acts of community development and pragmatic acts of self-preservation.

The final two papers offer case histories of very different sorts. The paper by Graziano makes it clear that scientific and humanitarian motives for clinical innovation are often inhibited by the desire for political power. The result, all too often, is *innovation without change* as Graziano clearly shows.

The "case history" offered by Kenniston—although it is a fantasy—provides us with still another picture of the possible future of the community mental health movement. Kenniston's fantasy reminds us that the balance of power between local citizen control and powerful centralized mental health professionals gaining totalitarian control is precarious. He asks us to consider the possible consequences of a community mental health movement, uncontrolled by and unresponsive to local needs, that crushes political dissidents in the name of mental health.

There are, then, at least three possible outcomes of the community movement. As Graziano suggests, attempts at innovation may ultimately result in paralysis and "innovation without change." Or, as Kenniston implies, mental health ideology may become a thinly disguised rationale for the control of political dissent. Or perhaps, as Freed and his co-workers have shown, a delicate balance between the interests, needs, and motives of the local community and pragmatic acts of self-preservation by mental health professionals can be achieved. Such a balance would require a working coalition of responsive professionals and local citizens.

There are a number of different forms that such a coalition could take depending on the dominant ideologies of both the professional and the community. In the postscript that follows this section, we attempt to analyze the ideologies of community intervention and consider several distinctly different models of community mental health that are responsive to the needs of people from various ethnic and social backgrounds.

THE CONCEPT OF COMMUNITY: THE SHORT-CIRCUIT OF THE MENTAL HEALTH MOVEMENT

17

Anthony F. Panzetta

Certain words have a way of taking on meanings never intended. Words of a high level of abstraction are like that. Because they touch so many diverse phenomena, these abstract terms are both practical and impractical at the same time. "Community" is an example of such a word. It can be applied in a variety of situations and so is versatile as a one-word concept. But it also is prone to multiple connotative meanings and so can be easily misunderstood (1).

In today's mental health vocabulary, "community" has taken a prominent position. To some, it rings a public health note; to others, it has a sociopolitical connotation. It may suggest a neighborhood, a district, or an ethnic grouping. It may generate a mood of warmth and togetherness, or one of pragmatic association. It has a current mystique, however, that transcends any of the usual denotative or connotative meanings. This is a mystique of value, an inherent sense of goodness attached to the various concepts of community. To be procommunity is to be virtuous; to be anticommunity is to be evil. Both assessments precede any attempt to clarify what is meant by "community."

Gemeinschaft and Gesellschaft

Sociologists have grappled with the concept of community since Comte and, before him, philosophers since Plato. It is unlikely that we shall settle on the ultimate choice here. There is a useful distinction for our purposes, however, that was elaborated by Tönnies in his use of the terms *gemeinschaft* and *gesellschaft* (2). A *gemeinschaft* community is characterized by an implicit bond that relates person to person. Like the extended family, such a community is held together by common values, affection, mutual dependence, respect, and a sense of status hierarchy.

Reprinted from *Archives of General Psychiatry*, 1971, 25, 291–297. Copyright © 1971, American Medical Association. Reproduced by permission. Dr. Panzetta is currently with the Health Sciences Center, Temple University Medical School, Philadelphia, Pennsylvania.

There are no formal rules of relationship, and the roles of the members of that community are set by the traditions and cultural expectations of the group. This type of community is becoming increasingly rare and depends for its existence on a rural or feudal type of social organization.

Today's dominant type of community is *gesellschaft* in nature (2). Here the bonds are formal and explicit. People relate to one another through formulated guidelines or even through rules and regulations. Affection and dependence on one another for survival is rarely operative. In the *gesellschaft* community, people come together through formal institutions, like their place of employment, their church, professional or civic organization, and so on. Very often, great blocks of time are spent in these vertical groupings (in institutions usually away from the area of their home), in contrast to the lesser blocks of time spent in horizontal groupings (in their home neighborhood).

It is the reality of the *gesellschaft* and the longing for the *gemeinschaft* that often lead to a misorientation of "community-minded" psychiatrists. While it is true that there are territorial commitments that all persons make to their "home," and while it is true that these commitments are apt to carry with them affective and durable qualities (3), it is anachronistic to program for a form of social organization that no longer exists (*gemeinschaft*). It would seem much more reasonable to program for the dominant form, that is, the *gesellschaft*. If there are existent *gemeinschaft* forms in the population, then these can be taken into account, but not to the exclusion of the more prevalent *gesellschaft* forms.

The visible manifestation of the *gemeinschaft* approach to community mental health planning is the "catchment area." Here, a geographic area is designated as target area, and all those who live within the specific boundaries are members of the mythical *gemeinschaft*. This horizontal approach to community makes sense from a limited public health point of view because it allows for the assignment of responsibility. But this goal, that is, the fixing of responsibility, is an operational accomplishment and does not speak to the issue of community.

There is a further paradox implicit in this approach. One of the ways a *gemeinschaft* group is maintained is by a radical provincialism. Remnants of such groups remain in some of the ethnic communities of Chicago, and they have been able to maintain this Old World coherence by inbreeding and careful exclusion of cultural values of the pluralistic community around them. They have resisted acculturation to an extent (although this is disappearing rapidly) and so are set apart. The Amish settlements of Pennsylvania and Indiana are better examples of the *gemeinschaft* community. But, again, in all of these examples, the *gemeinschaft* is preserved by a nonintegrative approach to the larger surround. The paradox in this rests with the black neighborhoods that, to some extent, have also maintained a *gemeinschaft* way of life but by enforced exclusion from the larger community. Since many, if not most, of the community mental health centers are in black areas, they are forced to program their services in such a way as to reinforce the separatist ethos of that area. Although this may fit into the plans of the militant black activist, it should be recognized as what it is, a closed market.

A visible remaining example of *gemeinschaft* living that persists throughout modern society (although under great pressure) is the family. It makes great sense to program for family-oriented services since this social form is naturally occurring and durable. But it is possible to program for family-oriented services without paying a great deal of attention to the horizontal community orientation.

This perspective, which differentiates the vertical (institutional) community from the horizontal (geographic) community and which separates the *gesellschaft* (formal) relationship from the *gemeinschaft* (mutually dependent) relationship, can and should clarify some of the inherent difficulties as mental health centers program for their assigned "community" (catchment area).

The resolution of this seeming dilemma lies in the careful application of logical definition. If the overriding consideration is the need for a system that fixes medical and paramedical resonsibility, then the catchment area concept may indeed be optimum. But to go further and equate catchment area with "community" is a nonsequitur. If the primary goal is to develop programs that fit the idiosyncrasies of a discrete community, then the catchment area concept is meaningless unless the boundaries of the catchment area coincide with the boundaries of an existing *gemeinschaft* community; and, if such a community is identified, then we must realize that our efforts may very well serve to reinforce the separatist and exclusionary character of the *gemeinschaft* community.

Where: Community as Catchment Area

In a clear way, the catchment area community is a "where" community. Its definition is dependent on street names, buildings, and general demography. It can be isolated on a wall map, which then becomes an impressive addition to one's office, particularly if there is a war games disposition. Colored pins can point out the structural parts of this community, and a sense of "my turf" is quickly established. The basic orienting grid to one's thinking becomes "those people living between Susquehanna and Diamond Streets." The great temptation is to assume that "those people" are like one another in their sense of community, that is, they share common beliefs, common problems, and common aspirations. What in fact is the reality?

There is a commonality that presents itself in the "where" community if that community is sufficiently oppressed. The social indicators of such a community are familiar in language today, that is, high death rates, high infant mortality, dilapidated housing, high crime rates, and so on. And so the common factors extracted from such a community become logical targets for intervention. These are the "symptoms" of the "where" community and hence the illusory logical target for the community psychiatrist. But the roots of these "symptoms" are not "where" in their vulnerability. A geographic approach may give topographic clues to what is between these boundaries, but it also fixes you to the outfield when the real action is in the infield. The dilapidated house on Diamond Street is a complex phenomena derived from City Hall, the money market, the suburban ethos, as well as from events and people within the catchment area. If we choose to define our mental health goals in this grand dimension, then we had better not assume a catchment area orientation in our programming.

The analysis of a "where" community is usually written in the language of demography and epidemiology. This defined population approach gives valuable information about the target population, but it is important to realize the type of information that is supplied. The information on incidence and prevalence, for example, is only as good as those criteria used for the identification of a "case." The more abstract these criteria, the more unreliable are the results. Because of the availability of rather discrete criteria for the identification of schizophrenia, this has become a favorite object of epidemiologic study (4), and the results of such studies have a higher degree of reliability than studies of more diffusely defined conditions, for example, the *Mid-Town Manhattan Study* (5).

The point of all this should be clarified here. If a community is defined in "where" terms, its analysis, that is, the dissection of its "problems," is biased in the direction of measurable and gross phenomena. What emerges is a picture of the social disorder of that area as reflected in incidence and prevalence rates of the high-visibility problems. Programming for the "where" community will therefore inevitably tend toward these high-visibility problems. This may or may not correspond with planning objectives derived from other considerations. It is reasonable to proceed from this point of view, providing one realizes what is happening. And again, what happens is that the high-visibility problems surface and become the crying targets for a "where"-oriented community program.

In my experience in a mental health center with a catchment area "where" approach, the above proved quite accurate. Although we initially programmed for general psychiatric disorders, we felt the pull toward the high-visibility problems of juvenile crime, unemployment, alcoholism, addiction, geriatrics, and mental retardation quite soon after we were operational. It led some to wish we had planned originally for these high-visibility problems, and it led others to frustration since few of these visibility problems are "attractive" or "responsive" to the psychiatric and parapsychiatric professions. So despite an earlier general orientation, the consequence of a "where" approach may shift the focus of attention elsewhere.

A collateral effect of this horizontal concept of community is to place a pseudosociologic aura to one's efforts. This may be an exciting prospect initially, as one becomes imbued with the sense of innovation and the illusion of being an instrument of social change. However, illusion it is, because entrance to the social institutions that create and devour the social condition requires skills, power, and time beyond the resources of the mental health center as a collective force or the psychiatrist as a well-meaning individual. The problem is that an aura does exist and it takes time before this aura is recognized for what it is. During the interim, staff and program may very easily be pulled down the road to its inevitable, disillusioning deadend.

When: Community as Epiphenomenon

One of the alternate ways to consider the concept of community is to place it into a dimension of time. We have all been aware, at one time or another, of a sense of community that comes and then goes. People commonly band together to accomplish certain discrete goals and then disband. Organizations often prove to be "when" communities as they bring people together in common pursuit over a period of time. If we wished to look back, with a reverent historical purview, to the feudal gemeinschaft communities, we would still note the dissolution of that communal form over time.

Time, of course, changes all things, or, more correctly, all things change in time. The great leveler of human grandiosity, history, has been able to chronicle, with predictable certainty, the demise of all sorts of social organizations. Civilizations and families alike are modified or terminated. But too great a preoccupation with the dimension of time becomes distressing and discouraging. After all, we must acknowledge our own temporal finiteness and the even greater temporal finiteness of our work. To feel that one's work must endure forever or to fear that one's work will be washed away immediately is to be equally absurd at either pole.

The hard-core reality of the temporal dilemma is that it is very difficult to estimate correctly (1) if the phenomenon we are observing is an artifact of the time or a durable reality and (2) if our response to the phenomenon is appropriate to its duration. Is it a short-range solution to a long-range problem or, conversely, a long-range solution to a short-range problem? The dilemma is more often than not worked out in retrospect.

When time is applied to concepts of community, it brings to them an element of uncertainty that should humble the community expert. Most so-called communities are so time-bound that they come and go like evanescent clouds. The conditions that create a community are themselves so fragile that community itself is more correctly an epiphenomenon than a primary reality in its own right. This concept of community as epiphenomenon is exceedingly important for anyone who is working in "community-oriented" work. An epiphenomenon is a phenomenon that occurs as a result of preexisting phenomena or set of conditions. An epiphenomenon is nothing unless the preexisting events occur. And, likewise, a community, in its "when" sense, does not exist unless certain conditions exist. Epiphenomenon, simply defined, is a secondary phenomenon accompanying another and caused by it. There is, for example, a theory of mind called epiphenomenalism, which states that mental processes are epiphenomena of brain processes.

These necessary conditions would seem quite important to be aware of; yet it is extraordinary to witness the degree to which they are ignored by "community-oriented" workers. There is probably no greater cohesive force by which people come together into an epiphenomenon community than that of oppression. The history of the Jews and now the black experience in this country are graphic documentation of this. To take away the oppression is to take away much of the binding power of the community. To take away the oppression is to dissolve the epiphenomenon.

Working classes after the Industrial Revolution learned the lesson well, and the organized labor movement in this country was the epiphenomenon of that capitalistic oppression. Even today, unions are maintained as organizations only as well as management is able to play the role of potential oppressors, or be placed in that role by union leaders.

Oppression is only one of two necessary conditions for the epiphenomenal community. The second is leadership. That sense of shared values, common goals, and kinship that is community must be articulated and transmitted to those persons who are to comprise the community. An oppressed people remain fragmented and isolated as long as no one stands to call them together, point out their common plight, articulate their frustration, and present a plan for joint effort. Community implies unity, and unity implies the condensation of many voices to one or few. Given the two necessary conditions, oppression and leadership, a community is born; take either of them away and the epiphenomenon vanishes.

A predictable objection arises here. Is it not so that there are examples of communities that persist without these two preconditions? Is not the family such a community? Again we must return to the distinction made earlier between *gemeinschaft* and *gesellschaft* communities. The *gemeinschaft* community exists only in rare instances outside family life. The traditions and way of life that nourished and sustained the *gemeinschaft* community are gone. And so we see as the prevalent form the *gesellschaft* community. It is my contention that there are episodic variations in the usual *gesellschaft* model that tend to take on the characteristics of the *gemeinschaft* community, and that these variations occur as a result of two major conditions coming together. The resulting "sense" of community lasts only as long as these conditions, and so the *gemeinschaft* community is not a durable *gemeinschaft* at all—but rather a fragile state that we can term an epiphenomenon.

There are several implications of this perspective for community psychiatry. Those community mental health programs that have developed in suburban or affluent areas are characteristically oriented toward the provision of services to individuals or families. Their community orientation is primarily geographic and a function of fixing responsibility for various services. They have inadvertently, but accurately, perceived the lack of *gemeinschaft*. Those community mental health programs that have developed in urban centers, with a predominantly black and oppressed constituency, have noted a sense of community and have tried in myriad ways to relate to that sense of community. It is here that the confusion is generated.

If a mental health center assumes that the community is bound together in an historical and romantic way and makes overtures for joint responsibilities, it will soon enough discover that the community will act and respond "as community" only in those issues directly related to oppression or related to the roles and prerogatives of their leaders. It will not receive a sustained community input on those more pedestrian issues that have to do with the delivery of psychiatric services. If the psychiatric services can somehow be brought into the oppression equation, then interest may exist, but it will be short-lived. Again, I must clarify this statement. Community interest—that is, the *representative* sentiment of a large group of persons expressed by responsible leadership— can be sustained only in those areas directly related to their binding power as a community, that is, the binding power of oppression and leadership. The interest in a mental health program can be generated in isolated "community" individuals who, for one reason or another, are interested in mental health matters, but do *not* assume that these interested individuals can represent a community in matters other than those related to their oppression. Even in the latter area representative views are difficult to identify.

The confusion is brought into stark relief when the community mental health center seeks to "find" its community. Who speaks for the community? is the plaintive cry. The answer, of course, is that there is no community out there, as there is no community out in the suburbs unless you are interested in getting to the epiphenomenal community, which is there for reasons already noted. In that case, their response is a relatively predictable one—and it is inexorably linked to issues of great social import. That community voice will speak to the mental health center about oppression and demand that the center take a role in their struggle. Many centers have and will attempt to get into that struggle. They are then epiphenomenal centers that will ultimately depend for their existence on the maintenance of an oppressed community.

If a center "turns its back to the community" and selects out those residents of the area interested in the center's conception of mental health services, then it runs the high risk of being identified as not truly a "community" mental health center.

How: Community as Instrument

If the foregoing concept of epiphenomenal community is plausible, then what remains to be discussed is the functional role of that tentative community. If there are urban communities, marked by oppression and secondary communal "togetherness," then how do they operate in their common goals? What is the basis of their instrumental effectiveness? Although there are many ways to address these questions, I shall select the following approach because it captures the reality of today's urban life.

The ultimate instrumental force with which a "community" may attempt to impose its collective will is that of confrontation. After all, there would be no "community" had there not first been a condition of oppression and, hence, a state of imminent conflict. The very creative force responsible for the emergence of community is itself a real or imagined threat and so the counter-force is its putative equal, counter-threat.

The point of this is to identify the fundamental force that, on the one hand serves as the community's power and, on the other, serves as a reinforcement of its sense of being an oppressed victim and, hence, a reinforcement of its sense of community. This force of confrontation must be analyzed into its various forms, and a would-be provider of "community mental health services" must accurately perceive its proper relation vis-à-vis these forms of confrontation.

A community has at least four levels of confrontation that it can mobilize: (1) as physical force; (2) as antiparticipant; (3) as franchiser; (4) as consumer.

Physical Force.

This leaves little to the imagination and essentially is a call to violent opposition. It has become a common device in today's urban brinkmanship and is characterized by a burst from threat to action. It should be clear that the relationship of a mental health center to its "community" cannot be fashioned after this type of functional community role. The "take-over" approach, wherein "community" members literally force institutional personnel out of offices, and so on, and then proceed to effectively close down the operation of the institution, is an example of the physical force approach. As a technique, for a community to impose its collective will upon an institution, it is the most dramatic. When applied to a fragile institution, like a community mental health center, it promotes confusion and dismemberment.

Antiparticipant.

A community may view an institution as sufficiently contrary to its needs so as to take a vocal stand in opposition to its existence. One can imagine the mental health center whose real or imagined program is thought to be a further instrument of societal oppression. With that provocation, a community could urge that no one participate as patient or employee or in support of the center. Again, this hostile relationship can hardly serve as a model for center–community interaction. It is a fact, however, that many centers are being described as instruments of social oppression and militant opposition has developed in many instances. But again let me draw out the important distinction. Although there may be articulate and militant opponents to a program, it is a nonsequitur to ascribe this opposition to the ubiquitous "community." Truly antiparticipant reaction from "the community," that is, a broad level, grass-roots opposition, could develop only if a center could (1) capture the attention of the entire community, (2) behave in a blatantly oppressive fashion so as to generate their cohesive opposition, and/or (3) through distorted charges of great magnitude, be incorrectly perceived as oppressor. These are extremely unlikely conditions and so also is a truly antiparticipatory response from the community.

Franchiser.

A community takes on a special relationship with a center if it is in the position of franchiser. This suggests ultimate sponsorship by the community, with consequent control (or "power" in today's vocabulary) of program, personnel, and funds. On the face of it, this would seem an ideal way for a community to "confront" an institution that attempts to provide it service (6). However, the magic of the word covers the underlying absurdity. A community, in its true sense, does not organize itself in such a way as to provide an authoritative control over an institution. It will not yield a "representative" body with the abiding interest and competence to "control" so idiosyncratic an institution as a mental health center. To be sure, isolated individuals from here and there, for this reason or that, will rise "on behalf of the community," but there is little reason to expect in them the mandate or wisdom of the people for whom they wish to speak. It very quickly becomes an argument based on the viscera . . . a little community is better than none at all, isn't it?

Let us assume, however, that a community has developed its own internal system of representative voice and action. There are communities of this type. Here, I am not referring to the usual governmental structures that in their own way are "representative," but rather referring to area organizations (such as in the Woodlawn area of Chicago) (7). Such organizations have a way of maintaining their identity for functions far removed from their original intent. An organization formed to deal with housing or education could conceivably provide the sponsorship of a mental health center, but to suppose that it is a "community" vehicle for control, support, and responsibility may or may not follow. If the level of communication and mutual trust between the people of the community and the representative organization is consistent and durable, then it may well be an ideal franchiser of mental health services. It would be naïve, however, to hope to create a new community organization concurrently with a new mental health center. Both require enormous inputs of dedication, sophistication, and organizational skill. To have two mutually dependent institutions go through their separate and idiosyncratic processes together is to invite their mutual dissolution.

Consumer.

The ultimate power of a community is the power inherent in those persons who, by common need, accept or reject the role of service consumer. If the goal of an institution, like a mental health center, is to provide a service, then there can be no greater control than that which operates in the decision of a consumer to use or not use the service. To be able to extend this "power" to "the community" necessitates a relatively free market atmosphere. It means the provision of alternative services and the right of patients to choose that service that more closely meets *their* idiosyncratic need. To close the options by creating catchment area boundaries is to imprison the people of that area and to insure their dependence on what could be an arbitrary mental health program, whether by professional design or by design of those "professional" community representatives who speak with neither mandate nor clear vision.

The dilemma becomes clearer, however, when we fully appreciate the impasse. Given a catchment area exclusivity, we find a community voice impossible or improbable in each of the four functional strategies open to it. This leaves us with a peculiar conclusion: A community mental health center is neither of the community, by the community, nor for the community.

Given the reality of today's catchment area approach, with the consequent closed market for the consumer, the only viable functional role left for "the community" is as franchiser. As already noted, however, this will only be possible in rare instances. Again, at the risk of being overly redundant, let me restate that the concept of community in the foregoing refers to the evanescent *gemeinschaft* still to be found in oppressed populations. It refers to their collective, and therefore representative, needs and demands and *not* the interpreted needs and demands of a pseudocommunity as articulated by self-appointed "representatives."

Community Control: Grassroots and Weeds

Community mental health centers face the same dilemma in relating to community as do all other service-oriented institutions. They are considerably more at risk because of connotations of terms like mental illness and mental health. Having been born into times of accelerated change, they can hardly succeed in forging a self-identity. People are now "seeing" irrelevance in all or most institutions, and so the wish or demand for institutional change runs rampant. "If they can't make their institution more relevant, we will!" So goes the cry from the people . . . or at least some of the people. "They" are usually thought of as alien, hostile, and malevolent, while "we" are dedicated, altruistic, and intrinsically instrumental. In today's heightened atmosphere of confrontation, the way to resolve a problem is to "confront" it, and so it is pure logic to confront the caretakers.

The balance to the above is that many institutions are, in fact, unable to meet increased demands. The demands are now quantitatively and qualitatively more complex. The charge of irrelevance becomes an issue and a fact as long as the "demands" are not carefully defined and as long as priorities within institutions are not set. An institution that says to a community "we shall attack mental illness" or "we shall promote mental health" is simply setting itself up for the rejoinder "you are irrelevant."

And so the issue of community influence, whether as the franchiser or as consumer, is integrally linked to the issue of program goals. Someone has to decide what these goals shall be. A community will never succeed in imposing its goals on a center that is unwilling to accept them, and a center will never succeed in imposing its goals on a community if there are no consumers. The commonplace "battle for control" is an exercise in futility for both combatants.

A starting point is imperative. Let us start at the community end. If the foregoing has any merit, we can anticipate two relevant community roles: (1) as franchiser and (2) as consumer. Either of these roles are possible, but their possibility depends on the extant nature of the particular community in question. As I have indicated, a franchising community necessitates an existing "representative" body. The "incorporation" of interested community persons is an exercise in illusion. The incorporated body is as much a *special interest group* as any institution. Their special interest will emerge from their own narrow perspectives. To be willing to relate to such a franchising group is no different than relating to any institutional franchiser. To relate to a true community franchiser is desirable but difficult to attain.

What seems a rational premise is that the search for the "community" be abandoned. A search for the Grail would be as rewarding. What then should a mental health center set about to do vis-à-vis its "community"? Contrary to the romantic readiness to do the community will, a mental health center must know, in advance, what it is it can do and wishes to do. Armed with this sense of identity and purpose, it can turn to "its community" and identify itself. As part of its process of deciding what it is and what it can and wishes to do, it must also decide to what degree it wishes to balance its internal decision-making processes by the inclusion of persons *identifiable* as (1) area residents; (2) vitally interested in the work of the center; (3) with the ability to conceptualize the types of problems and types of solutions involved; (4) with a willingness to participate and an ability to disagree as well as agree. This is "organizational sensitization," that is, the conscious internal process of keeping an organization open to the life-style and "needs" of its potential consumers. This is a process that should be initiated from within the center. It cannot easily be imposed from without because that breeds organizational coercion and not sensitization. If a center's leadership does not choose to support and welcome the voices of its potential consumers, then it simply will not have a sensitized organization. One may wish it to be otherwise, but the difference between rhetoric and performance lies within those who must perform. This is nowhere more true than in the highly personalized and complex task of intervening into human behavior. As long as an organization can maintain an internal system of self-regulation, so as to constantly focus and refocus on its task, it will remain viable. This internal system of self-regulation will not work well unless it is truly internalized, that is, unless there are multilevel consumer-oriented imputs. No consumer-oriented institution can survive unless it pays attention to its market. The market research department, within consumer-oriented industry, is a fundamental system that keeps organizational goals relevant to consumer needs. An analogic system within community mental health centers is critical. The dependence on external inputs, such as with the common use of an advisory board structure, quickly degenerates into a pro forma relationship if there is no internal system of consumer influence.

Some centers have been able to maintain organizational sensitization by carefully seeing to it that area residents with the aforementioned criteria are hired for "meaningful" jobs within the center. The indigenous worker trend may be more important because of its influence as an agent of organizational sensitization than for its more explicit manpower resource role. If this is working well, then good balance can come from an advisory board structure, providing the advisors and the internal staff have open communication with each other.

The point to all of this is to demythologize the term *community* and refocus the issue around organizational sensitization. Simply stated, this means the awareness of an organization of the multiple problems, some subtle and some not, related to doing its task. It implies neither a predetermined task nor a task arrived at by representative election. Presumably, there are some tasks for which persons in the mental health professions are particularly suited, and some for which they are not. Once those tasks are made clear and decided on as organizational goals, then, and only then, should an organization turn to its potential consumer for help in maintaining its awareness of the problems in reaching its goals. If those goals are not the ultimate goals for a "community" (presuming those could be discovered), then it will simply become a service institution for a population group, with a priority (or "relevance") less than ultimate. It means being willing to see oneself as less than the savior institution and being willing to say to "community" voices that the mental health center is not the grand instrument of social renovation.

Issue of Black and White

This dilemma about community must be placed into perspective, especially in regard to its racial implications. The popularization of the concept of community is a corollary to the entire social awareness reaction of the last decade. One of the fundamental catalysts of this social consciousness has been, and continues to be, the Negro struggle for equality. The tragic dimensions of this social revolution dwarf other processes involved in institutional renovation. Nearly every institution is caught up in its own attempt at renewal, but the contagion and drama of the Negro plight has attached itself to these various institutions. Their own future course now becomes enmeshed in the working out of the black identity process.

It is conceivable that, because community psychiatry has come into vogue in the wake of the black revolution, its own identity and working through will be confounded by the vagaries of the more historically profound movement. There is a double-edged sword here. On the one hand, the moral impetus of the black revolution has imbued the community psychiatry movement with an aura of moral righteousness, and therefore its personnel has been enthusiastic and committed. On the other hand, it has created a whole series of illusory goals, abstractly related to sacred concepts of mental health, and therefore may have sealed its own ultimate frustration. Highly committed persons in an inevitably frustrating task . . . therein lies the potential tragic element.

The movements are distinct and separate. One, the black revolution, is profound and touches the total fabric of our social structure. The other, the community psychiatry movement, is a moment in time, a transition stage between a narrow view of care to the mentally ill and a broader view with yet uncertain borders. Each has its own goals and processes. To begin to apply the jargon of mental health, developed to understand the individual, to institutions, communities, and value systems is to invite the collective wrath of those whose expectations will have been raised beyond our capacity.

There are so many red herrings with racial implications in the community psychiatry movement that it is common to see the staff of a large urban mental health center devour itself as it seeks some new guilt-reducing strategy. The amount of effort turned toward a therapeutic community approach becomes enormous. The irony, however, is that the object of this therapeutic preoccupation is the center staff *itself* and not those persons for whom, presumably, the center exists. To ignore the reality of racial bias and its effects on the personnel of a center would be naïve, but preoccupation with organizational cleansing is a trap as self-limiting as any.

REFERENCES

1. Arensberg, C. M., Kimball, S. T. *Culture and Community*. New York, Harcourt Brace Jovanovich, 1965.
2. Nisbet, R. A. *The Sociological Tradition*. New York, Basic Books, Inc., Publishers, 1966.

3. Ardrey, R. *The Territorial Imperative.* New York, Atheneum Publishers, 1966.
4. Pasamanick, B., Scarpitti, F. R., and Dinitz, S. *Schizophrenics in the Community.* New York, Appleton-Century-Crofts, 1967.
5. Srole, L., Langer, T. S., Michael, S. T., et al. *Mental Health in the Metropolis.* New York, McGraw-Hill Book Co., Inc., 1962.
6. Smith, M. B., Hobbs, N. *The Community and the Community Mental Health Center.* Washington D.C., American Psychological Association, 1966.
7. Kellam, S. G., Schiff, S. K. The Woodlawn mental health center. *Soc. Sci. Rev., 40:*255, 1966.

MAXIMUM PARTICIPATION OF THE POOR: ANOTHER HOLY GRAIL?

18

Stanley J. Brody

It may be a human trait or one previously restricted to the ancient Greeks or early English knights, but whatever it is, Americans have it obsessionally. This is the "holy grail" complex—the need to find a mythical solution to all problems. Social planners suffer from this condition pathologically; they have chased "holy grails" until they see a silver chalice under every bush.

Panaceas

One early panacea was public housing, because of which delinquency would vanish, full employment would occur, and venereal disease would disappear. In the forties there was Alinsky's Back-of-the-Yards movement (1). And for too many years, social welfare was sidetracked by an almost libidinous desire on the part of social workers to act like psychiatrists.

The next panacea was Cloward and Ohlin's "opportunity" concept, which was incorporated in the Juvenile Delinquency Act of 1961 (2). Paralleling this were the Manpower and Development Training Acts and a variety of massive retraining programs.

A few years later, the mental health planning legislation picked up an old World War II venereal disease control concept—that of comprehensive planning. This panacea took hold so effectively that there shortly developed comprehensive manpower planning, comprehensive mental retardation, comprehensive vocational rehabilitation, comprehensive health planning, the regional health plans euphemistically called the heart-stroke-cancer program, and comprehensive pediatric care for children in needy areas.

In short, true to our pluralistic nature, we have a veritable plethora of incomprehensive, comprehensive, and sometimes incomprehensible

This paper is a revised version of one originally presented at the APWA Conference, Boston, Massachusetts, September 5, 1968, and is reproduced here by permission of the National Association of Social Workers, from *Social Work*, Vol. 15, No. 1 (Jan. 1970), pp. 68–75. Stanley J. Brody is currently with the Department of Community Medicine, University of Pennsylvania, Philadelphia.

plans. The granddaddy of them all is the Model Cities program—a parlay of all health, welfare, education, industrial, and home construction comprehensive plans.

Under the Juvenile Delinquency Act of 1961 a few projects—the Neighborhood Service Center programs—were developed and analyzed based on the idea that juvenile delinquency is a symptom rather than a diagnosis. Such a center was to be

> . . . physically and psychologically visible, accessible and comfortable. Its services must be integrated, relevant, comprehensive and coordinated . . . [and] consistent with the values and life styles of the neighborhood. Its social action must be carefully planned and well executed, appropriate to local needs and related to the larger community; it must meaningfully involve neighborhood residents. (3)

Economic Opportunity Act

Out of these experiences and reflecting "the felt necessities of the times" (4), the Economic Opportunity Act of 1964 and its 1967 amendments evolved. They extended the opportunity concept from employment and training for youths to

> a full range of opportunities . . . [for] the poor. . . . The ultimate goal is to enable low-income persons to achieve self-sufficiency. In short, the community action program should move poor people through their own efforts into the mainstream of American life. (5)

The 1967 amendments to the Economic Opportunity Act retained the requirement of "maximum feasible participation of residents" (6) and also stated that these neighborhood residents must be represented on the governing board of the community action agency. Furthermore, they promoted the hiring of neighborhood residents as staff members and strengthened this practice by requiring not only maximum employment opportunity for residents, but also opportunity for further occupational training and career advancement. In addition, the amendments contained a new provision, which encourages the use of neighborhood-based delegate agencies at least half of whose governing board members are to be "residents of the area and members of the groups served."

Responding to the bureaucratic enthusiasm for the Neighborhood Service Center programs and for community participation, in August 1966 former President Johnson pledged to establish through administrative fiat "in every ghetto of America" a neighborhood center of the people who live there. The result was the Neighborhood Service Pilot Program, representing the cumulative efforts of the Departments of Health, Education, and Welfare, Labor, and Housing and Urban Development, the Office of Economic Opportunity, and the Bureau of the Budget. Fourteen cities were selected to demonstrate how well federal, state, and local human service agencies could work together in developing such innovative and integrated service delivery systems with "broad participation" by residents of the neighborhood.

At the same time, Congress was developing the Demonstration Cities and Metropolitan Development Act of 1966. Its purpose was to help cities "plan, administer and carry out coordinated physical and social renewal programs to improve the environment and the general welfare of people living in slums and blighted areas" (7). To do this, the act set up Model Cities that, as part of their demonstration program, would be required to have "widespread citizen participation in the program" (8). The policy statement of the Model Cities Administration emphasizes the following:

> (1) the constructive involvement of citizens in the model neighborhood area [and] (2) opportunities should be afforded area residents to participate actively in carrying out the demonstration. (9)

Major Thrusts

Currently, then, there are three major thrusts of federal legislation and executive direction aimed at the community. One requires broad participation of neighborhood residents; the second, widespread citizen participation; and the third, maximum feasible participation of area residents.

As contrapuntal themes to these activities, there are also federally funded community participation programs under the Juvenile Delinquency Act of 1961 (e.g., the Police–Community Relations Program in Philadelphia), the Children and Youth Pediatric Projects of the U.S. Children's Bureau, the OEO Neighborhood Health Centers, and some mental health and mental retardation centers, to name but a few.

The net effect in the community is a bewildering series of new programs based on citizen participation, funded independently for the most part by a variety of federal agencies, and administered by a rapidly revolving kaleidoscopic assemblage of federal personnel with enormous community and program case loads. These programs do not exist in a vacuum but are in communities that have been aroused to a new sense of worth and have high expectations.

It is suggested that rather than re-experience the past infatuation with public housing, psychiatry, and other program focuses, the current panacea should be examined critically and professionally. Bernstein states the problem succinctly:

> How do we transform administration in the delivery of social services

to achieve support and involvement from clients without losing the skill and decisiveness of administrators? (10)

This paper will be devoted to such an exploration. Since of the current crop of citizen participation programs those of the Office of Economic Opportunity are the most venerable, an examination of the "maximum feasible participation of residents of the area and members of the group served" may be the most profitable way to begin.

"Maximum"

One of the definitions of "maximum" is "the greatest quantity or value attainable in a given case" (11). Built into the definition, then, is not an absolute but rather a variable. This is borne out by the experiences of a local Community Action Program in attempting to use the election process as a method of achieving this maximum participation.

In Philadelphia in 1965, after a massive program to interest the community including full and enthusiastic support from the news media and voluntary and governmental agencies, 13,500 voters turned out to elect 144 representatives to the neighborhood boards making up the Philadelphia Anti-Poverty Action Committee at a gross cost of $56,000. The number of voters represented at maximum less than 5 percent of the potential electorate. In 1966, after an even greater effort and with the added asset of twelve existing neighborhood community action councils, 28,792 persons voted. The Philadelphia Anti-Poverty Action Committee notes that "every known technique for obtaining community participation and some new ones were employed to inform area residents of the elections" (12). The American Arbitration Association reported a total of 17,315 votes cast in the September 1967 election (13). In the last election, which took place in the spring of 1969, 16,507 votes were cast, at a cost of $80,000. As a comparison, it might be useful to note that during this period about 50,000 adults were receiving public assistance and perhaps another 75,000 adults would have been eligible to receive medical assistance. In the 1967 Philadelphia primary election approximately 270,000 persons voted out of 955,000 registered voters. Over 900,000 voted out of one million registerees in the 1964 presidential election (14).

Another and perhaps more definitive voting experience was that held in early 1968 for board membership in the Philadelphia Neighborhood Service Pilot Program. In that instance, 256 voted out of a population of 25,000, of whom half may be assumed to have been adults and therefore eligible to vote. A similar number voted in February 1969, despite the efforts of a dozen community workers.

It may be concluded that "maximum," which by definition is relative, when modified by "feasible" cannot be considered a valid index.

Certainly in the aforementioned case, it is clear that when less than 10 percent of the estimated eligible population voted, the requirement, no matter how vague, has not been met if election and choice of representatives are considered the controlling values.

"Participation"

"Participation"—"the action or state of taking part with others in an activity; . . . of partaking of something; . . . sharing" (15)—opens up wider areas for evaluation. The first aspect of this may be seen by comparing the number of persons employed and the number reached. In an undifferentiated count, the Philadelphia Anti-Poverty Action Committee reports 6,863 employed and 718,485 served over the two-year period 1965–67. If 400,000 people were affected in one year, then this might be considered a substantial number. However, the nature of the service rendered may severely modify the significance of this figure. As a comparison, in Philadelphia there are currently 145,000 persons receiving public assistance and another 110,000 receiving medical assistance, figures that describe specific, substantial services (16).

There is an even more important question than that of the number of persons who elect representatives and the number who are served. That question arises from the nature of the participation: What is its basic character?

The Poor

To find some indication of this, let us proceed to the third definition, that of the "residents of the areas and members of the groups served." By some public relations mystique, this has been interpreted to be the "poor." The *New York Times* credits an early morning inspiration of Adam Yarmolinsky (at that time painfully separated from the administration of antipoverty programs) for this interpretation. The dictionary defines "poor" as "lacking material possessions: existing without the luxuries and often the necessities of life: having little money" (17). It is submitted that this does not describe a homogeneous group, no more than does any other grouping of citizens by ethnic or political persuasion. It is suggested that the poor may be subdivided for the purposes of this paper into the upper-class poor, the middle-class poor, and the poor-poor.

The upper-class poor are not necessarily underemployed. Their special needs may modify their available income. Thus a person may be needy because of the expenses of psychiatric treatment, despite an income of $10,000. Other special costly medical needs, such as long-term chronic care or kidney dialysis, can deplete an otherwise substantial income. The middle-class poor are usually underemployed or have large families and, for the purposes of this paper, their income would be less than that needed by a workingman's family of four for a minimum standard of living. The poor-poor are considered to be those who are dependent on public and medical assistance payments. (In Pennsylvania the amounts would be $4,000 for medical assistance and $2,400 for public assistance for a family of four.)

Empirically it may be observed that the poor-poor are rarely visible on any community boards under any programs, federal or otherwise. Perhaps one of the characteristics of the poor-poor is their total isolation from the community, not only from the Establishment community, but from that of the ghetto as well. This separation is even more marked when measured by the static figures of those states that have matured medical assistance plans. For example, in Pennsylvania the number of persons using medical assistance has leveled off while the number receiving public assistance has grown, which indicates a hardening of a group that is a small percentage of the total population but is numerically large (18). At the same time, the mean income of families is steadily increasing, so that the financial gap between the poor-poor and the middle-class poor is rapidly widening.

Another indication of the isolation of the poor-poor is their nonparticipation in civil disorders. The Kerner commission's report, while admittedly sketchy, states that "the data show that rioters are not necessarily the poorest of the poor (19). In the Philadelphia disturbance of 1964, those apprehended did not include a single public assistance recipient (20).

A number of factors have led to this accentuated separation. The cumulative effect of inadequate public assistance grants, with the resultant nutritional deficiencies, creates a sense of apathy among recipients. The way public assistance has been administered acts as a further depressant. Minuchin notes that from a psychiatric point of view, poor-poor families are unable to relate objectively within the family unit to any problem (21). Thus the volatile feeling levels within the family contribute to the inability of its members to deal with community problems that require abstract considerations. The lack of adequate clothing and the sense of shame projected onto the public assistance family also add to this group's lack of participation in the ghetto community.

For the most part, the Office of Economic Opportunity's programs have not been related to the welfare programs. This is in part due to the lack of knowledge of those programs by OEO personnel and their a priori thinking, which has written welfare programs off as a viable resource. In Philadelphia until recently, most attempts to involve public assistance programs with the antipoverty program have not been received with interest.

The one visible involvement of the poor-poor has been through the National Welfare Rights Organization. This group, which had some initial public welfare and community support, is slowly and painfully becoming an effective force in the community. The NWRO, too, is sensitive to its exclusion from the antipoverty action movement and reports hostility and distrust from that group.

Control of Poverty Programs

As a result, the poverty movement is in the hands of the middle-class and upper-class poor who focus on those programs that respond to the motivated underemployed poor. Moreover, professionals who associate themselves with these programs have a tendency to control them, as do their fellow bureaucrats in the governmental Establishment and the ubiquitous consultants who skillfully manipulate citizens for their own ends. Some of these administrators follow the line of what Schlesinger calls the "new creed," whose "leading advocate" is Herbert Marcuse:

> As [Marcuse] sees it, any improvement in the condition of the powerless and the oppressed only plays into the hands of the rulers—and is therefore to be regretted. And the device of tolerance is particularly evil because it renders "the traditional ways and means of protest ineffective—perhaps even dangerous because they preserve the illusion of popular sovereignty." (22)

The community is normally made up of many organizations, each with its own interests, each jealously guarding its own sphere of influence. Since each federal community program carries with it the promise of jobs for the ingroup, the multiplicity of federal sponsorships increases the number of nonrelated competitive ghetto agencies. In the Philadelphia Neighborhood Service Pilot Program (NSPP) area alone, it is possible to identify six separate boards, each separately funded and each dealing with a different federal agency or configuration of agencies. In effect, the federal government has reproduced at the neighborhood level the same separate agencies and bureaucracy that it has sponsored at the state and local governmental levels. In the struggle for power the focus on services becomes inadvertently lost and community energies are dissipated.

With the introduction of the NSPP and the Model Cities program, the problem has been confused by differing interpretations of participation. Those federal personnel with OEO backgrounds see local participation as local control. The Department of Housing and Urban Development (HUD) personnel, having always dealt with advisory groups in urban renewal and other traditional housing programs, see participation as sharing. Indeed, the two laws—the Economic Opportunity Act of 1964 and the Demonstration Cities and Metropolitan Development Act of 1966—clearly reflect this difference between "maximum feasible" and "widespread" citizen participation. In the middle of this conflict are the Department of Health, Education, and Welfare personnel, with their focus on universal state-administered or supervised mandated programs with strict controls built into state plans. Neither OEO nor HUD had any intensive experience in working with states so that the early stages of the NSPP and Model Cities program did not seriously take into consideration the heavy federal and state investment in substantial welfare programs. Yet those welfare programs, however justifiably or unjustifiably castigated they may be, are the only programs that affect the poor-poor.

The Challenge

The challenge then is twofold. At the federal level there must be strenuous efforts to make more precise the nature and goals of citizen participation. It might even be useful for state personnel to provide training sessions for federal officials who are not familiar with state and local public programs. At the least, the ties of creative federalism must be less of a slogan and more of a reality.

In public welfare we must respond to Bernstein's challenge for

> . . . the establishment of mechanisms of participation for the poor with respect to programs that affect their lives. . . . We have to build this framework of fulfillment and inclusion for the disadvantaged at the same time that the counterpart capability of administration continues. . . . (23)

Commitment to the involvement of the poor-poor must never mean that the public agency abdicates its responsibility. The task is to create competence on both sides, not separation. The job is to extend the process of participation but not to divide power to the point of impotence.

Public officials at all levels must confront the definition of participation. Is it control? Lourie likes to pose the dilemma of what would happen if each neighborhood group wanted to establish its own sewerage system (24). Would that be acceptable? If participation means neighborhood control, are we in the process of complicating our already unworkable multigovernmental structure of townships, boroughs, cities, counties, district school boards, and the like?

However, there can be accommodations. If the Model Cities program has done nothing else, it is forcing this kind of dialogue among the various levels of government. There are positive strengths in the situation. Most of us in public welfare acknowledge the lack of involvement of the poor-poor in our programs and we recognize that we have as much to learn from them as they do from us.

One example with which we are currently experimenting is the use of the rental dollar for the purchase by responsible community groups of their own neighborhood centers. Public welfare agencies can rent space from these new neighborhood groups with day care and medical and public assistance moneys, which would enable them to purchase their own centers. We can explore with neighborhood groups new jobs and methods of screening so that public personnel giving services in these centers would be acceptable to the community. As much as possible, priority should be given to public assistance recipients from the community in hiring for these jobs. Neighborhood center social service review boards could be instituted, which would have a role similar to that of police review boards. NWRO members from the neighborhood could be hired as advocates for the clients to assure relevant and responsible delivery of services.

But in all this, we must recognize our professional role of constantly evaluating, analyzing, and challenging each old and new idea and not understate the complexity of the problems. We must be forthright in accepting responsibility for those things we can change. We must be just as forthright when we are unable to bring about change and must direct the community to where the power to change lies, be it in the municipal council, the state legislature, or in Congress.

Change is the way of the day, but all change is not necessarily for the better. As Peter Drucker has pointed out, we may only conserve by innovating—by stability in motion. We in public welfare have been motionless for too long. Let us move—with all our skills and integrity —but move *now!*

REFERENCES

1. For a discussion of Saul Alinsky and the Back-of-the-Yards movement, see Thomas D. Sherrard and Richard C.. Murray, "The Church and Neighborhood Community Organization," Social Work, Vol. 10, No. 3 (July 1965), pp. 3–14; and Saul D. Alinsky, Reveille for Radicals (Chicago: University of Chicago Press, 1945).
2. Richard A. Cloward and Lloyd E. Ohlin, Delinquency and Opportunity: A Theory of Delinquent Gangs (Glencoe, Ill.: Free Press, 1960).
3. Edward J. O'Donnell, "The Neighborhood Service Center," Welfare in Review, Vol. 6, No. 1 (January 1968), p. 12.
4. Oliver Wendell Holmes, Jr., The Common Law (Boston: Little, Brown & Co., 1881), p. 1.
5. Economic Opportunity Amendments of 1967, Senate Report No. 563, Sen-

ate Committee on Labor and Public Welfare, 90th Cong., 19th Sess., p. 45. This was earlier distilled in Sec. 202(a), Subsec. (3), of the Economic Opportunity Act of 1964, which requires that Community Action Programs be developed "with the maximum feasible participation of residents of the areas and members of the groups served."

6. Economic Opportunities Act of 1964, 88th Congress, 2nd Session, Sec. 202(a), Subsection 3.

7. House Report No. 1931, 89th Cong., 2d Sess., p. 4.

8. Demonstration Cities and Metropolitan Development Act of 1966, Sec. 103(a), Subsec. (2), 89th Cong., 2d Sess.

9. City Demonstration Agency Letter No. 3, U.S. Department of Housing and Urban Development, October 30, 1967. This is further spelled out in the Model Cities program guide, *Improving the Quality of Urban Life* (Washington, D.C.: U.S. Department of Housing and Urban Development, December 1967), which calls for a form of organizational structure, existing or newly established, that embodies neighborhood residents "in the process of policy and program planning and program implementation and operation."

10. Bernice L. Bernstein, "Urban Crisis and the Delivery of Social Services," p. 6. Paper presented at the New York City Department of Social Services Supervisors Dinner, New York City, May 2, 1968.

11. *Webster's Third New International Dictionary* (Springfield, Mass.: G. & C. Merriam Co., 1961), p. 1396.

12. *Progress Report* (Philadelphia: Philadelphia Anti-Poverty Action Committee, 1966), p. 29.

13. American Arbitration Association, "In the Matter of the Election," (Philadelphia: Philadelphia Anti-Poverty Action Committee, 1967). (Mimeographed.)

14. *Philadelphia Bulletin Almanac* (Philadelphia: The Evening and Sunday Bulletin, 1968), pp. 19, 20.

15. *Webster's Third New International Dictionary*, p. 1646.

16. "Summary Statistical Report" (Philadelphia: Philadelphia County Board of Assistance, June 1968). (Mimeographed.)

17. *Webster's Third New International Dictionary*, p. 1764.

18. *Public Welfare Report, 1967–68* (Harrisburg, Pa.: Pennsylvania Department of Public Welfare, December 1968), Table 13, p. 24.

19. *Report of the National Advisory Commission on Civil Disorders* (New York: Bantam Books, 1968), p. 131.

20. Personal communication to the author.

21. Salvador Minuchin *et al.*, *Families of the Slums: An Exploration of Their Structure and Treatment* (New York: Basic Books, 1967).

22. Arthur M. Schlesinger, Jr., "America 1968: The Politics of Violence," *Harper's*, Vol. 237, No. 1419 (August 1968), p. 21.

23. Bernstein, *op. cit.*, p. 5.

24. Norman V. Lourie, "Orthopsychiatry and Education," *American Journal of Orthopsychiatry*, Vol. 37, No. 5 (October 1967), pp. 836–842.

COMMUNITY CONTROL AND THE COMMUNITY MENTAL HEALTH CENTER: A VIEW FROM THE LINCOLN BRIDGE

19

Mel Roman

Two of the most controversial issues today are community power and the crisis in our nation's health services. Both reflect the growing cry for self-determination, for decentralization of authority, and community control of human services, and both offer ample evidence of breakdowns in old, overburdened, and outmoded urban structures.

Community control in its current political sense is a concept refined in minority group confrontations—Ocean Hill–Brownsville, the new medical school in Newark, the Harlem community's struggle with Columbia, and the recent Lincoln strike. "In the past twelve months it has been the ubiquitous rallying cry of advocates for decentralization, Jeffersonian democracy, Wallace segregationism, student revolution and black nationalism, not to mention Norman Mailer's independent city-state." [1]

Historically, the attempt to break political life down to more manageable neighborhood units came as early as fifteen years ago with the white exodus to the suburbs. And though community control exists aleady in many white areas, the idea of restructuring and bringing government and public institutions closer to home today calls up in the popular mind visions of the radically disenfranchised, mainly minority groups and the alienated young. Since communities with social options have community power already, community control is primarily beneficial to the disenfranchised.

We are pretty clear on who is politically disenfranchised. But when the issue turns to the crisis in health services, the issue of who is disenfranchised is not nearly so clear. Just as military–industrial factions have

This paper was originally presented at a NIMH staff meeting on Metropolitan Topics—Dilemma of Community Control: University and Community Relations, November 21, 1969, Washington, D.C., and is reproduced here by permission. Formerly Associate Director, Lincoln Hospital Mental Health Services, Mel Roman is currently Associate Professor of Psychiatry, Albert Einstein College of Medicine, and Director of Research and Development, Sound View–Throgs Neck Community Mental Health Center.

[1] Louise Kapp (Ed.), editorial, *New Generation*, Summer 1969, *51* (3), 1.

been regarded as usurpers of grassroots power in politics, so monolithic structures in the health field have resulted in an ignorance of, an estrangement from, and an inability to cope with current health needs, especially those of the poor.

Concern about the crisis in health care has created other reactions —among them, popular anger at the rising cost of hospitalization and medical insurance, an increased activism on the part of a new generation of medical students who see before them a morass of administrative mammoths, and the terrible inequality in health care for the poor, a breakdown in trust for a medical profession that has allowed all this to happen.

In the health area many are disenfranchised. But some are more disenfranchised than others.

The Lincoln Hospital Community Mental Health Center in the South Bronx was one of the first and one of the most successful centers developed under the impetus of that act. The program began at the peak of the convergence of the civil rights integration movement and the antipoverty program. It filled a major need, serving a Puerto Rican and black community that had one of the highest incidences of psychosocial pathology in the New York metropolitan area.

The program was first funded in 1963, through a contract with the City of New York, and operated by the Albert Einstein College of Medicine. The program then developed, over the next six years, during a period of intense political disruption and change. In the midst of escalation of the Viet Nam war, failures within the antipoverty program, the development of black militancy and a separatist ideology, riots and assassinations, and the erosion of trust in authority, the program nevertheless expanded under the impetus of increased funding from the Office of Economic Opportunity and the National Institute of Mental Health. From a planning staff of approximately fifteen with a budget of $80,000 it grew to a staff of three hundred and a budget of $4 million and earned itself a reputation as one of the most innovative and effective mental health centers in the country. It was in the forefront of social and community psychiatry, a new development in psychiatric theory in which individual patient pathology is regarded as a manifestation of the ecology of a community. Social psychiatry is built around the hypothesis that the environment itself must be changed in order to bring about significant individual change.

From its beginnings the Lincoln program was oriented as much toward social change and community development as it was toward traditional goals of psychiatric treatment. It organized tenants' councils and participated in voter registration drives and welfare rights demonstrations. It provided neighborhood-based services in storefront first aid and social crisis centers. It pioneered in the use of indigenous nonprofessional workers, training them within a new careers program for a variety of mental health roles. Lincoln's programmatic success was especially gratifying to advocates of community control. Even though the Health Services Administration of the City of New York had positioned itself against community control (fearing a repetition of the Ocean Hill–Brownsville school decentralization situation), Lincoln developed and implemented the first model of community control in the mental health field. This model involved a unique contractual arrangement between the City, the Albert Einstein College of Medicine, and a model cities community corporation.

In view of the program's success in restructuring mental health services, in developing new manpower, and in initiating collaboration with community organizations, the breakdown at Lincoln that began with an explosive strike of mental health workers and professionals in March 1969 and has resulted in an almost complete debilitation of the program there is even more appalling. Lincoln might appear to be an isolated social tragedy, but the odds are in favor of further crises of the same sort in community health and mental health centers across the country, especially in urban ghettos where conditions parallel those that precipitated the confrontation at Lincoln. Originally two thousand community mental health centers were projected for cities across the country, many in urban ghetto areas, fifty-one for New York City alone. Whether these will materialize under the changed priorities of the Nixon administration remains to be seen. Nevertheless, it is both necessary and valuable to examine the interaction of personalities, issues, and social forces that precipitated the Lincoln crisis and come to some judgments on how similar crises can be averted in the future.

The rumblings of trouble at Lincoln began well before the actual strike. From the outset we were plagued by the absence of adequate space and supplies, bureaucratic delays and paperwork, conflicts between professional and nonprofessional staff regarding evaluations, racial conflicts, and, most importantly, conflicts over ideological issues.

The problems of the medical school with which Lincoln is affiliated increased the program's vulnerability to disruption and contributed significantly to the erosion of staff morale. Throughout the course of our program, the medical school was in the throes of a financial crisis. Since the medical school is administratively responsible for the program at Lincoln and staffed the program with its faculty members, the problems of the school became the problems of the Center, and conversely the problems of the Center invaded the campus (a fact noted by the Dean when, during the Lincoln crisis, medical students were picketing, petitioning, and sitting in).

In the early years of the program the most disruptive issues were the absence of clear-cut personnel practices and grievance machinery and the irresponsible business and fiscal practices of Yeshiva University, the parent body and fiscal agent for all contracts and grants coming to the Albert Einstein College of Medicine. As Directors of the Lincoln program, we controlled neither our funds nor our personnel practices. For that matter, the medical school itself had no fiscal autonomy. All fiscal matters, payrolls, and payment of bills were handled through the business offices of Yeshiva University: Vendors and consultants were not paid for months; petty cash monies used for family emergency situations were inappropriately limited or withheld and often were obtained only after wasteful and enervating confrontations with business office administrators; there were frequent, inordinate delays and errors in paychecks.

A majority of our staff were black and Puerto Rican nonprofessionals who could ill afford being short-checked (through machine errors), much less go home without a paycheck. Such occurrences were immediately perceived as exploitative and racist, reinforcing the staff's distrust and resentment of the white establishment. For six years, the professional and nonprofessional staff, along with program administrators, fought unsuccessfully to change these practices. Nevertheless, during the first three years of the program very little happened to suggest that Lincoln would become the arena and victim of the internecine conflicts of a community struggling for power and demanding autonomy. The program received an enormous amount of favorable publicity and became a showpiece for the OEO as a demonstration of how a university-affiliated, hospital-based program could meaningfully address the myriad problems associated with ghetto life.

During the third year of the program a major issue arose around a conference about the use of nonprofessionals. The funds were provided by the OEO, and from the beginning the planning for this conference included the nonprofessionals. During the course of the planning a conflict arose over "whose" conference this would be. The professionals, while attempting to provide the nonprofessional group with major responsibilities in the planning and managing of the conference, were unwilling to relinquish the power of final approval. The nonprofessionals, although initially interested only in managing the conference, now demanded complete responsibility for the invitations, agenda, and operation of the conference, without any participation of professionals. Arguing that professionals were paternalistic and had exploited the nonprofessionals in advancing their own careers, the nonprofessionals insisted that, unless they had total control of the conference, they would take no part in it. As a result of the impasse created by this demand, the conference was canceled.

This confrontation was relatively muted, but it was a forerunner of the demands the nonprofessionals were later to make. With the issue of "whose" conference it was, the nonprofessionals had raised what was essentially a political question and thereby laid bare much of the rhetoric surrounding the program's use of nonprofessionals. Despite statements to the contrary, the number of professionals willing to give up some of the privileges of their position were few indeed. And further, there was an elaborate system of formal and informal practices that served to decree relative states of status and privilege. One of these was professional decision-making power. The nonprofessionals concluded that there were two organizational worlds and that the professional world, characterized by power and prestige, was not available and, in the absence of any massive programs to make access possible, was unlikely ever to be available to them.

The hostility over this reality perception was exacerbated by the unrealistic self-evaluations that had developed in the minds of the nonprofessionals, particularly as a result of the rhetoric of some of our senior staff. Told time and time again that the professionals had more to learn from the nonprofessionals than vice versa, it was not surprising that the nonprofessionals' sense of exploitation was aroused by their growing realization that their access to decision-making power was virtually nonexistent.

Although always posited as a professional–nonprofessional conflict, still other realities fostered a different meaning. The nonprofessionals were either black or Pureto Rican, lived in the ghetto, and were selected because they were poor or marginally employed. The predominantly white professionals lived outside the community and were conspicuously middle-class. Despite the professionals' view that the power differential was the result of their professionalism (credentials and experience), the nonprofessionals politicized the conflict, making it a question of different degrees of access to, and command of, organizational resources.

Attempts on the part of the nonprofessionals to undo the power differential began to take many forms. In one form it ranged from noncompliance to passive resistance around some programmatic decisions determined by professionals. At another level, the nonprofessionals actively and publicly demanded that administration alter the decision-making process, reverse the overwhelming dominance of white professionals, and provide means for upgrading, including access to credentialing. In the main, these actions were accepted as legitimate expressions around valid goals, even while we felt there was not sufficient appreciation of the complexities involved in effecting these changes.

As the nonprofessional staff experienced mounting frustration over the time it took to achieve even minimal change, their political activity increased, and their demands became more excessive. Whereas earlier the areas of concern were related to changes within the framework of medical school standards and procedures, the nonprofessionals now demanded status without benefit of additional credentials or experience, called for immediate replacement of white supervisors, and increasingly declared ethnicity to be the sole criteria for "legitimacy."

With the termination of our OEO demonstration grant in December of 1967 and the transfer of funding to NIMH auspices, difficulties in the program escalated. To begin with, the transfer itself was not orderly and occasioned a period of insecurity when we were not assured of funding continuity. Further, NIMH introduced an entirely new set of procedures and guidelines that required radical revision of staffing patterns and job categories. There was an interval when assignments and duties were ill-defined. The nonprofessionals' feelings of powerlessness and anger increased when it became apparent that as a result of the new grant, in the planning of which they played little role, there would be drastic changes in the program and in their own functioning. Their sense of powerlessness was further amplified when they found their union to be ineffective in resolving the many labor–management issues plaguing the program.

In May 1968 the nonprofessionals, convinced that neither the program directors nor the union had the power to effect change, took things into their own hands. They staged a sit-in in the business administrator's office at the hospital and demanded that all outstanding grievances be resolved immediately, that new payroll procedures be developed to avoid paycheck incidents, and, most importantly, that an education release-time and free tuition clause be built into the new community mental health center staffing contract. During the negotiations with the medical school and Yeshiva University, the directors and the professional staff supported the demands. The conflict was resolved quickly and constructively, in great part through the efforts of a new Associate Dean. The nonprofessionals had won a major victory and developed a political sophistication.

Two other major confrontations followed in rapid succession, this time on the part of senior faculty and professionals. The first was a "palace revolt" in which service chiefs and project directors demanded a major internal reorganization with greater delegation of authority and increased participation in policy making. Dr. P., the program's director, complied, and a task force was formed to develop a new organizational structure. In June, while the task force was still meeting, the professional staff staged a work stoppage when the Dean announced cutbacks in salary increments. The increments were subsequently reinstated. Both actions reflected the widespread discontent among professional and administrative staff. And both actions further radicalized an already militant staff.

Shortly thereafter the task force plan for reorganization was presented to the total staff. It was rejected for procedural rather than substantive reasons. Dr. P., under severe criticism for not having involved "all levels of staff," formed a new committee with representatives from all staff disciplines, professional and nonprofessional, charged with developing a policy planning and review board (PPRB). It was to have veto powers over the entire program. The next two months were spent in heated debate over the powers and composition of the proposed PPRB. Many argued that such a staff board could serve in an advisory capacity only, since it could not legally be given veto power over the program's officially designated director. The nonprofessionals, particularly one of the leaders of the black militants, took the position that the PPRB should be primarily composed of nonprofessionals, that it would have to have veto and policy-making power, and that it would serve as the program's board until a community board was formed, at which time the PPRB would dissolve itself. The nonprofessionals often argued that, as blacks and Puerto Ricans working with predominantly white professionals, they not only knew more *about* the community but could legitimately act *for* the community. My position was that the formation of such a board (PPRB) would significantly retard the development of community control through a viable community corporation because I doubted that the staff group, once having acquired such power, would be willing to transfer it to the community. More important in terms of principle, it seemed to me that the nonprofessionals, regardless of color or ethnic status, should, as providers of services, be responsible to a board composed of consumers.

In spite of some misgivings, Dr. P. supported the PPRB plan, although he indicated that its implementation would require the approval of the Dean. In September, after a summer's hard work, a plan for the PPRB was endorsed by the entire staff. It was promptly vetoed by the general counsel of Yeshiva University, who stated that the director had no authority to bring such a board into being and, further, that the action was in violation of our contract with the City of New York. The demise of the PPRB produced mixed reactions. Many nonprofessionals as well as professionals felt relieved, having viewed the PPRB as an administrative monstrosity and a power vehicle for a small militant faction. Many were angry, especially at Dr. P., who they believed had led them down the primrose path knowing full well the final outcome. An offer to implement the PPRB as an advisory group was angrily rejected by the nonprofessional workers association.

Clouds were on the horizon, but the storm did not break until March 1969. The months that followed the demise of the PPRB were surprisingly quiet and productive. Significant restructuring of the program did occur; business and personnel practices improved; project directors were given more authority and autonomy; increased efforts were made to recruit black and Puerto Rican professionals; and, despite the absence of specific guidelines for community participation, we developed and implemented the first model of community control in the mental health field. The community mental health center was shaping up and many of us among senior staff felt a renewed sense of optimism. The disruptions had diminished, and most people were again preoccupied with the tasks of the Center—the treatment and prevention of mental illness and the promotion of mental health.

Although things had quieted down somewhat internally, externally the South Bronx community was afire with political and racial turbulence. The teacher's strike had closed the schools in September, and in the months that followed the city was torn by conflict. The South Bronx community, united in its fight to keep the schools open during the strike, renewed its intracommunity warring once the strike was over.

In recent years, competition between black and Puerto Rican groups for political leverage and for control of antipoverty and model cities monies had become particularly intense, much of this spilling over into our program since many of the nonprofessionals on our staff were politically active community members. In the main, the Puerto Rican community had established a dominant position and had been much more effective than the black community in organizing and retaining political power.

In February 1969, a recently hired black nonprofessional mental health worker, whose mother also worked at Lincoln and was a core member of the black caucus, was fired. All the frustrations over pay and personnel snafus, the underlying—and never directly confronted—feeling that the blacks and Puerto Ricans were being manipulated by a white paternalistic administration interlocked with a black community power drive. All the workers knew, and would privately admit, that there were more than sufficient grounds for the firing of Mr. D., but some argued that administration had neglected to follow agreed-upon procedures. Mr. W. knew he had an issue and that he could draw upon the mother–son relationship to involve others in the black caucus in the fight. Still, before he was able to get major support, he had to find other issues, however ambiguous or fictional, to arouse wider interest. At first enormous pressure was put on the black supervisor who had evaluated Mr. D. negatively to change his evaluations. He refused to submit.

Shortly thereafter an administration offer of impartial review and binding arbitration was rejected by the nonprofessional workers. Then the storm broke.

On February 6, Dr. P., the program director, received a memo from Mr. M., chairman of the executive committee of the nonprofessional mental health workers association, demanding the immediate reinstatement of Mr. D. and of four other workers fired between October 1968 and February 1969. Their original firings had occasioned no comment. On February 14, Dr. P. responded in a memo to the mental health workers organization, saying that the firings were legal and in accordance with union procedures. He further indicated the availability of grievance machinery. There were rumblings about an imminent strike, but some observers who had the confidence of members of the nonprofessionals' association were told that there was not yet enough support for a move to pull the workers out.

On February 17, an eighteen-page statement of uncertain sponsorship ("State of Crisis") was distributed to the staff. It accused the mental health services administration of racist practices, malfeasance, and misuse of funds and generally denounced the affiliation of New York City hospitals with medical schools and teaching institutions. This document's material was taken from a report by State Senator Thaler regarding city hospitals in general, which had in fact indicated that Lincoln was by far the best of the affiliated hospitals. The Thaler report never concerned itself with our mental health services; yet the document made it seem that the charges had been leveled at our program. It was distributed with a four-page supplement that contained eleven recommendations. A great number of professionals, psychiatrists, psychologists, and social workers joined the nonprofessionals in signing a petition endorsing the eleven recommendations. When questioned as to why they had endorsed such an obviously plagiarized and distorted document, they indicated they were not endorsing the "State of Crisis" document but rather the recommendations. On February 27, the recommendations and the accompanying signatures were sent to Dr. P. (the critical recommendations are reproduced below):

1. The four black workers that were terminated be reinstated immediately with retroactive pay to their former positions.
2. Immediate staff election and implementation of the policy planning and review board agreed to by staff and Dr. P.
3. Immediate steps be taken by the PPRB to meet with Dr. M. (administrator) and the community lay hospital board and the community board steering committee to establish a meaningful community board to have significant powers and responsibilities over the administration and Lincoln Hospital Mental Service.
4. Immediate implementation of the union contract, the agreements,

declarations of the LHMHS to upgrade community mental health workers due promotions based on seniority, job experience, and so on.

5. The reclassification of community mental health workers to community mental health therapists.

6. The immediate establishment of a system of steps and/or grades within the titles of secretaries, clerks, typists, maintenance men, messengers, telephone operators, and so on, to provide for upgrading, appropriate salary adjustments, based on seniority and job experience.

On the following day 60 to 70 percent of the staff occupied the entire administration building, locked out nonsupporters of their strike, and announced that they would continue to maintain services under the auspices of the strike. Mr. W., in a memo to all staff and the press, designated himself the new director of the Lincoln Hospital Mental Health Services. Other strikers followed suit, and soon all the divisions had nonprofessionals as chiefs of service. These services included the out-patient services, the day and night hospital, consultation services, research, and training. It was a theater of instant competence created by memoranda.

Professionals supporting the "work-in" and agreeing to accept the authority of Mr. W. and the newly designated administrators were allowed to continue in their services as consultants. All service chiefs except three rejected the authority of the dissidents.

Signs went up declaring the program the "People's Mental Health Center." SDS's Mark Rudd made an appearance, and the Black Panthers lent some support to the dissident staff. Local 1199, the mental health workers' union, refused to support the takeover, declaring it illegal and in violation of union contracts. Inside the occupied building, it became clear that the action was not representative of the community, which was 70 percent Puerto Rican. As one community organizer remarked, "Baby, this is some people's revolution. You got white shrinks from Westchester, the VC flag, posters of Che and Malcolm, but there ain't a Puerto Rican button in sight."

On March 6, Dr. P., noting the impossibility of effective liaison between the service-maintaining professionals at Lincoln and the administration-in-exile at Jacobi Hospital (some miles away), notified Hospitals Commissioner T. that, under the circumstances, he could no longer be responsible for patient care. At 5:00 P.M. the City closed the mental health services at Lincoln.

That evening Dr. M., Assistant Commissioner of Hospitals for New York City and administrator at Lincoln Hospital, convened an emergency meeting of the Lincoln Hospital Community Advisory Board (a group comprised of representatives of some two hundred community organizations) to discuss the crisis and suspension of services. The community advisory board (CAB) formed an ad hoc committee to meet with all parties concerned in an attempt to resolve the crisis. On Friday, March 7, after having met privately with all groups, the CAB committee organized a negotiating session that was terminated because of repeated disruptions by members of a black militant faction among the dissidents. Finally, the committee reported that it could no longer continue in its efforts to mediate since the strikers themselves seemed not to trust their representatives.

On March 9, the CAB sent a telegram to Commissioner T. stating that they, and not the dissident staff at Lincoln, were the designated representative body to speak for the community on issues pertaining to the delivery of health and hospital services in the South Bronx. The CAB rejected the action of the dissidents and supported the duly authorized professional directors of the program. On March 10, Mr. W., angered by the statement of the CAB, an organization he regarded as unrepresentative of black interests, led a delegation to the Bronx Borough President's office in an attempt to create city-wide interest and support through an escalation of the conflict. The Borough President agreed to use his good offices to try to resolve the crisis.

On March 15, two days and countless meetings after negotiations had reached an impasse, the Puerto Rican caucus of the dissident staff adopted Mr. V. as their spokesman, accepted our formula for an interim Policy Advisory Committee, and agreed to return to work. On Monday, March 17, the mental health services at Lincoln were reopened, and by Tuesday most of the staff had withdrawn from the strike and returned to work. About eighty remained out. On Wednesday, March 19, a joint statement was issued by the City's Health Services Administration and Albert Einstein College of Medicine implementing our recommendations for resolving staff grievances, including the convening of the community policy advisory committee. The memorandum further stated that all staff who did not return to work would be suspended without pay. On the 20th, twenty-three members of the staff staged a sit-in in the clinical services, interfering with patient care. They were arrested and, along with others who did not report for work, were suspended without pay. According to an official accounting on Friday, March 21, sixty staff members, including the three psychiatrists who were service chiefs, had been suspended.

On March 24, the Steering Committee of the faculty organization informed the Dean that the faculty handbook indicates faculty members cannot be suspended without pay. Unable to reconcile the inequality in the reinstatement of salaries for suspended faculty without equal consideration for nonfaculty, an offer was made to lift all suspensions and to accept without prejudice all staff who returned to work by Monday, March 31. By Tuesday, April 1, all but thirty had returned to work.

Although all the services were now functioning, the situation was still very unclear. Thirty of the staff were still out; the interim advisory committee was beginning to meet, but its authority had not been spelled out; the schisms in the staff were severe; and personal animosity between those who worked and those who struck was intense. Staff who once worked well together stated they could no longer do so, and many asked for reassignment. At this point, Dr. K. and I, as acting co-directors of the community mental health center, took the position that without the authority to fire and transfer staff, and without the College's explicit and public support of our position favoring community control of the Center, we could not provide the leadership necessary to pull the program together. Although supported in this request by Dr. R., chairman of the department of psychiatry, Dr. C., chairman of the department of community health, Dean G., and many others, the Dean would not support a policy of community control and could not authorize the firing of faculty. Being unable to obtain what we considered to be the necessary authority and support to run the program, Dr. K. and I requested reassignment to other work in the department of psychiatry.

In the weeks that followed, things went downhill at an ever-increasing pace. Almost all of the senior professional staff left, including two of the three striking psychiatrists. Many others requested reassignment and were planning to leave. Dr. P. resigned, and an interim director was appointed. Some months later, he too resigned, in part because of staff demands that he do so. The services were almost at a standstill. Community groups were battling for recognition and control of the proposed policy board, and a once vital community mental health center now resembled a ghost town.

At this writing (October 1969) a new director acceptable to the community and college has been appointed, and efforts are again underway to revitalize the program.

The troubles of the Lincoln Hospital mental health program pose many problems, leave many questions unanswered. Let us discuss the events and issues from two perspectives: first, from the specifics of the Lincoln program and its social–political context, and then from a broader view of issues pertaining to community health and mental health programs in general.

As administrators, we were expected to assume responsibility without adequate authority to fulfill expectations. We did not control our funds, nor did we have the *final say over the hiring and firing of staff*. We were, in effect, middle management, operating a highly innovative, technically and administratively complex program, beset by unforeseen political conflicts and made especially vulnerable by the irresponsible business/fiscal/personnel practices of AECOM–Yeshiva. Most important, we were hamstrung by the absence of explicit guidelines concerning community participation from the city, the state, or the federal funding agencies. Lest this sound like an apologia, let me state what I consider to have been the major defects in the program's leadership. We had serious programmatic overcommitment, coupled with inadequate consolidation of existing programs, an inability to delegate authority and to distribute the rewards of success, and the tendency to aggrandize nonprofessionals at the expense of the professional. We grew too fast; the community and its militancy changed as fast as we grew. But, most pertinent to the escalation of conflict, *we initiated the program without organized and coherent community support and sponsorship.*

Against this backdrop of widespread staff discontent and in the context of the rising expectations of nonprofessionals, the slow pace of upgrading and institutional change, and the growing militancy of the community, it is important to state that the crisis at Lincoln was not precipitated by conflict over community control. The action was a grab for power on the part of a small dissident group, led by black militants attempting to use the program as a base from which to compete with Puerto Rican groups politically dominant in the community at large, and supported by the anger of white professionals toward program administrators and AECOM–Yeshiva University. In the main, the white support derived from the envy and anger of pseudoradicals intent on "doing in" the establishment and, on the part of many, from a desperate need to identify and ingratiate themselves with militant blacks.

After the initial phase of the crisis, factional conflicts within the dissident group and their need to find community support and legitimacy led the dissidents to make the issue one of community control. In fact, however, it was from the start a demand for staff control presented in the guise of community control; even when the community control issue became primary, the black staff faction clearly wanted to control the control of the community.

Throughout the crisis there was enormous confusion about goals and issues, much fashionable rhetoric about community control, revolution, and people power, without any felt necessity to be clear or specific. At no time were the dissidents able to develop meaningful community support. Most of the support that evolved came from left/liberal or radical groups outside the community, ignorant of the issues and developments and unmindful of the potential negative consequences for the community. Some, like the Panthers and SDS, were involved primarily in an effort to radicalize staff and community; others such as the New Careers Development Center exploited the crisis for image building of their own. No one seemed to have much interest in the wishes of the community itself nor in the community's critical need for services.

The speed with which the conflict spread was not only unanticipated by the dissident leadership; it was beyond their most ambitious expectations. But it is easier to start a conflict than to control it, and pretty soon the dissidents, frightened by the unexpected developments, found themselves playing the game of brinkmanship. It was a pseudo-radical and opportunistic strategy for change, and it had disastrous consequences.

The tragedy was one of major proportions to the South Bronx community; it might have been averted if the timing had been different. It occurred during a mayoral election year, so that local and city officials made decisions based on their search for political support. The marked ambivalence toward saving the program that was exhibited by everyone at all levels of government (NIMH made no site visit during the crisis) —and their profound unwillingness to take a position, however responsible, that might result in blame or criticism—might have been the result of the growing awareness that the Nixon administration was showing signs of disavowing many programs and policies that had been in operation under Johnson. People who stood to lose either political support or funding were keeping a low silhouette in 1969.

If not for these political factors, courageous and honest decisions might have been made that might have saved the program. It is noteworthy that while the student–faculty body at Harvard saw fit to discipline those students who disrupted the educational process, the AECOM–Yeshiva administration has not felt it necessary to discipline those physicians, psychologists, and social workers who disrupted patient care and jeopardized the very existence of the community's mental health services.

From a broader point of view, the strike demonstrates that all planned change, no matter how successful, is subject to the vagaries of unanticipated and unintended consequences. In retrospect it seems clear that much of what occurred was directly related to the ideology and strategy of the program and the nonprofessionals' attempt to turn them to their advantage. Further, it seems evident that the specific programmatic innovations—decentralization of services, utilization of indigenous nonprofessionals, participation of the poor, when combined with a new community militancy for self-determination—lead logically to the demand for community control.

The difficulties encountered at Lincoln are to be anticipated in all similarly innovative community based programs. The central point here is that *community control is both the problem and the answer*. Power to the people translated into workable and effective models of community control can and must be developed. The difficulties in achieving and implementing such models are considerable, especially as they often involve entrenched institutions unwilling to relinquish power and protected by the ambiguity of federal, state, and city guidelines. Two other considerations are relevant to the problems of transfer of power. First, the political competitiveness that exists and will continue to exist in ghetto communities orients itself more and more to the control of service institutions and invades the agency itself through the use of indigenous manpower. And second, most of the institutions providing health services to ghetto communities (municipal hospital systems and medical schools) are racked by overt dissension and conflict and are themselves in the process of major reorganization. Health and hospital systems are in a precarious financial state, especially with the recent Nixon cutbacks. Many will not survive. Medical schools are equally precariously funded and are undergoing major structural change, the final forms yet to emerge. Given the political and structural instability of both the community and health care systems, it is unlikely that meaningful transfer of power will occur quickly, in an orderly manner, and without violence. Nevertheless, such transfer of power is essential. For unless new structural forms can be developed that will protect life-maintaining institutions from becoming victims of factional fights, ghetto communities will be increasingly deprived of crucial services.

COMMUNITY ACCOUNTABILITY AND
MENTAL HEALTH SERVICES
20
Sheldon K. Schiff

The turmoil at Lincoln Hospital (5, 7, 8, 24, 25, 27, 28, 32, 37), the activities of black mental health professionals at recent professional meetings (22, 23, 31, 33, 34, 35), and the New York teachers' strike of 1968 (18) would seem to indicate that there is a special problem in the relationship of the white professional working in a black urban community. It would be more accurate, however, to see these occurrences as merely highlighting the problems and ambiguities that surround the emerging collaborative relationship between mental health professionals and the communities they serve.

The mental health professional's responsibility to the community—

Reprinted from *Mental Hygiene,* April 1970, *54*(2), 205–214.

Sheldon K. Schiff, M.D., is Director, School Intervention and Training Program, and Associate Professor of Psychiatry at The University of Chicago.

The author is particularly grateful to the Woodlawn Mental Health Center Board for providing him the opportunity to enjoy the most personally satisfying and productive years of his entire professional career. Neither the program nor the work of the Woodlawn Mental Health Center would be possible without the Board's support and active participation. The Board has been fundamental to the work of the Center.

The author is especially indebted for the support given the program by the Chicago Board of Education and by Dr. Benjamin C. Willis, former General Superintendent of Schools, and Dr. James Redmond, currently General Superintendent of Schools; Dr. Curtis C. Melnick, Area A Associate Superintendent; Dr. Donald Blyth, Superintendent of District 14; Mr. Michael R. Fortino, Superintendent of District 21; and Rt. Rev. Msgr. William F. McManus, Superintendent, Archdiocesan School Board.

The Honorable Richard J. Daley, Mayor of the City of Chicago; Dr. Samuel L. Andelman, former Commissioner of Health, and Dr. Morgan J. O'Connell, former Commissioner of Health, Chicago Board of Health; Dr. Melvin Sabshin, Head of the Department of Psychiatry, University of Illinois College of Medicine, and Dr. Daniel X. Freedman, Professor and Chairman, Department of Psychiatry, Pritzker School of Medicine, University of Chicago, have each provided important support and cooperation in this work.

This program is supported by Research Grant No. 2–3301–9296 from the National Institute of Mental Health, and grants from the Maurice Falk Medical Fund, the Wieboldt Foundation, the van Ameringen Foundation, and the Field Foundation.

as opposed to his responsibility to the individual patient—has traditionally received little recognition in professional training and practice until recently. The events of the past few years, and particularly those of recent months, have served to greatly emphasize and confound the racial aspects of a long-standing problem—what the relationship should be between professionals and the community.

The great majority of reports describing implementation of large-scale mental health programs of study or intervention prior to the events at Lincoln Hospital revealed that similar difficulties have been encountered by white professionals in white, nonurban communities (1, 4, 13, 15, 26). Because of today's pervasive intensities, the historical roots of these difficulties have been obfuscated, and our perspective of the problem and its solution has been distorted. However, the role of the community in effecting professional change in mental health has historically been related to societal change and conflict (2, 38, 42).

If one looks at two of the earliest community–professional relationships developed following passage of the community mental health centers' legislation, that of the Woodlawn Mental Health Center in Chicago and Lincoln Hospital in the Bronx (New York City), there are certain differences and similarities that have been sources of major problems contributing to the tensions reported in both experiences.

Both, for example, are municipal facilities affiliated with private universities; both are substantially funded by additional governmental and private sources; both are located in urban ghetto communities; and both are directed by white professionals. At Lincoln Hospital, tensions partly attributable to these characteristics led to the disruption of program activities; the Woodlawn Mental Health Center, on the other hand, has operated continually over a period of six-and-a-half years.

There are three distinctions basic to any discussion of the ongoing, though not untroubled, operation of the Woodlawn Mental Health Center and the recent discontinuance of Lincoln Hospital's mental health program: (1) the nature of the mutual responsibility defined in the professional community contract and its mechanism of implementation; (2) the nature of the professional's primary professional and institutional bases and their effect upon the content of this contract and its implementation; (3) the effects of the contract upon the role of the professional and the nonprofessional.

The Professional–Community Contract: The Woodlawn Mental Health Center Board

The early difficulties of the Woodlawn Mental Health Center were related largely to the professionals' inadequate training in community involvement, their inexperience, and their lack of understanding of the professional–community relationship (9, 11). The community itself suggested what was probably the most important mechanism developed to meet this problem—a community advisory board.

The Center's advisory board included approximately twenty-five community citizens who related to the professional directors of the Center with only informal powers of consent. However, from the beginning it was mutually understood that this board would not only provide community sanction for the Center's programs but play a central role in planning the use of nonprofessional community resources. The commitment of the Center's professional staff was to discuss with this board all major decision making necessary to the Center's operations.

During the few years of the board's advisory status, one of the co-directors assumed the chairmanship of board meetings. As the board became more intensely involved in the Center's developing programs, and as the Center gained increasing acceptance in the community, the chairmanship became a source of some controversy. Board members came to feel that having a mental health professional as chairman vitiated their own roles—particularly with respect to their responsibility to the community groups many board members represented.

As time went on it became clear to everyone that the board had moved to a more autonomous position. The chairmanship was subsequently assumed by a board member, and shortly thereafter the group framed a constitution that described the formal structure of a full-fledged community board with powers to advise and consent. This included all aspects of the professional staff's involvement with their university departments, the city board of health, and other community agencies (43).

The Contract at Lincoln Hospital
and Its Effect on Community Support

The Lincoln Hospital operation included no mechanism for community involvement. Although Lincoln Hospital is a municipal facility, through a contract with the City of New York, Albert Einstein College of Medicine was designated as the responsible fiscal and operating authority. Subsequent funding from federal agencies, largely the National Institute of Mental Health and the Office of Economic Opportunity, was also administered through the university business office. At no time was there any effort to involve a constituency of concerned citizens in the planning and implementation of the hospital's programs. Community boundaries, program goals, and even more important—program priorities—were all determined by the professional staff. As a result, the nonprofessional became the only conduit to the community—initially as part of a rationale, and later by default and the momentum of events.

Despite a substantial financial base amounting to a budget of $4 million a year and widespread professional endorsement, the Lincoln Hospital operation was critically vulnerable with regard to its professional–community contract. It was the ambiguity and indirectness of this contract that was to surface ultimately as the critical flaw. As one of the directors candidly stated, the single most potent factor pertinent to "the escalation of the conflict" was the professionals' initiation of the program "*without organized and coherent community support and sponsorship*" (37).

The Professional's Primary Base and His Community Contract

The professional's vulnerability to being politicized is perhaps greater than that of the nonprofessional. The mental health professional engaged in the development of innovative programs often finds it difficult to resist the inducements of academic title and security, rapid professional recognition, political power and station, or a role in local community policy making.

Both the Woodlawn Mental Health Center and Lincoln Hospital have similar sources of funds. In contrast to Lincoln Hospital, the Woodlawn Mental Health Center's budget from city and state grant-in-aid funds has been small. For the first four years it remained unchanged —$125,000 a year. As a result of the board's intervention, this amount has been increased slightly, but remains less than $200,000 a year in useable funds.

The directors of the Center made the deliberate decision to be funded by the local public health structure rather than be dependent from the outset on grant funds. Also, since the determination of program priorities was a function of the board, the directors made no effort to secure grant funds until the first program focus was specified. Only after the board had made its decision to develop a program for young children primarily concerned with prevention did the directors seek supplemental grant funds.

Thus, the first two grant awards supported the development of a mental health program for all the first-grade children entering the twelve Woodlawn elementary schools each year (10, 12, 40). These grants supported the program of prevention and early treatment,[1] its

[1] A grant from the State of Illinois Department of Mental Health, Research, and Training Authority, DMH No. 17–322, awarded for a three-year period beginning July 1, 1965. (Principal Investigator: S. G. Kellam, M.D., and Co-Principal Investigator: S. K. Schiff, M.D.)

evaluation of effectiveness, and associated studies.[2] In the meetings devoted to these grant applications, the board insisted upon the right to review all future reports of this work prior to publication and upon their primary rights of ownership—with due respect to medical confidentiality—of all the original information and data collected in connection with these efforts. It was the board's contention that their activities in obtaining community support and cooperation were based upon their own accountability to the Woodlawn residents for what resulted. The directors of the Center agreed to both of these conditions.

Grant funds awarded to the Center were administered from the very beginning by the university,[3] just as they were for the Lincoln Hospital staff. During the early years, perhaps because the amounts and staff were small, there was little of the kind of fiscal administrative problems described at Lincoln Hospital (37). However, in recent years similar problems have been encountered more frequently.

These developments have paralleled the increased grant support and program expenditures, and the growth of the Center's staff. They have been associated also with the expansion of part-time staff from the community, comprised mainly of parents and teachers (41), and the geographic separation of the Woodlawn Mental Health Center from its university medical school department—a problem the Center shares with Lincoln Hospital.

The problems experienced by a department of psychiatry and its faculty as a result of its association with innovative programs are mutually discomforting. In an article published in 1964, the Chairman of the Department of Psychiatry at Albert Einstein Medical School commented on the not entirely pleasant impact of such programs upon training and upon his own values with regard to psychiatric practice (39). In such innovative contexts, the academic goals of study and instruction can be confounded by those of social welfare and the need for social action (29). The enthusiasms of the teaching staff may then become merely ideologic and exhortative in nature. Also, departmental chairmen engaged in the arduous tasks of maintaining and building a department may see such developments as competitive. A number of psychiatric department chairmen have expressed these and still other concerns about these kinds of program associations (6, 16).

[2] A grant from the National Institute of Mental Health 5-RO1-MH-14807, awarded for a five-year period beginning January 1, 1966. (Program Director: S. K. Schiff, M.D.; and Co-Director: S. G. Kellam, M.D.)

[3] For the first three years of its operation, the Woodlawn Mental Health Center was affiliated with the University of Illinois Medical School Department of Psychiatry. Since that time it has been affiliated with the University of Chicago Pritzker School of Medicine, Department of Psychiatry.

While not unhappy about the funds or the publicity that attends these efforts, most medical schools and their universities are rightly concerned about the possible disadvantages and dangers of such experimental innovations. Certainly they raise the specter of an expensive service commitment that is neither in keeping with department staff capacity nor ideal for an adequate academic standard of teaching commitment.

It is, however, the concept of community participation and community prerogatives that is most threatening to both department and university alike. For many universities located in urban ghettos, the possibility of ghetto area residents organizing and demanding a redefinition of their mutual relationship with the university is viewed with considerable caution and uneasiness.

A well-designed, specific professional–community contract is certainly a key factor in transforming this threat into a positive force for effective programming. The construction of such a contract, however, must also take into account the many practical realities of administering the service programs. For the community this is an issue that is integrally related to their concern with the prerogatives defined by such contracts. Ultimately, service is one of the crucial factors in their wanting the right of accountability.

The Effect of the Contract upon the Nonprofessional

In the event a professional–community contract is faulty and fails, the most adverse consequences with regard to staff fall upon the nonprofessional. Members of this group, consisting of previously untrained residents of poor communities, are acutely aware of the newness of their occupation, uneasy about the responsibilities they have assumed and their ability to carry them out, and concerned about how they are viewed by the professionals and patients with whom they work. As a result, their potential to be "politicized" is directly related to the ground rules set by their professional supervisors.

The source of many of the actions and statements of the nonprofessional staff during the difficulties at Lincoln Hospital can be traced to the training and supervision by the staff professionals. First, the nonprofessionals were hired both as staff and as community citizens, with little if any distinction made between the two roles. Indeed, the use of Community Mental Health Workers as a source of community information, program feedback, and a kind of public relations liaison was part of the early concept of the nonprofessional role. Certainly, in the absence of any independent citizen board, the nonprofessionals were preeminently more qualified to "speak for the community" than were the professionals; but the duality of their function was a serious fault.

Second, the first director of Lincoln Hospital's storefront program directed too much of his training toward efforts to make the student comfortable and confident in his new role (37). The nonprofessional student's abilities were oversold by comparing his unique attributes—a result of his cultural background and community residence (both important employment criteria)—to the patent lack of the white middle-class professionals in this area. Hence, the confidence and comfort of the nonprofessionals at Lincoln Hospital was secured at the expense of the professional's role and areas of competence. The result was the negation of what should have been a respect for the mutual expertise and background of both professional and nonprofessional.

Third, the "new careers program" for nonprofessionals offered a solution to the problem of their occupational future (30, 36). It was interpreted as providing entry points into the professional's hierarchical ladder, thereby securing for the nonprofessional status and financial reward on a par with the professional. In light of the first and second points, it is easy to see how this experimental innovation was conceived. It was an unfortunate experiment for many reasons. The legitimate question—never fully entertained at Lincoln Hospital at any point—as to the true effectiveness of the nonprofessional's role and function was sidetracked. While this question is, in the main, unanswered for the professional, it is vital to the nonprofessional's self-respect.

Although it is clearly recognized today that the mental health professional's credentials are no guarantee of "cure" for all problems, this is not to say such credentials are without significance. The nonprofessional does not have professional credentials and should not be endowed with identical license. It is plain that the Lincoln Hospital program dismissed the professional's expertise too lightly (37), viewing his societal rewards as simply and totally issues of social powers not related to a highly marketable competence. This view had the grave disadvantage of polarizing the broader professional community against the nonprofessional and casting him in a pejorative self-seeking role which is largely unwarranted.

The Woodlawn Mental Health Center, because of its current organization of programs, is not entirely free from this serious and potentially fatal development—a politicized nonprofessional staff. There have been efforts by individual staff members, community groups, and others to influence the hiring and dismissal of staff members. However, the formal procedure of introducing each prospective nonprofessional staff applicant to the board for final approval after they have been interviewed and screened by the responsible professionals has been a great help. The board's Executive, Personnel, and Grievance Committees, constituted to resolve such problems, have been extremely successful. The Committees are available to any staff member who wishes to present a grievance or have a dismissal reviewed.

With the help of the board and its growing awareness of its singular responsibility in this area, further plans are under way to eliminate the weaknesses that still exist.

Discussion

The term *community control* has been eschewed deliberately in this paper in favor of *community accountability*. The most compelling reason for this distinction is that community control, as defined by the usage of both its advocates and its opponents, has broad negative connotations. Community accountability, on the other hand, is not only a less emotionally-charged term, but is, in fact, a more precise description of the real issue to be discussed.

The recent experiences at the Woodlawn Mental Health Center and at Lincoln Hospital have shown clearly that those most vehement in their demands for community control have been members of the professional and nonprofessional staffs employed by community agencies, schools, and, in only a few instances, community organizations. With rare exceptions, they have not been the parents and other resident citizens of the respective communities. The parents of the more than ten thousand first graders who have been involved in the Center's school mental health program have been and continue to be primarily interested in the current and long-range effects of the program and the school system on their children.

One of the major responsibilities of the Center's board is to insure that the staff of the Center and the schools are accountable to every parent and neighborhood resident. The board is committed to providing every Woodlawn resident the right to be "heard out," regardless of the nature of the concern and without any *a priori* judgment of its legitimacy.

The board has been crucial also in resolving the tensions generated by the demands for community control by the professionals and nonprofessionals. It was through the active participation of board members at public and private meetings with school faculties, staffs of other agencies, and community organizations that the fundamental question of who constituted and should represent the "Woodlawn community" was resolved. Members of the board recounted the history of their relationship to the co-directors, their investigation of the directors' views as white psychiatrists, how the directors' professional relationship with the community was defined, and the nature of that relationship. In many instances, these were the same questions being advanced to Center staff by groups concerned with the "interests" of this black community. The board forged a bridge of working understanding and successfully clarified the definition of the community and its citizens, making the distinction very clear. The buttressing of this bridge is a continuing process.

With few exceptions, the various staff members advocating community control did not live in Woodlawn. They resided in nearby, more middle-class neighborhoods and, by their education and income, clearly belonged to a different socioeconomic class than the Woodlawn resident. It became very apparent that in feeling qualified to "speak for the community," they also expected to become the direct possessors of "community control." These were important issues to define and resolve—and neither could have been accomplished by the Center staff alone or by any programmatic design.

It is not the intention of this paper to present the Center's professional–community contract or the Woodlawn Mental Health Center Community Board, the mechanism by which it is implemented, as being without serious flaw. The experiences of the Center and its board— particularly those of this past year—have made it clear that this design does not eliminate the possibility of policy actions that are in direct conflict with the primary mental health aims to which the professional staff and members of the community board are mutually committed. A variety of parochial self-interests of individuals, community groups, professionals, or affiliated institutions can threaten the fulfillment of this contract. Only by maintaining the unencumbered commitment of each board member, together with the board's ongoing participation, can capitulation to one or another of these self-interests—by either staff or board—be prevented.

It has been the intention of this paper, however, to point out that community control is not only far from being a solution in itself—a position that is not uncommon these days—but it represents a concept that seriously threatens the ability of poor minority communities to realize those rights of accountability guaranteed by our Constitution and already available to the citizens of white middle-class communities. If this kind of control is obtained, it will undoubtedly be the result of the decision by the pertinent vested interests that they no longer want it—not because control has been wrested away by successful strategy. Control over a bankrupt enterprise pockmarked with a multiplicity of complex problems and fiscal needs would be a Pyrrhic victory indeed.

There have been a number of reports describing the failure of community action programs (3, 17, 19, 20, 21). Some have revealed a disturbing pessimism about the ability of poor communities to effectively alter their own condition (17, 20). Few of these reports address themselves to sources of failure other than the community citizen. Culpability for these failures must also be assessed in the light of the problems presented by local government, agency professionals, and, in the private sector, the role of the university and large foundations (3, 18, 19).

Unless serious attention is focused upon these other sources of failure, the consequences for both the recipients of mental health services and those who provide such services (nonprofessionals as well as professionals) will be disastrous.

There is great likelihood that the role and function of the mental health professional will be fixed into rigid, traditional modes that allow little more than token experimentation and innovation. Similarly, graduate and professional schools responsible for training mental health professionals will be less likely to support investigations, programs, and teaching efforts that have major public health commitments rooted in the community rather than in the hospital–clinic context.

The nonprofessional's future will be even more imperiled. For these new career lines to develop in directions complementary to the professional's inexorably specialized role, there must be the kind of professional freedom that is now only minimally available, but that will be almost totally curtailed by the fearful, defensive reactions to community control.

With the exception of the Communist countries (14), the difficulties experienced in developing effective professional–community contracts in poor communities are magnified in poor nations around the world. The advantages of the democratic principles embodied in our Constitution, the number of professionals available and the capacity to train such professionals, and a gross national product sufficient to develop human services—particularly those largely professional oriented—are almost nonexistent in most of these nations.

It is for these reasons that the innovations now being tested, such as community mental health centers, community school districts, and others that utilize large numbers of nontraditional professionals, represent an immense promise. The premature and unwarranted rejection of these innovations, then, has even larger implications.

The academic professional and the university, because of their traditional role and mission to pursue new knowledge through free inquiry and the preservation and transmission of knowledge already gained, have a unique responsibility. They represent a singular capacity for independent and objective examination of community service programs and their sources of failure. Regardless of their increasing burden of conflicting self-interests, critical investigation of these failures by the academic professional and the university is greatly needed. Without their contribution, it is doubtful that an effective solution to this problem will be obtained.

REFERENCES

1. Aberle, David F. Introducing Preventative Psychiatry into a Community. *Human Organization*, 9:5–9, Fall 1950.
2. Bloom, B. The Community Mental Health Movement and the American Social Revolution, Keynote Address delivered at the Third Rocky Mountain Psychological Association Professional Development Institute, Albuquerque, 1969.
3. Clark, K. B. *Relevant War against Poverty: A Study of Community Action Programs and Observable Social Change.* New York, Harper & Row, 1969.
4. Cumming, Elaine, and Cumming, John. *Closed Ranks.* Cambridge, Mass., Harvard University Press, 1957.

5. Fraser, C. G. Community Control Here Found Spreading to the Field of Health, *New York Times*, March 9, 1968.
6. Grinker, R. G. Psychiatry Rides Madly in All Directions. *Archives of General Psychiatry*, 11:228–237, 1964.
7. Harper, T. S. The Lincoln Hospital Protest: Community Mental Health Leadership as the Agent of Ghetto Imperialism, (mimeographed).
8. Hicks, N. Lincoln Facility in Bronx Opens: But 100 at Mental Health Center Continue 'Action,' *New York Times*, March 18, 1968.
9. Kellam, S. G., and Schiff, S. K. *The Social Service Review*, 40:255–263, 1966.
10. Kellam, S. G., and Schiff, S. K. Adaptation and Mental Illness in the First Grade Classrooms of an Urban Community, Psychiatric Research Report No. 21, American Psychiatric Association, 79–91, April 1967.
11. Kellam, S. G., and Schiff, S. K. An Urban Community Mental Health Center. In *Mental Health and Urban Social Policy: A Casebook of Community Actions*, edited by L. Duhl and R. Leopold, San Francisco, Jossey-Bass, 1968.
12. Kellam S. G., Schiff, S. K., and Branch, J. D. The Woodlawn Community-Wide School Mental Health Program of Assessment, Prevention and Early Treatment, Midwest Annual Regional Conference, Reports from the Rockton Conference, 1968, Rockton, Illinois.
13. Kiessler, F. *More Than Psychiatry—A Rural Program, in Mental Health and the Community: Problems, Programs and Strategies*, edited by M. Share and F. Mannino. New York, Behavioral Publications, Inc., 1969.
14. Kiev, Ari, ed. *Psychiatry in the Communist World*. New York, Science House, 1968.
15. Klebanoff, L. B., and Bindman, A. J. *American Journal of Orthopsychiatry*, 32:119–132, 1962.
16. Kolb, L. C. *American Journal of Psychiatry*, 126:39–48, 1969.
17. Lowi, T. J. *The End of Liberalism: Ideology, Policy and the Crisis of Public Authority*. New York, W. W. Norton, 1969.
18. Mayer, M. *The Teachers Strike, New York 1968*. New York, Harper & Row, 1969.
19. Moynihan, D. C. *Commentary*, 46:19–28, Aug. 1968.
20. Moynihan, D. C. *Maximum Feasible Misunderstanding; Community Action in the War on Poverty*. New York, Free Press, 1969.
21. Moynihan, D. C. *The Public Interest*, No. 5:3–8, Fall, 1966.
22. Newsletter, American Orthopsychiatric Association. Blacks Demand APA Action on Racism. Dec. 1969, p. 5.
23. Newsletter, American Orthopsychiatric Association. Confrontation at Annual Meeting. Dec. 1969, p. 2.
24. *New York Times*. Bronx Health Units Shut After Revolt, March 7, 1968.
25. *New York Times*. City Health Service Protested in Bronx, March 5, 1968.
26. *New York Times*. Community Balks Aid to Retarded, Dec. 26, 1966.

27. *New York Times.* Some Cross Picket Lines at Lincoln Hospital Center, March 19, 1969.
28. *New York Times.* 23 Seized at Sit-In in Lincoln Hospital, March 21, 1968.
29. Peck, Harris B., Kaplan, Seymour, and Roman, Melvin. *American Journal of Orthopsychiatry, 36:*57–69, 1966.
30. Peck, H. B., Levin, T., and Roman, M. *American Journal of Psychiatry, 125:*74–81, 1969.
31. *Psychiatric News,* American Psychiatric Association. Blacks Attack Psychiatry for Ignoring Ghetto Needs, May 1969.
32. *Psychiatric News,* American Psychiatric Association. Indigenous Workers Sieze Mental Health Services, May 1969.
33. *Psychiatric News,* American Psychiatric Association. Physician Lauds Radicals for Ortho Confrontation, Dec. 1969.
34. *Psychiatric News,* American Psychiatric Association. Radical Protests Upset Psychologists Convention, Oct. 1969.
35. *Psychiatric News.* American Psychiatric Association. Use of Indigenous Workers Paid to Exploit Blacks, Nov. 1969.
36. Riessman, F., and Popper, H. *Up From Poverty: New Career Ladders for the Nonprofessional,* New York, Harper & Row, 1968.
37. Roman, M. Community Control and the Community Mental Health Center. A View from the Lincoln Bridge. Paper presented at a NIMH staff meeting on Metropolitan Topics, Washington, D.C., Nov. 21, 1969.
38. Rosen, G. History of Medical and Applied Sciences. *19:*388, 1964.
39. Rosenbaum, M., and Zwerling, I. Impact of Social Psychiatry. Effect on a Psychoanalytically Oriented Department of Psychiatry. *Archives of General Psychiatry, 11:*31–39, 1964.
40. Schiff, S. K., and Kellam, S. G. A Community-Wide Mental Health Program of Prevention and Early Treatment in First Grade. Psychiatric Report No. 21, American Psychiatric Association, 92–102, April 1967.
41. Schiff, S. K., Turner, D. T., and Kaufman, R. V. Woodlawn School Mental Health Training Program: A Community-Based University Graduate Course, unpublished manuscript.
42. U.S. Congress House Select Committee on Lobbying. Report and Recommendations on Federal Lobbying, 81st Congress, 2nd Session, H.R. 3239, 3, 1951.
43. Woodlawn Mental Health Center Board Constitution, adopted Nov. 21, 1968.

COMMUNITY PARTICIPATION IN MENTAL HEALTH SERVICES: A CASE OF FACTIONAL CONTROL

21

Harvey M. Freed, David J. Schroder, Beatrice Baker

One of the most complicated tasks facing social welfare administrators today is that of developing services in conjunction with the residents of a particular community. Difficult as the task may be, it is seen by many as the most promising means of improving ineffective services. In this paper, we examine one of the potential outcomes of involving community residents in the planning and development of services: factional control.

The authors of this paper had their ideas shaped by the experience of participating in and observing the development of one community mental health program on the Near Southwest Side of Chicago. Called the Community Mental Health Program of the Medical Center Complex, the program is sponsored by the three training institutes of the Illinois Department of Mental Health (the Illinois State Psychiatric Institute, the Institute for Juvenile Research, and the Illinois State Pediatric Institute) and the Department of Psychiatry of the University of Illinois College of Medicine. The senior author of this paper has been Director of the program since its inception in 1966.

This particular program was guided by the ideology that the development of a mental health service should serve as a vehicle for the further development of the community. One of the main problems of the community was seen as a lack of political power or influence. It was the community's relative helplessness that was seen as the main focus of the mental health program rather than the individual psychopathology of some of its separate members. To be sure, many of the residents were in need of clinical treatment for emotional illness, and such services were

Reprint from *Mental Health in Rapid Social Change* (Louis Miller, Editor) Jerusalem, Israel: Jerusalem Academic Press, 1970. Harvey M. Freed, M.D., is Director of the Medical Center Complex Community Mental Health Program, Chicago, Illinois. David J. Schroder, M.A., was a Research Sociologist for the program. Beatrice Baker, M.A., is currently a Fellow in Political Science at the University of Glasgow, Glasgow, Scotland. The authors want to thank the following people for reading and commenting on earlier drafts of this paper: Rue Bucher, Harold Demone, Danuta Ehrlich, Richard Ford, Jay Hirsch, Louis Miller, Pertti Pelto, and Melvin Sabshin.

heretofore relatively unavailable. But the delivery of such services alone seemed only a small part of the necessary task. To the Program Director, the problem was much broader and required placing equal priority on the delivery of service and community organization.

The strategy chosen to involve community residents was to attempt to organize a broadly based, representative advisory committee that would collaborate in program development. The Program Director felt that this advisory group should include community leaders who had taken or were prepared to take action to alleviate some of the community's detrimental social conditions.

Finally, the host community itself was segmentalized. At least three major factions can be identified: militants, moderates, and brokers. The three factions were not in agreement as to goals or objectives, and certainly not as to strategy. What followed was a stormy process resulting in the development of a subcontract with the militant faction of the community. The case history describing the process was compiled by the authors from several sources, including field notes, minutes of meetings, recollections, and interviews. Heavy reliance was placed on interviews with and the the the recollections of the Program Director.

Case History

In the summer of 1966, four large mental health institutions decided to collaborate in the development of a community mental health program. This model service program was also to be used as a field laboratory for many training programs.

The primary responsibility for the development of the program was vested in a psychiatrist engaged by one of the institutions for that purpose. The first year was spent in planning the program together with many staff members from the institutions and with selected community leaders formed into an advisory board of twenty (1). An application for an NIMH staffing grant was submitted at the end of that period, and funding began on October 1, 1967. Since the area served by the program was populated by 130,000 people separated into four relatively discrete ethnic and racial communities, it was decided to develop storefront-based programs in each, backed up by the resources of the Medical Center. Operations began in the Mexican community in December of 1967 with plans to expand into the black and Central-Eastern European sections as soon as possible. As work began in the first storefront, the Advisory Board felt it had little to offer because so many members were from other communities. It was decided to abandon the board, to organize a separate board for each community as the programs developed, and subsequently an overall board with representatives from the former.

In April of 1968, the community organizer for the program was asked to make contacts in the black neighborhood preparatory to the initial invitation to an advisory committee meeting. While the composition of the board would be open to all comers, *special* invitations were extended to about twenty people by personal contact followed up by letters. The first meeting was held the night of June 26, 1968, in a conference room at Psychiatric Hospital. Twenty people attended from the community.

It should be noted that this community, which we will call West Side, consists of 25,000 people, almost entirely black. The area is quite poor by all statistical indices. There are few viable agencies; two settlement houses, some churches, and a YMCA. While the institutions had historically served many people, they had not attempted to tackle the major social problems facing the community.

A significant factor in this area is the development of two community organizations. The first was started in the early 1960s by a city-wide religious society. Originators of the project were both white and black, but the white ministers early took a back seat in an effort to promote the development of local leadership. A handful of black men, all ex-convicts, formed the nucleus of this group. A conflict with a local laundry brought it prominence and set the stance as militant. In the last six years, it has developed expertise in the housing and welfare systems and has helped numerous citizens to obtain better service. Likewise it has focused on job placement. While having connections with wider civil rights activities (Martin Luther King was headquartered here in the summer of 1966), it is less interested in broad social action and more interested in working with local citizens to promote their individual development. We will call it West Organization (2).

The other organization is of more recent vintage. At the time of Dr. Grant's initial conversations with community leaders in the winter of 1966–1967, the group had not yet risen to prominence. Composed mostly of younger men, it is led by a charismatic, often charming, but controlling and explosive leader. The group, which we will call Black Students, is affiliated with the YMCA, and some of the young men are enrolled in a YMCA college. It has been successful in encouraging the Medical School to open a local health center to serve the people of its neighborhood.

The two organizations have divided West Side in half, and they control the neighborhoods east and west of Ash Street. While both groups prefer separate identities, they respect each other and cooperate in certain ventures. In recent months these two organizations have combined with three others to form a neighborhood corporation, designed to develop businesses and social programs. The West Organization already runs a Shell gasoline station and a small factory in the area.

Three other organizations deserve mention. The first, One Community, consists of local women for whom West Organization is too militant. The second, XYZ, is a coalition of some agencies, business leaders and citizens. However, both Mrs. Green and Mrs. Elson, leaders of the two groups, have ties with Mr. Ronald, Director of West Organization. Likewise, the third group, predominantly women and called Concerned Citizens, has ties with Mr. Lawrence, leader of Black Students.

With this by way of background, let us return to the first meeting of the advisory committee held in late June 1968. The twenty people in attendance included one of the leaders of West Organization, although not Mr. Ronald, both Mrs. Green and Mrs. Elson, some women working as community representatives from the schools, some community workers for one of the settlement house, a staff member from the YMCA, the community liaison person from the University, a local minister, a local public school principal, several nuns from a local Catholic School, and the director of the local branch of CORE, now relatively defunct. The meeting was held at Psychiatric Hospital at the suggestion of those invited.

While the meeting was called for 7:30, it did not begin until after 8 P.M. Dr. Grant chaired the proceedings and opened with a very brief review of program developments to date. Insistent questions were asked about the number of people from the community to be hired, the salaries, the degree of community control, what had been accomplished in the Mexican community thus far, and what the stance of the program would be with regard to going beyond service with patients to efforts to change the social institutions causing the problems. Both the Director of CORE, Mr. Craft, and Mrs. Elson played active roles.

The next meeting, in late July, was quite similar in style. This time, however, a few of the staff members who were to work in the program were in attendance. Plans had been to move a few of the staff from the Mexican area into West Side in a temporary location and on a temporary basis until a permanent site could be found and permanent staff members recruited with the involvement of the advisory board.

No meeting was held in August, as several people were out of town. The meeting scheduled early in September marked the first time that Mr. Lawrence and three of his colleagues were present representing Black Students' Organization. The meeting began with a report from the Administrative Assistant to the effect that she had located a temporary site for the center in a Park District Fieldhouse. It was proposed that the staff begin working there the following Monday. The proposal met with silence, followed by the exchange paraphrased below and reconstructed by notes from a secretary:

Mr. Lawrence: What do you mean, "temporary . . ."?

Mrs. Kate (Administrative assistant): Until we can find quarters which are more suitable. It's difficult to locate true owners of buildings and to find adequate space for sixteen people. Urban renewal is a problem.

Mr. Lawrence: Uh huh. Will people from our side be able to use it?

Dr. Grant: I didn't hear you.

Mr. Lawrence: [loudly] Can our people use it? What's the matter, don't I speak plain? J. W., you hear me?

Mr. J. W. Wright: Yeah, I heard you.

Dr. Grant: Sure, it'll be available to everyone in the area. It's probably not the best location, but I think it's important to begin offering direct service to people as soon as possible.

Mr. Lawrence: What's direct service?

Dr. Grant: Working with people who have mental problems and trying to help them.

Mr. Hairston (West Organization): Say, Dr. Grant, are you going to work with kids?

Dr. Grant: Sure, we'll work with people of all age groups.

Mr. Hairston: You think kids from black neighborhoods are sick?

Dr. Grant: There are sick kids here as well as elsewhere. I know what you mean—social conditions are worse here, and a lot of the kids just need a chance.

Mr. Hairston: So this is just whitey's way of controlling the kids.

Dr. Grant: No, no, that's not . . .

Mr. Lawrence: Say, what is your program? What is psychhi-atry?

Dr. Grant: Well our goals are to treat those people who are mentally ill and to work to try to promote the mental health of the people of the community. If people have problems, we'll try to help them. If the problems stem from social factors, we may try to deal with them, for example, police, housing, unemployment. We may not always succeed, but we're going to try . . .

Mr. Lawrence: What do you mean?

Dr. Grant: We feel that often people need someone to talk with about their problems. Sometimes it takes more than that.

Mr. Wright: Are the problems psychological or sociological?

Dr. Grant: Both.

Mrs. Person: (Acting storefront director): Take the schools; often teachers have the wrong attitudes or school policies are . . .

Mr. Lawrence: We know the conditions. What are you going to do about them?

Dr. Grant: Each problem is an individual one . . .

Mr. Wright: Tackle the psychological problems—they come first.

Mr. Lawrence: You think you know how to handle all the problems?

Dr. Grant: You're baiting me.

Mr. Lawrence: Dammit! Don't tell me what I'm doing. Nobody else has to tell Lawrence what he's doing.

Dr. Grant: I think . . .

Mr. Lawrence: You don't think! You do what I tell you to do. You want to come into our community, you do what we say. We do the talking here.

Mrs. Person: We aren't sure what we can do. This is a new thing. In the Mexican community we've tried all kinds of things that none of us have done before. Some worked and some didn't. Depends on what's needed.

Mr. Wright: Another experiment. Always experimenting with black folks.

Mr. Craft: We heard you say you wanted to help and something about what you wanted to do. Will the state back you up?

Dr. Grant: We don't know. This is a new ballgame which nobody has much experience with. We're certainly willing to try, and we hope you buy this idea. Let's decide the best way for these resources to be used.

Mr. Craft: Will you recommend whatever changes are necessary to officials in order to do the job? . . . I mean if you find something wrong with the schools, for example.

Mr. Hart (Onlooker from Medical Center): Will you make professional recommendations?

Mr. Craft: Can we have an answer from you, Doctor?

Mrs. Elson: If the community said that *this* was the problem and you concurred, what would you do?

Dr. Grant: I see our job as feeding information to the various community groups for them to do with as they wish.

Mrs. Elson: Would you repeat that?

Dr. Grant: We'd feed such information to community groups, and we might try to effect the necessary changes—I don't know; it would depend on the situation.

Mrs. Person: You're dealing with us as individuals and as an organization. We have to keep in mind that some actions would get us thrown out on our ear.

Mrs. Elson: Are you afraid?

Mr. Craft: Then the mental health program will not be accountable to the community.

Dr. Grant: I think we'd be in a much better position to do some of those things if we had strong community support—your support. As for what Mr. Craft says, there is no such thing as exclusive community control. As long as we aren't paid by the community, we have to balance things.

Mrs. Person: I resent some of this. I was involved in the earliest boycott marches, here and elsewhere. We certainly want the community in on this thing, or I, for one, wouldn't be here.

Mr. Craft: We have to be careful this isn't a facade.

Mrs. Porter (Local school principal): Control comes in the way the community uses the service.

Mrs. Elson: We have enough nonfunctional agencies.

[At this point Mr. Lawrence and his three colleagues from Black Students got up and walked out of the meeting.]

Dr. Grant: What are you asking of us? If we find there's a problem, we'll try to act on it. In the meantime, we have to care for people who are mentally ill. There are many areas in which we may be able to help by pointing out some of the problems—schools, welfare, and so on.

Mr. Hairston: How come you don't know what you're going to do, and you get all this money, and when we make a specific proposal from West Organization for federal funds, we don't get a penny?

Mrs. Elson: Where?

Mr. Hairston: You know, under Title II. We haven't been funded.

The meeting continued for some time in the same vein. Finally, Mrs. Elson brought up the subject of a black male vocational rehabilitation counselor who had been dropped from the staff that was to work in the community. This was discussed at length, with several people from the neighborhood complaining that, whatever the staff objections to this man, he seemed to be competent, and perhaps the staff was not best qualified to judge who could be effective in this area and who could not. As a result, a personnel subcommittee was proposed that would review all personnel transactions, would become actively involved in recruiting and screening all applicants for positions, and, specifically, would review the case of the particular counselor mentioned above for further discussion at the next meeting.

After this meeting, the staff moved into its temporary quarters at the Park District Fieldhouse and began to see patients from the area. Some of the women who were community representatives for the local schools and who had attended the meetings, dropped by to wish the

staff good luck. They were pleased to see that "something was happening besides all that talk." "Besides," they said, "people there don't represent our point of view. We need services badly in this area. Those
people shouldn't bother you—don't let'em get on your back. That Mrs.
Elson don't even live here." Thus began a theme that would be heard
repeatedly over the next few months: a challenge to the "representa-
tiveness" of the spokesmen at the advisory board meetings.

Over the next few months there were several developments. Permanent quarters were located in a building adjoining one of the settlement
houses. A black man, with no graduate degrees, but with community
and administrative experience, was recruited by the Advisory Committee to head the program. The personnel subcommittee (three citizens—
two staff) agreed to rehire the previously discharged vocational counselor. There was also constant pressure to increase the number of
community workers (initially there were to have been nine professional
and four community workers) and the salaries. Finally, an agreement
was made to hire, automatically, people recommended by the two community organizations for the community worker positions.

During this period, initiative shifted from Mrs. Elson and Mr. Craft,
who, informally, had been directing the Advisory Committee, to Mr.
Lawrence and the Black Students. Lawrence, typically, would fly into a
rage during the meetings, stage a walkout, and leave those behind to negotiate a compromise.

As the New Year was ushered in, things seemed to be progressing.
More staff was recruited with the assistance of the Advisory Committee,
and now had a leader in Mr. Worth, the newly hired director. A permanent site had been located at Lighthouse Annex, and the staff had
moved in. The first advisory committee meeting of 1969 was to be held
in the community, in a room provided by the Lighthouse Settlement
House. More than fifty people were in attendance by the time the proceedings got under way, including representatives of almost all the organizations and agencies mentioned above. A rather festive air marked the
occasion as the newly appointed Advisory Committee Chairman was de-
layed in arriving and neighborhood residents spent more than an hour
chatting and exchanging greetings.

The meeting began with a discussion about job applicants but
hadn't progressed very far when Mr. Lawrence interjected that the discussion was hung up on qualifications: "Tonight we're not walking out;
we're staying to the end, so you're just going to have to deal with us.
Been playing games with us long enough." He also implied that some
people like Mrs. Elson had been getting money "under the table." Mrs.
Elson responded angrily and the two of them began to argue. Rev.
Harrison, of the West Organization, broke in and suggested that Mr.

Lawrence let the other organizations talk. After a brief discussion, Mr. Collins of West Organization called for a Black Caucus, to include black staff members present. Dr. Grant and the three or four other whites present left the room for the "ten minute" caucus. An hour later they were called back into the meeting room.

Mr. Worth broke the icy silence by standing up and saying that the group was demanding that the community workers be hired immediately at a salary of $6700 a year. Dr. Grant protested that personnel regulations would not permit this, but that he would be happy to work with the group to try to get things changed or for special dispensation. Mr. Lawrence replied, "Honky can always do things if he wants to." Dr. Grant felt cornered, angry, alone, and, for the first time, frightened. There had been implied threats such as, "Think you're going to get out of here tonight?" and so on. Looking around the room at this moment, it appeared as if there were no friends in sight. After what seemed like an endless quiet, Dr. Grant said that he thought there might be a way of doing what was asked but he would not do it unless everyone in the room knew exactly what was happening. To this, Mr. Darling of West Organization said, "If you want to go to jail, Doc, that's your bag. Black folks have done enough time on their own." Mr. Collins of West Organization then rose and made a speech about all the people who had died for the civil rights movement and suggested that this was important as an indication of how far people were willing to go in order to do what was necessary. Finally, Dr. Grant agreed to the $6700 salary. The meeting ended precipitously.

As Dr. Grant left that night he was furious. He returned home in a rage about what he felt he had been forced to do. His immediate response was to contact the Director of the Medical Center and to insist on the support and assistance of the Directors of the four Medical Center institutions. While those four men had comprised a Policy Committee under whose direction Dr. Grant was to have functioned, in actual fact the group had not met for some months for a variety of reasons. The urgent demands of the community now forced the issue.

Over the next several weeks the pace quickened. The Policy Committee entered the picture actively and, after one exposure to the entire Advisory Committee, insisted on meeting with a smaller negotiating team. The two organizations developed a team composed exclusively of their leaders and pushed this through the Advisory Committee. There were some objections from the women present at the meeting where this was done, but Mr. Darling of West Organization quashed them with an impassioned speech about how black women had dominated black men for too long. Others were too frightened to speak up. After two and three meetings a week, culminating in a final walkout by Black Students from a Sunday morning session and the closing of the storefront for one week, the two organizational leaders met with Grant in mid-May and handed him a proposal. It suggested that the Medical Center subcontract with the two organizations, and that the staff consist primarily of local people as counselors, dealing with the hard-core problems of the West Side, that is addiction, alcoholism, and so on, which had been avoided by mental health programs in the past. It proposed working with the people who in the past had been "outside the reach of most community mental health programs . . . too long . . . associated with social service agencies staffed by outsiders."

Dr. Grant's immediate response to the proposal was positive. From the middle of May until the middle of November the time was spent in working out the details of the plan and in securing the approval of all the necessary authorities. The plan was unique in that it marked the first time that the Department of Mental Health agreed to subcontract in this manner to local community organizations staffed by local people.

Discussion

The discussion is organized to answer two questions: Why did the process take the direction it did? How desirable is the outcome of subcontracting for service with two community organizations?

Program Ideology and the Institutions

The Program Director began with the assumption that the major problem confronting the community was the disenfranchisement of community residents, both in the political sense as well as in many other areas of decision making from which they were excluded. This assumption led him to place as few restraints as possible on the process established to seek community representation and participation in the development of the Program. As far as possible, he hoped that the natural course of events would lead to a balancing and compromising of the various viewpoints in the community just as he expected it would, ultimately, between the community and the Medical Center (3). While there were certain requirements as stated by the funding sources such as, for example, the need to provide certain clinical services, he was prepared to consider delegating these to other components of the Center if the community were to decide on this course of action. He did not, however, expect that the community would make such a judgment because to him it seemed unreasonable. In other words, he had considerable faith in the natural political process that had been set in motion to churn out the community leadership and to determine the correct course of action. The important thing was to impose as few constraints on the process as possible.

One of the factors that enabled him to establish such an unstructured process was the freedom given him by the sponsoring institutions. At times he had mixed feelings about that freedom and would have preferred that certain expectations be clearly stated or that an organizational structure be developed that would have placed limits on the process. But in general he felt that freedom was critical in seeking, identifying, and working with the community leadership in such a way that its impact on the program could be real.

For their own part, the institutional leaders were inexperienced in community transactions, were at an early phase in the development of a collaborative relationship among themselves, and were sufficiently committed to the task of developing a community mental health program to follow the lead of the Program Director. Further, there were enough internal struggles over priorities to prevent them from setting tighter limits on the process.

The Community

Participating in this process were several community people who seemed to be divisible into three camps, each with its followers and assumptions: the "militants" (West Organization and Black Students), the "brokers," seasoned veterans of previous civil rights confrontations but seen by the others as outsiders (predominately Elson and Craft); and the "moderates" (school principals, teachers, school–community representatives, settlement house staff, and clergymen). It should first be noted that the "militants" and the "brokers" were politically sophisticated as a result of previous community confrontations and participation in civil rights activities.

In retrospect, the "militants" seemed to be operating on the assumption that social programs had always been a failure. Therefore the central task was not to "participate in the planning" of useless social programs but to get their hands on the money or to get jobs for local residents. The latter was the consistent theme through the long months of the negotiations. At least if jobs were provided for some community people, the money would not be entirely wasted. They seemed to be much more dubious that any social good might come of the program itself.

By contrast, the "moderates" seemed to believe that the program might provide real service to the neighborhood, which had been virtually without resources of any kind. They were most anxious to get over the wrangling and to recruit staff to see patients. They were pleased to see the storefront opened rapidly, albeit temporarily, at the Park District fieldhouse.

The "brokers" seemed somewhere in the middle. They believed in the importance of providing service to the community, but felt that community control or involvement in the service was critical. It is important to remember that they were few in numbers and outsiders, a substantial disadvantage in a community such as this in which people are so suspicious of those they don't know (4).

In addition, the paralysis of the black staff of the storefront needs a closer look. At one time there were at least ten members of that staff, some of whom were experienced professionals. That they never played a major role in the negotiations and confrontations was undoubtedly because of the difficult position that they were in, caught between the demands of the black community with which they strongly identified and the professional values that they had worked hard to achieve. In a particularly tenuous position was Mr. Worth, the storefront chief. He had grown up in the neighborhood, had gone on to college and prominence as a basketball player, and had subsequently worked in an administrative capacity at a nearby agency. But his approval by the Advisory Committee was capped by comments from Mrs. Elson, "The only reason I question his appointment is because you people (Dr. Grant and the staff) like him!" and by Mr. Lawrence, "We'll be able to deal with him!" Mr. Worth did not want to be seen as a "Tom"; and yet as storefront director his salary was paid by the hospital, and he worked for Dr. Grant. That these staff members were paralyzed by their conflicts was evidenced by their relative inaction and the fact that most of them resigned by the time the negotiations were completed in late spring.

The two community organizations then used confrontation tactics effectively enough to gain the day. There were few attempts by community people to challenge their leadership. Initially the "brokers" dominated the advisory committee, but they were unseated on the night of the Black Caucus, when the entire group united behind the leadership of West Organization and Black Students. On another occasion, Dr. Grant was invited to meet with a group of mothers and teachers who were dissatisfied with the direction the advisory group had taken. Both the chairman of the Advisory Committee and the Storefront Director accompanied him, and all three encouraged this dissident group to speak up at the next meeting of the group. When they did so, as noted above, a speech by one of the leaders of West Organization about the dominant role of women in black society quieted them. Finally, after the decision to subcontract with the two organizations and after the period of the case history, the Director of one of the settlement houses wrote to the Governor decrying the outcome. But he had been relatively inactive in the process that had taken place in the community itself, and his pleas were to no avail.

The Outcome

How are we to view a situation in which an attempt to foster a democratic process to seek community representation goes awry? Do we insist on democratic rules and refuse to recognize those who have emerged victorious? Some have argued cogently for such a choice (5). It seems to us, however, that it depends on the goals to be achieved and on how undemocratic the tactics used. Wolfe has pointed out that in confrontation tactics whites representing institutions are never in real danger because of the recognition that such tactics would not achieve the desired goals (6).

In the process described in the case history, violence was never used. Threat tactics were prevalent, but negotiation, discussion, speech making, and compromise were also demonstrated. Moreover, it was apparent that people from other factions of the community agreed with much that the community organizations were trying to do. Speeches or comments by leaders of the organizations often met with nods of approval by others present in the meeting, and the group did unite behind the organizations' leadership on several occasions.

In addition, it must be remembered that an early contention of the Program Director was that these two groups were central to his strategy of community development. They had taken an active stance in the struggle for jobs, services, and people's rights in the past, and he felt that such a position was necessary in view of the social and political conditions facing the community. Thus when it became apparent that these two organizations were coming to dominate the process evolving in the community, he was unwilling to intervene, both because he feared that such intervention would not succeed and because he feared that the organizations would be driven away if it did succeed.

The ultimate test, of course, is the effectiveness of the program developed with the two organizations, that is, whether the Program can provide effective services to the community and whether it can provide community residents an experience of having a meaningful impact on one social program. One might argue that, with regard to the latter, only the few community residents involved in the process would be affected. The task is to try to encourage the organizations to foster the participation of others in such a process.

An area of concern for many people is that psychiatric services delivered to the community under such auspices will be ineffective or incompetent. The first line of defense will be local counselors selected by the two organizations from residents of the neighborhood. Most of these have had a high school education or less and have had little training in dealing with the emotionally disturbed. The denigration of professionalism so apparent at the two organizations will contribute further to this. There is, however, another side to this. Mental health professionals, recruited by the organizations, work alongside the counselors on a regular basis. In fact there is now a request for more professional time. Patients posing difficult problems are readily discussed with these professionals or referred to the Medical Center institutions for further work. Reports are that the counselors are more willing to use professionals than in the beginning. Training programs have not been nearly so effective as on-the-job supervision and discussion. The professional staff is impressed by some of the difficult problems that have been handled very effectively by the counselors. Only time will tell us how effective this approach is, but the working together of professionals and counselors is the important ingredient in determining the outcome.

A second objection is that the resources will be diverted from their "proper" use to tasks deemed more critical by the organizations. Salvador Minuchin made an important point in this regard when he noted that while professionals often welcome nonprofessionals into their systems for the many worthwhile reasons often cited, what they do not bargain for is the degree to which the system will be changed in the process (7). In mental health, such an arrangement brings with it the conceptualizations cherished by nonprofessionals, one of which is that mental illness is more a function of a rotten social fabric than of early life experiences. Professionals are willing to be broad-minded about certain things; but when it comes to challenging the very concepts on which the mental health professions are based, that is going too far. "Open housing, school desegregation, and so on, OK—but not our cherished ideas!" If resources are diverted by the two organizations from work in the classical mode with patients and their families (however much disguised by newer or more relevant techniques) to work on the social fabric, that is heresy. Or is it? As Minuchin suggests, ultimately the solution must rest on a new conceptualization and a functional division of labor based on a confrontation of ideas, however painful.

There are other risks as well. Such an approach may foster division within the community by supporting one group at the expense of another. Or the community organizations may be co-opted and thus diverted from their main task of speaking for the people. Or a social program may risk being abolished by conservative forces that denounce the use of funds in such a manner.

Measured against these risks, however, are considerable gains. These have to do with the provision of services and programs that deal with core issues as defined by the community leadership. They also include the incorporation of mental health goals by that same leadership. Another advantage is opening up social institutions so that they may focus more centrally on societal and individual problems. In addition, the theories and practices held by professionals will be tested severely; if sound, they will emerge strengthened. If not, they will be altered as a result of the new data. Most basic, however, is what is to be gained by opening society as a whole to "intruders" who have been heretofore excluded. In the process, the struggle will be monumental. The outcome should be that the emergent social fabric will be different, but strengthened.

REFERENCES

1. Freed, H., and Miller, L. "Planning a Community Mental Health Program: A case history." *Community Mental Health Journal,* 7, pp. 107–117, 1971.
2. Ellis, W. E. *White Ethics and Black Power,* Chicago, Aldine Publishing Co., 1969.
3. Banfield, E. G. *Political Influence,* New York, The Free Press of Glencoe, 1961.
4. Suttles, G. D. *The Social Order of the Slum,* Chicago, The University of Chicago Press, 1968.
5. Walzer, M. "The Obligations of Oppressed Minorities," *Commentary,* 49, pp. 71–80, May 1970.
6. Wolfe, T. "Mau-Mauing the Flak Catchers," in *Radical Chic and Mau-Mauing the Flak Catchers.* New York, Farrar, Straus & Giroux, 1970.
7. Minuchin, S. "The Paraprofessional and the Use of Confrontation in the Mental Health Field," *American Journal of Orthopsychiatry,* 39 (5), pp. 722–729, October 1969.

COMMUNITY DEVELOPMENT AND POLITICS IN THE ORGANIZATION OF A DRUG ABUSE PROGRAM

22

Harvey M. Freed, William Gschwend, Bruce Denner

The literature of community mental health tends to underemphasize the gap between theory and implementation. Yet administrators know that translating ideas into action is more difficult than finding the ideas themselves. The intense politicking engaged in by administrators in any setting means convincing, persuading, cajoling, and pressuring people in order to achieve desired objectives. Working in the community, however, adds another complex dimension to the already complicated task.

It is much easier to sustain one's own morale, interest, and perseverance when you have control over the forces in any particular situation. This is more likely to be the case in clinical work since the clinician is usually the only change agent working with the individual, family, or group, and so on. Similarly, the administrator of a mental health program that is not community-based usually deals with fellow mental health professionals who speak the same language, even if they don't always agree. But in community work one must work with community leaders, groups, or institutions who have other priorities, who view the invading professionals with suspicion, and who are jealous of their "obviously unlimited" resources. Community mental health work involves engaging such people, sometimes influencing them, but just as often being influenced by them. Under such circumstances one must cope with the constant counter-pressures and resistances brought to bear on any plan, and one must continually compromise and bargain but without stripping the initial program plan of so much of its substance that it is alive but not well. An acquaintance responsible for developing drug

Dr. Freed is the Director of the Community Mental Health Program at the Illinois Mental Health Institutes of the Illinois Department of Mental Health and Associate Professor of Psychiatry in the Department of Psychiatry of the University of Illinois College of Medicine. Mr. Gschwend is the Director of Community Children's Services, Institute for Juvenile Research of the Medical Center Complex of the Illinois Department of Mental Health. Dr. Denner is the Director of Staff and Program Development of the Community Mental Health Program at the Illinois Mental Health Institutes of the Illinois Department of Mental Health and Associate Professor of Psychology in the Department of Psychiatry of the University of Illinois College of Medicine.

abuse programs in an urban area recently told me his goal was simply to "get a program going and get out alive."

To illustrate the process we will present a case history of the development of a drug abuse program by a community mental health program (CMHP) with a strong commitment to community development. By that we mean a commitment to seek out, to work with, and to support the development of community leadership that can promote the development of planning and action by community people to meet their needs.[1] We hope the case history will illustrate some of the complicated forces a mental health worker actually meets with.

Case History

In the fall of 1969, the CMHP was site visited by its funding agency, the National Institute of Mental Health (NIMH) and was reminded of the priority of drug abuse. But the Center, like most others in their early years, had been preoccupied with its own survival. Making the paper resources a reality had been a full-time job, described elsewhere (1, 2, 3). In short four institutions served a population of 130,000, divided into relatively segregated blocks of Mexicans, blacks, and Central-Eastern Europeans. An outpost had been open for close to two years in the Mexican area, and another was just getting under way in the Central European area. Both were staffed with professionals and nonprofessionals in the usual manner. In the black community, however, there was a subcontract arrangement with two community organizations, West Organization and Black Students, whose militancy had forced the issue. That outcome, while a pragmatic political solution, had nevertheless been consistent with the ideology of supporting community leadership and of capturing the attention and involvement of the men of the area whose energies and talents seemed critical to the task of rebuilding the community (2).

The site visit had come at a time only a few months after the first annual subcontract had been negotiated on July 1, 1969. The process leading to the subcontract had dragged on for a year, was arduous, and had led to intense and bitter feelings on all sides. Dr. Grant, the CMHP Director, could hardly contemplate dealing with drug abuse in addition to all else.

[1] The rationale for this approach is that in some very deteriorated or impoverished communities the development of service programs of any kind is like trying to fill the proverbial leaking bucket. Thus the service programs should be developed in such a way as to promote community development because local residents ultimately have much more responsibility for and stake in the welfare of the community than do outsiders.

He therefore seized the opportunity presented to him when the Director of the State Drug Abuse Program (SDAP) called a few weeks later proposing collaboration. Dr. Grant visited the SDAP offices and was impressed, but insisted on involving West Organization in the planning. He then spoke with Mr. Darling, of West Organization, and suggested that the former visit SDAP himself.

In retrospect, this was a critical decision. It must be understood in the context of the long, painful year of negotiations with the black community that led to the subcontracts. Dr. Grant was anxious to develop effective working relationships with the two organizations. And since his working assumption was that the main problem with drugs in the catchment area was in the black neighborhood, it seemed reasonable to involve one of the organizations from the beginning. Since the constant use of abrasive, disruptive confrontation tactics by Black Students during the preceding year had been such an irritant to Dr. Grant, he chose to work with West Organization. The latter, while itself no patsy, had used confrontation tactics that, while militant, were not so abrasive.[2] In addition, West Organization was clearly the more established, more mature organization with an already proven track record, and often wound up in the role of mediator between Black Students and the CMHP.

When a few weeks had passed and West Organization still had not made the visit, Dr. Grant inquired and learned that aside from the usual scheduling problems, West Organization leaders had taken some time to learn about SDAP through their network of contacts in the city. They learned that SDAP seemed research-oriented, was centrally controlled, and was not as concerned with community involvement as with the expansion of service programs. Under more prodding from Dr. Grant, a meeting was finally arranged but ended without plans for collaboration because of the disagreement in philosophy between West Organization and SDAP. Dr. Grant was puzzled and annoyed because he had not anticipated West Organization's refusal to cooperate. He therefore had a private conference with Mr. Darling, who had led the West Organization negotiating team, to discuss the matter. During the conference he expressed his annoyance at not knowing what West Organization had had in mind and said that he would have to be brought into West Organization's confidence if they were to collaborate effectively. In return he learned that West Organization felt it was critical to have control over any programs it was to be involved in. He also learned that West Organization had prepared and submitted grant applications previously, and had been refused funds, only to learn of other organizations being

---

[2] While confrontation tactics are often effective in forcing change when other strategies have failed, extreme militancy may cause a reaction.

funded for similar programs. Dr. Grant left the conference with a better understanding of West Organization's motivations and of Mr. Darling, and with greater personal commitment to continue to work with West Organization to develop a drug abuse program despite its insistence on control.

The insistence on control, however, did pose some problems for him. How would Black Students react to not having a major voice in the planning of the program? Mr. Darling reassured Dr. Grant that West Organization had an understanding with Black Students and that there would be no trouble. Nevertheless, Dr. Grant took the trouble to tell Mr. Lawrence, leader of Black Students that, while he was working with West Organization on a drug abuse program, he would subsequently work with Black Students on an alcoholism program. While this was a sincere gesture, it came more immediately from the need to forestall an angry response from Black Students than from careful program planning.

Shortly thereafter, Mr. Mitchell, a person known to West Organization, showed up and announced himself as a candidate for the directorship of the drug abuse program. He was a fifty-year-old black ex-addict with a long history of addiction followed by successful rehabilitation at Lexington and elsewhere. He had learned of the developing program through the grapevine, had contacted West Organization, and inquired about the position. Mr. Darling had made some inquiries about him, had learned that he had been employed as one of the first staff members of SDAP, had left because of a disagreement with other staff, and was now employed at another drug abuse program in the city. Dr. Grant agreed to Mr. Mitchell's appointment primarily because of his growing confidence in Mr. Darling, who supported Mr. Mitchell's request.

With Mr. Mitchell now on the CMHP payroll temporarily as a community worker until special funding could be obtained, two developmental lines began to occur simultaneously. Together, all three men continued to plan for the preparation of a grant request, while Mr. Mitchell assumed the initiative in beginning to organize a clinical program with existing resources.

During the winter of 1969–1970, the three men educated themselves about drug abuse. Both Mitchell and Darling knew the issues at the street level and were convinced that an approach that combined medical and psychological treatment with community work was essential. Grant knew very little about drug abuse at all but was eager to learn. Reading whatever information was available, visiting hospitals and community centers, working with addicts, obtaining consultation from experienced professionals, and exchanging ideas, the three men began to formulate a plan. At the same time, contacts were made with potential funding agencies. Federal, state, city, and private agencies were all involved in discussions. While all were sympathetic, since the new program was to be connected with a community mental health program, most of the agencies advised that additional NIMH community mental health center funding seemed to be the best route. At the same time, matching funds would again be necessary (the state provides the matching funds for the CMHP), and in any case all applications for drug abuse grants would have to filter through a committee at the state level anyway. It seemed obvious that the next step was to put the plan on paper and to submit it to the State Department of Mental Hygiene, ultimately the agency to which the CMHP was responsible and which had an important influence on the state-wide review committee on drug programs.

By February a preliminary program plan was on paper and distributed to a number of people and agencies for comments. By that time three patients at a time were being detoxified in the hospital in three beds made available on the CMHP unit for that purpose. Dr. Grant left for a vacation in March, pleased with the progress thus far. He returned to a hornet's nest.

During his absence there had been growing dissatisfaction in the other communities served by the CMHP about the drug abuse program. Questions were raised about the appropriateness of West Organization sponsoring a program to serve the other areas. In fact, a few Mexican addicts were threatening to split off from the core group and to develop an independent program.

To complicate matters further, the hospital was experiencing a number of problems with the addicts. Detoxification was not proving successful, as addicts were returning to the community and to heroin immediately on discharge. In addition, since addicts did not see themselves as mentally ill, and staff tended to agree with them, at best they did not fit in with the milieu on the ward and at worst they were disruptive. There were also the problems of an increase in thefts in the hospital (attributed to the addicts), addicts using the hospital as a refuge, charges that passes were being made at nurses, and so on, all of this exaggerated by the stereotypes and projections of hospital staff. In part, this was a recapitulation of what was experienced earlier in the history of the CMHP when "community patients" began to be admitted to the hospital in droves. Those patients had been seen as dirty, chronic, untreatable, and so on. These patients were likewise caricatured as conniving, dangerous, thieving, and so on.

In short there was a breakdown of the program on two fronts: in the community as well as in the hospital. The response of Mr. Mitchell, and the developing cadre of addicts and ex-addicts around him, on the one hand, and the West Organization, on the other, made the situation potentially very explosive. The latter saw the criticisms as racist attacks, based on the idea that blacks were not competent to develop a program that would serve others; the former had similar views but were perhaps more responsive to their identification with the addiction culture, seeing themselves once again threatened with ostracism, disappointment, and isolation.

As far as the community was concerned, the task was to see that the interest of all groups was protected, while at the same time to mollify the intense anger building in the West Organization and among the addicts. To illustrate the intensity of the anger, suffice it to mention that Mr. Lawrence of Black Students broke up a meeting with some consultants from the NIMH drug abuse staff by storming in, shouting his disapproval, and walking out. Shortly thereafter his staff threatened and badly beat one of the ex-addicts working closely with Mr. Mitchell in an effort to learn more about the supposed funding of the developing program. (Mr. Mitchell was still the only staff member whose salary was paid by the CMHP.) Mr. Lawrence was especially angry because the promised alcoholism program was nowhere to be seen.

Several months were spent in trying to solve the political problems posed by the drug abuse program. Much of the necessary groundwork was done by Dr. Grant in individual meetings with Mr. Darling and the directors of the outposts in the Mexican and Central-Eastern European communities. Mr. Darling and Mr. Mitchell worked with Mr. Lawrence and Black Students. An incident of major import occurred shortly thereafter. In June of 1970, the man who was appointed by Mr. Lawrence to direct the mental health program at Black Students was convicted of a murder and was imprisoned. This event threatened Black Students' existence, but CMHP, after much soul-searching, decided to continue its support. Under the circumstances, however, Mr. Lawrence was in no position to press his luck.

Toward the end of July, an agreement was reached among all parties that called for an advisory board to Mr. Mitchell, the Director of the Drug Abuse Program. It was to be composed of two representatives from each neighborhood served by the CMHP—one from the community and the second to be the outpost director or his designate. As for the relationship between West Organization and the CMHP re the drug abuse program, a contract was to be written between the two parties defining their relationship, which was to be enforced by the Director of the CMHP. It called for a one-year contract with a thirty-day cancellation clause, presumably the ultimate weapon of the CMHP Director. The agreement, while completely satisfactory to no one, did permit the continued development of the program, which had been blocked for some months by the discord. To a great extent, it was negotiated because of the insistence of the CMHP Director, the mounting pressure on all sides for some kind of a settlement, and the weariness of all parties. In fact the advisory committee was never developed, and the agreement did not prevent a splitting off of the Mexican group, which began to develop an independent program.

As for the problems on the hospital front, the pressure was relieved to some extent by the decision to abandon inpatient detoxification. The CMHP Director applied for and received an IND number that permitted detoxification and methadone maintenance on an experimental basis for outpatients. Mr. Mitchell and his volunteer staff, however, took squatter's rights to some of the vacant offices and an empty ward in the hospital. The program was attracting adherents because of Mr. Mitchell's charisma and because no programs had been developed in the city's large West Side. There was increasing unrest on the part of hospital administration and staff because the drug abuse program seemed to be expanding despite all efforts to contain it. Its volunteer staff was not beholden to the hospital authorities and would sometimes flaunt its opposition to hospital regulations when they seemed arbitrary and oppressive. There was a tendency for addicts to see the hospital as rich with resources but ungiving, and to ignore the many pressures the hospital faced. Both Dr. Grant and Mr. Mitchell had numerous meetings with hospital officials and department heads, as well as with addict patients, in an effort to increase understanding. Fortunately, the Director of the hospital was also the Medical Center Director, and was fully committed to the CMHP. While the drug abuse program posed innumerable headaches for him, his support was the bedrock on which all negotiations, meetings, and agreements took place. Gradually, hospital administration and staff, and the drug abuse program staff and patients, began to work out a modus vivendi, again, completely satisfactory to no one but sufficient to ease the pressures considerably.

By August, Mr. Darling of West Organization, Mr. Mitchell of the Drug Abuse Program, and Dr. Grant of the CMHP began again to work in earnest on a funding proposal. This time, however, it had become clearer that West Organization had some sanction from the CMHP and its various outposts to develop the drug abuse program for the CMHP. A proposal was drafted by September 1, 1970, and was submitted through channels to the Department of Mental Hygiene. The proposal asked for $260,000 for West Organization to develop a neighborhood-based "Drug Abuse Rehabilitation and Training Center." The plan was to rehabilitate a building that would serve as a base for community work, psychological and medical treatment. The idea was to involve a number of social systems, including the health, educational, welfare, and criminal justice systems, among others, at the local level. The Center would develop teams with expertise in the field who would fan out and provide educational workshops and training to all those on the Greater West Side and elsewhere who were interested in the problem of drug abuse. It was to employ local people and ex-addicts wherever possible. While a major interest was to serve the addicts of the black community, the proposal cited as its boundaries those of the CMHP catchment area, with secondary priority given to a larger area that was predominantly black.

The formal proposal was rejected by the Department of Mental Hygiene, based on the fact that all of the funds allocated for drug abuse programs for the fiscal year had already been spent. This response was not unexpected, but it paved the way for a direct appeal by the CMHP Director and the Medical Center Director to the Director of the Department of Mental Hygiene. Meetings were held, first without the Director of the SDAP, and subsequently with him. While he still had misgivings about the community approach West Organization was proposing he finally agreed to offer to fund the program with $40,000 to begin with, but insisted on tying it into the SDAP via the reporting procedure. In essence, the program would be similar to the many programs throughout the state that SDAP had already subcontracted with. The Director of SDAP had the full support of the Director of the Department of Mental Hygiene in this plan; both felt strongly that funding could only come under the SDAP umbrella because of legal and fiscal requirements.

Dr. Grant was disappointed but tried to convince West Organization to begin with the $40,000 and to build on that. Mr. Darling, however, thought that the price to be paid for the money was too much. He noted that West Organization would be controlled by SDAP after all; one year of effort to develop a community-run drug program would have failed and the community approach to the problem would not have been given a chance. A couple of meetings were held between Dr. Grant, Mr. Darling, Mr. Mitchell, and the Director of the Department of Mental Hygiene, but neither side would compromise. These conversations lasted through most of the winter of 1970–1971, finally ending without result.

By this time West Organization was more determined than ever to find other sources of funding. Mr. Darling and others contacted private foundations, representatives of several levels of government, and so on. These efforts were without the assistance or even consultation of Dr. Grant, who was now, to some extent, considered persona non grata. Since Dr. Grant had not produced, Mr. Darling felt that he had "sold out" to the professional system when the chips were down and had refused to press hard enough for community control. In addition, West

Organization was working without the collaboration of Mr. Mitchell and his staff; to a degree they were "tainted" by their location in the hospital and their close working relationship with the CMHP staff. West Organization worked alone, using friendships and political pressure wherever possible. At one point during the spring of 1971, Dr. Grant tried to dissuade Mr. Darling from continuing the search for funds. Grant argued that Darling would only be discouraged, and he was particularly vexed with some of West Organization's "friends" in positions of political leadership who had promised funding. He tried to encourage Darling to begin the job with existing resources and to build slowly. All of this was to no avail, however. Mr. Darling was determined.

The addict patients and Mr. Mitchell and his staff were also discouraged. They felt trapped between the CMHP, which had, they felt, offered relatively little in the way of substantive support, and the West Organization, which had refused to compromise. The dissatisfactions were intensified by another NIMH site visit in January of 1971 in which the site visitors were "appalled" by the fact that the CMHP had been able to provide such little support to the drug program. Space, medication, some laboratory and medical support, and three salaries were all that had been supplied. The patients now numbered over one hundred; many people had volunteered their time, had chipped in some funds from their earnings, had sold chicken dinners, and run benefits in an effort to keep the program alive. The turn of events had been very discouraging. At West Organization the same site visitors had been told that the CMHP could "go to hell" if the drug program was not funded.

Nevertheless, during the spring of 1971, addicts continued to be served by the program; the CMHP waited to see whether West Organization would be successful in obtaining funding—little could be done in the interim; West Organization worked furiously, contacting people, writing proposals, altering them to suit the needs of the various funding agencies, and visiting officials in the state and national capitals.

In the Mexican community, however, the independent program had now developed on its own and was seeking support, both financial and otherwise. Whereas initially fewer than ten Mexican addicts had expressed dissatisfaction with the developing program, by now the number had grown considerably. There was disappointment that the Advisory Committee and agreements about the existing program serving all communities had not worked. Whereas West Organization was willing to serve Mexicans, and had included some Mexicans on the small staff of its program, the Chicanos now wanted their own separate program. This had to be understood in the context of the "Brown Power" movement that was sweeping the country and to which certain Mexican community leaders were linked. The Mexican addicts had by this time split completely from the West Organization program, had incorporated, calling themselves ARRIBA, and were obtaining their methadone from a Mexican physician at a nearby Catholic hospital. They were running their own program based in the CMHP outpost in the Mexican community, and were growing in size. Dr. Grant was invited to a special meeting in a local settlement house with representatives of ARRIBA and some of the leadership of the Mexican community to discuss the needs of the new organization. He explained the history of the drug program to date, explained why he had supported the efforts of West Organization to develop a single program for the entire catchment area, and outlined the situation, namely that West Organization was seeking funds independently for the drug program. He felt that there was little that he could do for either group at the moment because he had no additional resources. He encouraged ARRIBA leaders to talk with West Organization leaders. He did, however, agree to include ARRIBA in any future planning. ARRIBA was loathe to collaborate with West Organization; instead a grant proposal was prepared and submitted to a federal agency, but was not funded.

West Organization, on the other hand, after close to two years of effort, finally succeeded in obtaining funding for three years from the Social and Rehabilitation Service of the Federal Government. Funding was in the neighborhood of $210,000 for each of the three years, and called for an emphasis on the rehabilitation of addicts and job placement. The medical and psychiatric support services would have to be negotiated with the CMHP or other medical agencies, according to the funders. This time, however, the West Organization proposal placed first priority on a larger west side area, which was primarily black, and second priority on the catchment area of the CMHP. Shortly after that, a new Director of SDAP was appointed (a man more committed to the concept of community involvement) who came to West Organization to negotiate an additional contract for $40,000, with a promise of more to come if all went well.

The only fly in the ointment remained the dissatisfaction of ARRIBA. Its leadership had approached the new Director of SDAP for funding of their own, and he had refused, based on his already having negotiated an agreement with West Organization to provide services for the entire catchment area of the CMHP. Under no circumstances did he want to abrogate his responsibility to West Organization since he felt that it held the key to the development of other services on the city's populous west side.

Dr. Grant, under pressure from the Director of his outpost in the Mexican area who was working closely with ARRIBA, called the Director of SDAP to discuss the matter. In response to the Director's inquiry as to the significance of the splinter group, Dr. Grant indicated that it would be difficult to argue that a group of Chicanos was less able to speak for the Mexican community than a group of blacks. While Dr. Grant had initially hoped that the groups would be able to work together, West Organization's insistence on control, coupled with the hardening attitude of the Chicanos in the same direction, precluded that possibility.

The question now was how best to serve both groups. It seemed that the only solution was to promote the development of completely independent programs, giving the individual addicts free choice in determining which program to participate in. The question was, how to fund ARRIBA without alienating West Organization. Together, Dr. Grant and the Director of SDAP thought of a solution. SDAP was prepared to invest additional funds to provide West Organization with the wherewithal to buy its pharmacy and laboratory support from the Medical Center parent of the CMHP (which West Organization wanted) in return for a release from West Organization, which would enable SDAP to negotiate independently with ARRIBA.

This is the proposal that Dr. Grant made to West Organization. Mr. Darling was hesitant to accept the trade-off, as it might imply that West Organization was unwilling to serve the Mexican community. Dr. Grant told Mr. Darling that he understood and respected that position, and yet it could be maintained by giving the individual patients the opportunity to select the program of their choice.

Just prior to the formal negotiations between the CMHP and West Organization regarding support for the drug abuse program, ARRIBA went to the regional office of HEW to complain about not receiving adequate support for its program. As a result of this, NIMH became involved again and put pressure on Dr. Grant to resolve the issue. Dr. Grant mentioned that he hoped the aforementioned trade-off would result from the negotiations. However, when West Organization came to the negotiating table, it had succeeded in obtaining other sources of revenue to support its request for pharmacy and laboratory support from the Medical Center. West Organization was adamant in its refusal to give up exclusive rights to the entire catchment area.

At the time of this writing, ARRIBA was in the process of preparing another grant request to NIMH for independent funding. This was at the suggestion of the NIMH drug abuse division in Washington, which said it would support such a request, in view of the circumstances. By now, most observers had come to the conclusion that the only viable solution was two independent programs. Importantly, however, West Organization still expressed the hope that ARRIBA would not try to develop an independent program but would negotiate with it about the services in the Mexican community. The regional office of NIMH, on the other hand, while reluctantly supporting the development of independent programs, was unhappy about the prospect of potentially overlapping or uncoordinated drug abuse programs.

Discussion

Throughout this history the goal of the community program was to develop a drug abuse program as well as to support community development. The probable outcome will be the development of two separate, independent drug abuse programs by black and Mexican community groups. And these two programs will be run by community organizations that are independent of the CMHP. How do we understand the process that led to this outcome, and what inferences may be drawn from it?

Two separate drug abuse programs serving different segments of the catchment area population are clearly not what the planners had in mind at the outset. Such an outcome is not consistent with the community mental health principle of coordinated services. Nevertheless, the outcome is consistent with the greater priority that this particular community mental health program places on community development. That is the important fact. For example, in the case history above, the emergence of ARRIBA as a force was not anticipated. When, however, ARRIBA did arise, the question was whether to insist on ARRIBA working with West Organization or to permit the group to develop an independent program. An approach that places a high priority on encouraging people to plan for themselves, such as this one did, would be likely to favor the independence of various groups. Perhaps later, after a sense of identity and self-determination has solidified in both groups, they will be more willing to work with each other.

Other major actions on the part of the CMHP administrators were also consistent with the idea of encouraging community groups to plan and implement programs to meet their needs. The early decision to support West Organization's refusal to work with SDAP, the many hours spent meeting with hospital personnel to explain the program, the decision to support West Organization's wish to seek independent funding rather than go through the CMHP—all of these and more are examples of carrying out the approach of community development.

And yet, what occurred was much more than simply carrying out a plan of action based on a particular approach. For example, the decision to support ARRIBA's wish to be independent of West Organization was also based on the important fact that ARRIBA's wish was backed up by the leadership of the Mexican community and their absolute refusal to work with West Organization. Even if the administrators had wanted ARRIBA to work with West Organization, there is probably very little that they could have done to bring that about. That a CMHP administrator is sometimes in a position where there is very little that he can to do influence a process once it has begun to unfold is an important point that needs emphasis.

In describing how important political decisions were made in a major city in the early 1960s, Edward Banfield (5) noted that the system of forces could be described as a pluralistic one. The banks, the press, major industries, the hospitals, and so on, all were part of that system. On any particular issue, however, some of these components were very involved, while others had less at stake. The mayor had the alternative of waiting to see how the forces would line up and then entering on the side of those with more power and influence, or of playing a much more active role by throwing his weight behind one side early in the contest in an attempt to help it gain the day. Actually, the mayor played an intermediate role, using what Banfield described as a "mixed" model, sometimes waiting and sometimes leading.

While a community mental health program is ostensibly a tighter administrative unit than a city can ever be, the analogy holds. A CMHP, like a city, is a system. Its components are not limited to its funded units or to its Table of Organization. They likewise include various community groups or constituencies, such as patients, funding bodies, private agencies, governmental units, and so on. Using the example of the Drug Abuse Program, it may be seen that NIMH took the lead in making the problem an issue in the first place. Dr. Grant then followed up on this by pursuing the opportunity offered to him by the Director of SDAP for collaboration. He next decided to involve West Organization in the process and even to support it in its early decision to refuse to collaborate with SDAP. He likewise took an active role in forging the compromise among the various contending community forces that permitted West Organization to continue its attempts to develop a program to serve the entire catchment area. As time went on, however, it became more apparent that the Mexican group, in particular, was dissatisfied, and after his attempts to obtain funding from the Department of Mental Hygiene failed, he decided to wait and see what would develop. At this point he shifted from a much more active leadership role to a much more passive one, awaiting the outcome of West Organization's quest for funding and the results of ARRIBA's dissatisfaction. In any case, by this time West Organization no longer offered him an opportunity to play as active a role in program development. This was just as well because by now ARRIBA had become established and was becoming more resentful at his working on behalf of West Organization but not for ARRIBA.

During this phase he did nothing but hold the same ground, telling the Mexicans that he could do no more while awaiting the outcome of the West Organization grant proposal. When, however, the West Organization proposal was funded by a federal agency, *and* the new Director of SDAP hurriedly negotiated an additional contract as well, the situation was different. The entire system was too much out of balance, with West Organization having two contracts and ARRIBA none.

CMHP administrators must attend to keeping the system in balance. The various components of a CMHP will all press for their individual needs, and the Director must often respond to issues that at that moment are most pressing. In the case history above, the greatest strain on the system, in the beginning, was the bad relationship between the black community and the CMHP. Likewise the insistence by NIMH on the development of a drug program was an issue in that NIMH was the funding agency. Subsequently, the resentment expressed by the communities toward West Organization's control of the drug program, West Organization's anger at not being funded by the State Department of Mental Hygiene, and most recently, ARRIBA's anger at being excluded, each in turn put great strain on the CMHP as a system.

What may seem like rank opportunism, namely, responding to "the squeaky wheel," is actually a time-honored political way of being responsive to the various constituencies that any program director must satisfy. It seems that the challenge of leadership is to try to walk the tightrope between moving a system in the direction of desired objectives and responding to the very real needs of the people who make up that system.

REFERENCES

1. Freed, Harvey M., and Miller, Louis, "Planning a Community Mental Health Center: A Case History," *Community Mental Health Journal*, 7, 107–117, 1971.
2. Freed, Harvey M., Schroder, D. J., and Baker B., "Community Participation in Mental Health Services: A Case of Factional Control," *Mental Health in Rapid Social Change*, Jerusalem Academic Press, 1971.
3. Freed, Harvey M., "Subcontracts for Community Development and Service," presented to American Psychiatric Association at the May 1–5, 1972, annual meeting in Dallas, Texas.
4. Ellis, E. W. *White Ethics and Black Power*, Chicago, Aldine Publishing Co., 1969.
5. Banfield, E. G. *Political Influence*, New York, The Free Press of Glencoe, 1961.

CLINICAL INNOVATION AND THE MENTAL HEALTH POWER STRUCTURE: A SOCIAL CASE HISTORY

23

Anthony M. Graziano

The 1960s have been a decade of increased involvement by social scientists and educators in the problems and welfare of society. Turning their professional acumen to the very old problems of employment, housing, education, poverty, mental health, and others, many have heard the repeated call to "innovate" creative and "bold new approaches" to our vexing social problems. The ensuing increase in new programs, all actively seeking humanitarian goals, has led many of us to suspect that humanitarian aims and scientific methodology have finally come together and melded into a broad new mobilization of the previously unfocused humane and scientific strengths of our culture. In the field of mental health we have seen new developments in the use of subprofessional manpower, the development of behavior-modification approaches to therapy, and plans to develop new comprehensive community mental health centers designed to increase the scope of services.

The common sound in those approaches is "innovation"; it is in the air, and in these conceptually fertile sixties many innovative ideas have been conceived and put forth. However, it should be clearly noted that the *conception* of innovative ideas in mental health depends upon creative humanitarian and scientific forces, while their *implementation* depends, not on science or humanitarianism, but on a broad spectrum of professional and social politics!

The main points of this paper are (1) that these two aspects, conceiving innovation through science and humanitarianism on the one hand, and implementing innovation through politics on the other, are directly incompatible and mutually inhibiting factors; and (2) our pursuit of political power has almost totally replaced humanitarian and scientific ideals in the mental health field. Innovations, by definitions, introduce change; political power structures resist change. Thus, while

Paper presented at the meeting of the Eastern Psychological Association, Washington, D. C., April 1968. Reprinted from the *American Psychologist*, 1969, 24, 10–18. Copyright 1969 by the American Psychological Association, and reproduced by permission. Anthony M. Graziano is at the State University of New York at Buffalo.

the cry for innovation has been heard throughout the 1960s, we must clearly recognize that it has been innovative "talking" that has been encouraged, while innovative *action* has been resisted. It has been the "nature of the sixties," as it were, to simultaneously encourage and dampen innovation in mental health. A major question for the next decade is: Following this "reciprocal inhibition" of both innovative and "status quo" responses, which of the two will emerge strongest, and what are we, as psychologists, doing about it?

The following discussion is an attempt to trace the progress of innovative ideas to the level of action, by examining a single case history in which a group of people with new ideas about the treatment of severely disturbed children encountered the resistance of the local mental health power structure. The developments, which cover some eleven years, are briefly described, and, recognizing the danger of generalizing from the single case, we nevertheless do so and attempt to suggest conclusions about our contemporary mental health professions.

The Case History

About eleven years ago a small group of parents sought treatment for autistic children and found available only expensive psychiatrists or the depressing custodialism of back-ward children's units at the state hospital. Local clinics were of little help since they operated on the familiar assumption that their services were best limited to those who could "profit most" from therapy, and, given a choice between a rampaging psychotic child and one with less severe behavior, the clinics tended to treat the latter and send the others off to the state hospitals. Unwilling to accept either deadly placement (private therapists or state hospitals), parents cast around and were eventually referred to the "experts," that is, the same clinics and private-practice psychiatrists who had previously failed to help those children. They were nevertheless still considered to be the proper agents to carry out a new program, now that a few determined *lay* people had thought of it. This is an important and recurrent point, suggesting that any new mental health service or idea, regardless of its origin, is automatically referred back into the control of the same people who had achieved so little in the past, perhaps insuring that little will be done in the future. The territorial claims of professionals, it seems, are seldom challenged, despite what might be a history of failure, irrelevance, or ignorance.

Following some two years of work, the lay group arranged with a local child clinic to create special services for autistic children. The result, a psychoanalytically oriented group program, operated uneasily for four years, amidst laymen–professional controversy over roles, responsibility, finances, and, finally, the program's therapeutic effectiveness. The lay people, rightly seeing themselves as the "originators" of the program, felt that they were being "displaced" by the professionals. The professionals, on the other hand, saw the laymen as naïve, not recognizing their own limitations and trying to preempt clearly professional territory. Threatened and angered, both sides retreated to positions that were more acrimonious than communicative. "Don't trust the professional!" and "Beware the layman!" were often heard in varied ways.

Hostilities grew, the groups split, and, after four years of their cooperative program, these two groups, the "insider" professional clinic with its continuing program and the "outsider" lay group, now determined to have its own program, were directly competing for the same pool of local and state funds.

The clinic, embedded within the professional community, had operated for some twenty-five years and espoused no new, radical, or untried approaches. It argued that it was an experienced, traditional, cooperating part of the local mental health community; that it was properly medically directed; that its approaches were based on "the tried and true methods of psychoanalysis." The clinic based its arguments on experience, professionalism, and stability as a successful community agency, and offered to continue the accepted psychoanalytic methodology.

The "outsiders," having acquired the services of a young and still idealistic psychologist who was just two years out of graduate school, contended that because psychoanalytic approaches had not resulted in significant improvement for autistic children the community should support many reasonable alternative approaches rather than insist upon the pseudoefficiency of a single program to avoid "duplication of services." One alternative was proposed, the modification of behavior through the application of psychological learning theory, that is, *teaching* adaptive behavior rather than *treating* internal sickness. Further, because this approach was psychological, it therefore would properly be psychologically and not medically directed.

Thus they criticized the establishment and proposed change, attempting new approaches based on a psychological rather than medical model and insisting on including poverty children in the program. Naïvely stepping on many toes, they said all the wrong things; one does not successfully seek support from a professionally conservative community by criticizing it and promising to provide new and different services that are grossly at odds with accepted certainties, essentially untried and, in many respects, ambiguous. Early in 1963, to offer psychological learning concepts as alternatives to psychoanalytic treatment of children and to insist that traditional clinics had failed to help low-income children was not well received. From the beginning, then, this group, henceforth referred to as ASMIC (Association for Mentally Ill Children), were cast as "radicals" and "trouble-makers."

Hoping to avoid competing within the clinical structure, ASMIC proposed to the local university in 1963 a small-scale research and training project to develop child-therapy approaches from learning theory, and to select and train nondegree undergraduate and master's level students as child group workers and behavior therapists. It was hoped that, after a year or two of preliminary investigation, federal support would be available through the university. Approved by the chairman and the dean, the proposal was rejected at the higher administrative levels because (1) the project was too radical and would only create continuing controversy; (2) the local mental health professionals had already clearly indicated their opposition to it; and (3) the university, always cognizant of town–gown problems, could not risk becoming involved.

The message was clear: The project was opposed by the local mental health professionals; it had already caused controversy, would create more, and the university was no place for controversy! [sic]

Thus denied the more cloistered university environment, ASMIC moved to compete within the closed-rank mental health agency structure, where they soon encountered what we shall refer to as the United Agency. That agency's annual fund-raising campaign is carried out with intense publicity, and donating through one's place of employment seems to have become somewhat less than voluntary. Operated primarily by business and industrial men the United Agency had some million and a half dollars to distribute to agencies *of their choice,* thus giving a small group of traditionally conservative businessmen considerable power over the city's social-action programs.

Having been advised that ASMIC's proposed program could not long survive, the United Agency's apparent tactic was to delay for a few months, until ASMIC demised quietly. That delaying tactic was implemented as follows:

1. The United Agency listened to ASMIC's preliminary ideas but could not act until they had a written proposal.

2. A month later the United Agency rejected the written proposal because it was only a "paper program"!

3. ASMIC's program was started and expanded but after six months of operation was again denied support because it had been too brief a time on which to base a decision. The group was advised to apply again after a longer period of operation.

4. After a year of operation, ASMIC's next request was denied on the basis that the program had to be "professionally evaluated" before the United Agency could act. And who would carry out the evaluation?

The local mental health professionals, of course. ASMIC objected to being evaluated by their competitors but agreed to an evaluation by the State Department of Mental Health, although they, too, had previously refused to support the program. This was to be the "final" hurdle and, if the evaluation was positive, the United Agency would grant funds for the program.

5. Completing its professional evaluation the State Department returned a highly positive report and strongly recommended that ASMIC be supported. Apparently caught off guard, the United Agency was strangely unresponsive, and several months elapsed before the next request for funds was again deferred, on the basis that the question of "duplication of services" had never been resolved.

6. After additional state endorsement and high praise for the program as a *nonduplicated* service, the United Agency rejected ASMIC's next request, replying that if the state thought so highly of the program, then why did not *they* support it? "Come back," they said, "when you get state support."

7. Six months later and nearly three years after starting the program, ASMIC had a state grant. The United Agency then allocated $3,000.00, which, they said, would be forwarded as soon as ASMIC provided the United Agency with (1) an official tax-exemption statement, (2) the names and addresses of all children who had received ASMIC's services, and (3) the names of the fathers and their employers.

For three years ASMIC had met all of the United Agency's conditions; they had provided a detailed proposal, launched the program, had successfully operated for three years, had expanded, had received high professional evaluations, had resolved the duplication-of-service issue, had provided the tax-exemption voucher but could not, they explained, provide confidential information such as names, addresses, and fathers' places of employment.

The United Agency, however, blandly refused support because ASMIC was, after all, "uncooperative" in refusing to supply the requested information.

ASMIC's final attempts to gain local mental health support was with an agency we will call "Urban Action," whose function, at least partly, was to help ameliorate poverty conditions through federally supported programs.

Arguing that the city had no mental health services of any scope for poverty-level children, ASMIC proposed to apply and evaluate techniques of behavior modification, environmental manipulation, and selection and training of "indigenous" subprofessionals, mothers, and siblings, to help emotionally disturbed poverty-level children.

The written proposal was met with enthusiasm but, the agency explained, in keeping with the concept of "total community" focus, more than one agency had to be involved. They therefore suggested inviting the local mental health association to join the project, even if only on a consultant basis. The mental health association, of course, was comprised of the same professionals who had opposed ASMIC's program from the beginning. Skeptical but nevertheless in good faith, ASMIC distributed copies of their proposal to the mental health association, again referring something new back to the old power structure. Five months later a prediction was borne out; the mental health association returned the proposal as "unworkable" and, in its place, submitted their own highly traditional psychiatric version, which was ultimately rejected in Washington. Those poverty-level children who received no mental health services in 1963, still receive no services, and there are no indications that the situation will be any different in the next few years.

The "outside" group, its new ideas clashing with the professional establishment, repeatedly encountered barriers composed of the same people and never did receive support from the local mental health agencies, the United Agency, the university, or the Urban Action Agency. For the first two years it subsisted on small tuition fees and a spate of cake sales organized by a few determined ladies, and eventually did receive significant state support from the Departments of Education and Mental Health. Thus it carried out its programs, in spite of the opposition and lack of support of the local mental health professionals.

This case history of an innovator ends on two quite ironic points. Moving into its fifth year, ASMIC had successfully overcome all major external obstacles and, having been evaluated by both the State Department of Education and Mental Health, was receiving significant support. The first irony is that having successfully overcome the external opposition, the agency began to disintegrate internally. Having achieved some status, success, and continuing support, it no longer had the cohesive force generated by battling an external foe. Its own internal bickering, previously overshadowed by the "larger battle," now became dominant, and the agency splintered, again along laymen–professional lines. The precipitating factor this time was the professionals' insistence on including poverty-level children, who were nearly all Negro and Puerto Rican. A few lay persons, actively supported in their anger by the professional director of an actively competing agency, objected to the "unfairness" of allowing Negroes into the program "free," that is, supported through a grant, while their "own" children had to pay a small fee. Poverty funds could not be used to support the more affluent white children, as the lay people demanded, and the professional staff was then faced with two main alternatives: (1) abandon the poverty program and work with only middle-class white children or (2) resign from the agency and continue the program under other auspices. The staff decided on the latter alternative.

The second irony is that, while the staff successfully continues its behavior-modification group program, neither the originally sponsoring agency, ASMIC, nor the opposed, traditional, and still well-supported child clinic has been able to maintain its group program for autistic children!

Thus, turning innovation *concepts*, that is, group behavior therapy and the inclusion of low socioeconomic-level children, into actual programs required a good deal more than humanitarian beliefs and scientific objectivity. The eventual reality of the program depended upon its ability to maintain its integrity throughout all of the political buffeting. The program continues today, well supported by the state, but no support was ever obtained from the local mental health area.

Local Agencies as a Field of Parallel Bureaucracies

In spite of the expressed support of the state and of many "outside" professionals, the local traditional agencies, such as the hospital, the clinic, the mental health association, United Agency, city clinics, and Urban Action, all maintained a closed-rank rejection of the program. It seemed apparent that a workable set of relationships among the various mental health agencies had developed over a period of years. In fact "interagency cooperation," ostensibly in the service of clients, seemed also to provide important reciprocal support for the agencies.

Despite overlap, the agencies were differentiated according to major functions: Some were referral sources (schools and churches); some provided services (the hospital, the clinic, the center for retarded children); some were financial supporters (United Agency, Community Chest); some acted as community planners (the Mental Health Association); some had dual functions such as the State Department of Mental Health and the antipoverty agency, both involved in community planning and in funneling federal money to agencies of their choice.

Each agency had its own administrative structure with its own bureaucracy, decision-makers, and line personnel. Thus there existed several autonomous, parallel bureaucratic structures, some larger than others, but all trying to deal with some aspect of human health. Their work was clinical, practical, dealing with issues of immediate reality. On the assertion of too much pressing immediate work, these agencies had no use for research of any kind, and therefore no adequate evaluation of the few available services was ever made. The agencies tended to give support to each other through their mutual referrals, and maintained an uncritical acceptance of the various territorial claims, never openly questioning the value of their own or other agencies' work.

Gradually another level of interagency cooperation became apparent; for example, the director of the leading mental health agency that received funds was also a ranking member of the major mental health planning group, which made recommendations about what agencies would receive funds; some persons were not only important members of agencies that allocated money, but also of agencies that received the money; some sat on boards of several agencies; some positions were held concurrently, while some people "rotated" through the various agencies. In a period of four years, the same relatively few people were repeatedly encountered in various roles associated with one or another of the agencies and making the major decisions regarding local mental health services. In other words, while the parallel bureaucracies that made up the "mental health community" were ostensibly autonomous, each with its own demarcated area of functioning, interagency sharing of upper-level decision-makers occurred, and the situation approached that of the "interlocking directorates" of big business.

There was yet another way in which the parallel bureaucracies cooperated: Based on some immediate issue or problem, temporary agency "coalitions" were formed. The composition varied according to the nature of the issue, and the coalition relaxed when the issue was resolved. One such coalition was the original cooperation of ASMIC and the clinic, while the United Agency stood opposed. Later, when conditions had changed, a new set of coalitions formed, this time finding the United Agency and the clinic together.

Thus the active mental health field in this city was made up of parallel bureaucracies, that is, various social agencies that, by virtue of their "expertise," had been granted legitimate social power by the community in the area of mental health. Despite the essential autonomy of the bureaucratic structures, they closely cooperated in several major ways that tended toward mutual support and perpetuation of the existing bureaucratic structures. This cooperation occurred through (1) normal and clearly legitimate professional channels, such as reciprocal referrals of clients; (2) tacit uncritical acceptance of agency "territories" and functions; (3) interagency "sharing" of upper-level decision-making personnel; (4) temporary variable-composition coalitions that briefly intensified agency power in order to deal with specific issues.

Mental Health Power Structure

We have thus far described the practice of the mental health professions as a legitimized special interest segment of a community. That segment, or field, was composed of parallel bureaucratic agencies that, by virtue of their control over professional and financial resources, cooperated in their own mutual support and tended to maintain decision-making power within that field. There thus existed a definable and relatively stable social structure through which agencies shared leadership, made cooperative decisions, and wielded legitimized social power that tended to support, strengthen, and perpetuate the viability of the structure itself. Schermerhorn (1964) notes, "The power process frequently crystallizes into more or less stable configurations designed as centers or structures of power [p. 18]." Clearly what has been described as a *power structure*, a "temporarily stable organization of power resources permitting an effectual directive control over selective aspects of the social process [p. 24]."

Polsby (1963), who takes issue with the prevalent "stratification" theory of authority power structures, nevertheless notes that

> By describing and specifying leadership roles in concrete situations, [we] are in a position to determine the extent to which a lower structure exists. High degrees of overlap in decision-making personnel among issue-areas, or high degrees of institutionalization in the bases of power in specified issue areas, or high degrees of regularity in the procedures of decision-making—any one of these situations, if found to exist, could conceivably justify an empirical conclusion that some kind of power structure exists [p. 119].

We have tried to show that such conditions did obtain and therefore conclude that there existed a viable *mental health power structure* that made all major decisions in the "mental health field" of this community. Never static, the mental health power structure continues to react to new pressures, and to maneuver, in a changing world, in order to maintain and further strengthen itself. In so doing, it becomes a defender of its own status quo. It is our contention that local mental health power structures across the country have become so thoroughly concerned with maintaining themselves, that the *major portion* of their commitment has been diverted from the original ideals of science and humanitarianism, and invested instead in the everyday politics of survival.

Selznick (1943) writing about bureaucracies noted,

> Running an organization as a specialized and essential activity generates problems which have no necessary (and often opposed) relationships to the professed or "original" goals of the organization. . . . [these activities] come to consume an increasing proportion of the time and thoughts of the participants, they are . . . substituted for the professed goals. . . . In that context the professed goals will tend to go down in defeat, usually through the process of being extensively ignored [p. 49].

Thus we maintain that contemporary mental health practice is carried out within power structures that are primarily concerned with justifying and maintaining themselves, while they pay scant attention to the scope of mental health services and even less to the objective evaluation of quality or effectiveness. They maintain their own self-interest, which conflicts with humanitarian ideals, science, and social progress. Such conflict is clearly evident in the power structures' relationships to (1) their clientele and (2) to any intruding innovator.

Relationship to Clients

Because of the proliferation of agencies with their territorial claims on one community, there must be some means of parceling out the available client pool. Some agencies deal with children, others with adults; some deal with poor children, some with retarded children; some with Catholics and some with Jews; some with immigrants and others with unemployed. None deals with just people, but all deal with "certain kinds" of people who are categorized and parceled out. To whatever category he might be assigned, it is implicit that the client is, in some way, a failure; that he has folded up and dropped out; that he is marginal; that he is not as bright as "we," or as well adjusted as "we," or as well employed as "we," or as nicely colored as "we." There is always an implicit and very real distance that separates the clinician from the client. And at the upper end of this breach is the righteous and very certain knowledge of the professional that he is behaving nobly, in a humanitarian cause. While the clinician focuses on each "client-failure," society is busy producing several more. We too often fail to recognize that our individual internally focused ministrations have little if anything to do with the amelioration of those social conditions that have shaped up the individual's disorder in the first place. To say that the mental health professionals have failed to recognize the crucial importance of external *social conditions* in shaping disturbed behavior is another way of saying that *professionals refuse to recognize that we labor to rebuild those lives that we, in our other social roles, have helped to* shatter. Nowhere is this more obvious than in the area of civil rights, where a clinician might occasionally help some poverty-level minority group member, and later go home to his restrictive suburb, attend his restrictive club, play golf on a restrictive course, and share a restrictive drink in a restrictive bar with businessmen who hire Negroes last, in good times, and fire them first in bad times. By fully accepting the "official" power-structure view of the "sick" individual in an otherwise fine society, we clinicians never admit the validity of such nonscientific analyses as Kozol's (1967) shattering "Death at an Early Age"; and we therefore need not admit that the restrictiveness of our own lives has anything to do with the frustrations of someone else, in another place.

The power-structure clinics tend to limit their services to white middle-class children with mild to moderate disturbances, that is, to those children with the best chances of improving even when left alone; those children whose parents would be most cooperative in keeping appointments, being on time, accepting the structure, and, of course, paying the fees; those children who do not present the vexing and, to the middle-class clinician, *alien* problems of lower-class minority groups. Certainly a clinic is much "safer," much "quieter," more neatly run, when it limits itself to the most cooperative clientele and, we might suggest, when it *selectively creates a pool of cooperative clients.* The waiting list is one of the selective devices used to weed out the impatient and retain the most docile clients. By insisting on the incredibly lengthy and largely irrelevant traditional psychodynamic study, the clinics refuse to deal immediately with a client's problems. Instead they artificially create a waiting list that then serves as an objective validation of the continuing "need" for clinic services over the next year or so. The length of the waiting list is, in fact, often seen as a positive indication of the value of the clinic. Thus, in some perverse manner, the slower and less efficient the clinic and the longer its waiting list, the greater is that clinic's claim to importance and to increased money and power! It would not be surprising to find that a clinic that efficiently handled all new referrals within an hour would be considered of dubious quality because it had no customers waiting at the door.

Thus the structure, responding primarily to its own needs for self-perpetuation, has created a mythical client beset by dramatic internal conflicts, hidden from himself, but who is apparently little affected by the realities of external social conditions. The professional, with his role clearly delimited by the power structure, continues his myopic psychodynamic dissection of individuals and never perceives the larger social, moral, or, if you will, *human* realities of that client's existence. The power structure, further insuring its own perpetuation, carefully selects clients who best meet the structure's needs and rejects the great majority who do not. The "most hopeful" but still doubtful psychiatric services are offered mainly to bright, verbal, adult, neurotic, upper-class whites. In the context of contemporary social reality, the mental health professions now exist as expensive and busy political power structures that have little relevance for anything except their own self-preservation. In this process, we suspect, the client might too often be exploited rather than helped.

Response to Intruding Innovations

The mental health power structure, committed primarily to its own preservation, is alertly opposed to any events that might change it. Thus, when innovation intrudes, the structure responds with various strategies to deal with the threat; it might incorporate the new event and alter it to fit the preexisting structure so that, in effect, nothing is really changed. It might deal with it also by active rejection, calling upon all of its resources to "starve out" the innovator by insuring a lack of support.

The most subtle defense, however, is ostensibly to accept and encourage the innovator, to publicly proclaim support of innovative goals, and while doing that to build in various controlling safeguards, such as special committees, thereby insuring that the work is always accomplished through power structure channels and thus effecting no real change. This tactic achieves the nullification of the innovator while at the same time giving the power structure the public semblance of progressiveness. The power structure can become so involved in this pose that the lower-line personnel come honestly to believe that they are working for the stated ideals such as humanitarianism, science, and progress, while in reality they labor to maintain the political power of the status quo.

This has occurred in civil rights and antipoverty programs where federal money has been poured into the old local power structures that have loudly proclaimed innovation, improvement, progressiveness, while all the time protecting themselves by actually nullifying those efforts. After several years of public speeches and much money, it becomes clear to the citizens of the deprived area that nothing has changed. Then, frustrated and angry, many submerge themselves into nonprotesting apathy, and others, perhaps the more hopeful ones, erupt into violence, smashing their world, trying, perhaps, to destroy in order to rebuild.

Hence, while the power structure continues to proclaim innovation, it expends great energy to insure, through its defensive maneuvers, the maintenance of its status quo. Innovation is thus allowed, and even encouraged, as long as it remains on the level of conceptual abstractions, and provided that it does not, in reality, change anything! The hallmark of this interesting but deadly phenomenon, of spending vast sums of money and effort, to bring about no change, all in the name of innovation, might be summed up in what I recently suggested as a motto for one of those agencies, *Innovation without Change!* This motto reflects a central tendency of mental health services in the 1960s: maintaining our primary allegiance to the power structures, rather than to science and

humanitarianisms, and continuing our busy employment, creating innovations without changing reality.

Every community has its built-in safeguards that, in the mental
health field, guarantee rejection, neutralization, or at least deceleration
of any new approaches that do not fit the prevailing power structure.
Significant progress in mental health, then, will not be achieved through
systematic research or the guidance of humanitarian ideals since they
are neutralized by being filtered through the existing structure. In order
for those scientific and humanitarian conceptual innovations to remain
intact and reach the level of clinical application, they must avoid that
destructive "filtering" process.

Likewise, progress will not be initiated by or through the power
structure, but will depend upon successfully changing or ignoring that
structure. It does not seem possible at this point to join the structure
and still maintain the integrity of both areas, that is, the essentially political power structure, and the humanitarian and scientific ideals. The
two areas are incompatible; science and humanitarianism cannot be
achieved through the present self-perpetuating focus of the power structure.

A case in point is the present interest in the development of comprehensive mental health centers. When a community commits itself to
the vastly expensive reality of a mental health center, and then *refers
control of that center back to the existing power structure*, it has created
"innovation without change." The major result might be to enrich and
reinforce the old power structure, thus making it vastly more capable of
further entrenching itself, and successfully resisting change for many
more years.

Our personal experience in contributing to the planning of comprehensive mental health services led us to the conclusion that the comprehensive centers would provide only "more of the same." Instead of
trying to determine the needs of the people in the urban area, and then
create the appropriate approaches, the planners asked questions such as:
"How can we extend psychiatric services to treat more alcoholics?"
"How many beds do we need for acute cases?" "How can we increase
our services to schizophrenic children?" "How can we pool our resources for more efficient diagnostic workup of cases?" and so on. The
questions themselves assumed the validity of the existing power structure and were aimed at *extending old services* rather than determining
needs and *creating new services*. Only the scope and not the relevance
or effectiveness of existing approaches was questioned.

Thus, surrounded by the modish aura of "innovation," the existing
structure not only remains intact, but becomes enriched, and continues
its existence irrespective of the real and changing needs of its clients. By

allocating a great deal of money to the existing power structures, whether through mental health centers, antipoverty programs, special education, or other action, we are playing the game of the "sixties," "Inovation without Change," and, win or lose, we run the risk of insuring our own stagnation.

In summary we have maintained that contemporary United States mental health professions have developed viable community-based professional and lay power structures that are composed of mutually benefiting bureaucracies. Scientific and humanitarian ideals are incompatible with and have been supplanted by the professionals' primary loyalty to the political power structure itself. By virtue of their focus on self-preservation, these power-structures (1) maintain a dogmatically restrictive view of human behavior and the roles of the professionals within that structure and (2) prevent the development of true innovations. The basic self-defeating weakness in the variety of current attempts at innovative social action is their unintended strengthening of the existing power structure, which is incompatible with innovation. Thus, future advances in the practices of mental health will most readily occur outside of the current mental health power sturctures.

Contemporary American mental health professions base their major decisions neither on science nor humanitarianism, and certainly not on honest self-appraisal, but on the everyday politics of bureaucratic survival in local communities. As Murray and Adeline Levine (1968) have pointed out, while the professions operate to maintain themselves, society changes, and the two grow farther apart. Eventually the mental health professions become grossly alienated from the human realities of the very clients they purport to help, and the professions soon achieve the status of being irrelevant. Admitting no need for critical evaluation, the professional continues to provide services that are, in fact, of limited scope, questionable value, and extremely high price. As long as we continue uncritically to refer all new developments back into the control of the old power structure, we will continue to insure "innovation without change." Then, as professionals, we can all continue going about our business, keeping our private lives out of phase with our professional pose, and keeping both of them alienated from larger social realities. In this way, we need never allow the restrictiveness of our lives to mar the nobility of our profession.

REFERENCES

Kozol, J. *Death at an early age.* New York: Houghton Mifflin, 1967.
Levine, M., and Levine, A. *The time for action: A history of social change and helping forms.* Unpublished manuscript, Yale University, 1968.

Polsby, N. W. *Community power and political theory.* New Haven: Yale University Press, 1963.

Schermerhorn, R. A. *Society and power.* New York: Random House, 1964.

Selznick, P. An approach to a theory of bureaucracy. *American Sociological Review,* 1943, 8, 47–54.

HOW COMMUNITY MENTAL HEALTH
STAMPED OUT THE RIOTS (1968-78)

24

Kenneth Keniston, Ph.D.

One day, after I gave a lecture in a course on social and community psychiatry, a student asked me whether I thought community mental health workers would eventually be asked to assume policing functions. I assured him that I thought this very unlikely, and thought no more about it.

That night I had the following dream: I was sitting on the platform of a large auditorium. In the audience were thousands of men and women, some in business clothes, others in peculiar blue and white uniforms that seemed a cross between medical and military garb. I glanced at the others on the platform: Many wore military uniforms. Especially prominent was a tall, distinguished, lantern-jawed general, whose chest was covered with battle ribbons and on whose arm was a blue and white band.

The lights dimmed; I was pushed to my feet and toward the podium. Before me on the lectern was a neatly typed manuscript. Not knowing what else to do, I found myself beginning to read from it. . . .

Ladies and Gentlemen: It is a pleasure to open this Eighth Annual Meeting of the Community Mental Health Organization and to welcome our distinguished guests: the recently appointed Secretary for International Mental Health, General Westmoreland [loud applause], and the Secretary for Internal Mental Health, General Walt [applause].

This year marks the tenth anniversary of the report of the First National Advisory Commission on Civil Disorders. And this meeting of representatives of 3483 Community Mental Health Centers, 247 Remote Therapy Centers, and 45 Mobile Treatment Teams may provide a fitting occasion for us to review the strides we have made in the past decade and to contemplate the greater tasks that lie before us. For it was in the past decade, after all, that the Community Mental Health movement proved its ability to deal with the problem of urban violence, and it is

Reprinted from *Trans-action*, July–August 1968, 5(8), 21–29. Copyright © by *Trans-action* magazine, New Brunswick, New Jersey. Kenneth Keniston is Professor of Psychology at Yale University, New Haven, Connecticut.

in the next decade that the same approaches must be adapted to the other urgent mental health problems of our society and the world.

Review of Past Decade

In my remarks here, I will begin with a review of the progress of the past decade. Arbitrarily, I will divide the years since 1968 into three stages: the phase of preparation; the phase of total mobilization; and the mop-up phase that we are now concluding.

In retrospect, the years from 1968 to 1970 can be seen as the time of preparation for the massive interventions that have since been made. On the one hand, the nation was faced with mounting urban unrest, especially among disadvantaged sectors of the inner city, unrest that culminated in the riots of 1969 and 1970, in which property damage of more than $20 billion was wrought, and in which more than five thousand individuals (including twenty-seven policemen, National Guardsmen, and firemen) were killed. Yet, in retrospect, the seeds of "Operation Inner City" were being developed even during this period. As early as 1969, the Cannon Report—a joint product of Community Mental Health workers and responsible leaders of the white and black communities—suggested that (1) the propensity to violence was but a symptom of underlying social and psychological pathology; (2) massive federal efforts must be made to identify the individual and societal dysfunctions that produce indiscriminate protest; and (3) more effective methods must be developed for treating the personal and group disorganization that produces unrest.

From 1968 to 1970, a series of research studies and demonstration projects developed the basic concepts that were implemented in later years. Indeed, without this prior theoretical work by interdisciplinary teams of community psychiatrists, sociologists, social workers, and police officials, Operation Inner City would never have been possible. I need recall only a few of the major contributions: the concept of "aggressive alienation," used to characterize the psychosocial disturbance of a large percentage of inner-city dwellers; McFarland's seminal work on urban disorganization, personal pathology, and aggressive demonstrations; the development, on a pilot basis, of new treatment systems like the "total saturation approach," based upon the concept of "antidotal (total) therapy"; and the recognition of the importance of the "reacculturation experience" in treating those whose personal pathology took the form of violence-proneness. Equally basic theoretical contributions were made by those who began to investigate the relationship between aggressiveness, alienation, and antisocietal behavior in other disturbed sections of the population, such as disacculturated intellectuals and students.

After the riots of 1969, rising public indignation over the senseless slaughter of thousands of Americans and the wanton destruction of property led President Humphrey to create the Third Presidental Task Force on Civil Disorders. After six months of almost continuous study, Task Force chairman Ronald Reagan recommended that massive federal intervention, via the Community Mental Health Centers, be the major instrument in action against violence. Portions of this report still bear quoting: "The experience of the past five years has shown that punitive and repressive intervention aggravates rather than ameliorates the violence of the inner city. It is now amply clear that urban violence is more than sheer criminality. The time has come for America to heed the findings of a generation of research: *inner-city violence is a product of profound personal and social pathology. It requires treatment rather than punishment, rehabilitation rather than imprisonment.*"

The report went on: "The Community Mental Health movement provides the best available weapon in the struggle against community sickness in urban America. The existence of 967 Community Mental Health Centers (largely located in communities with high urban density), the concentration of professional and paraprofessional mental health workers in these institutions, and their close contact with the mood and hopes of their inner-city catchment areas all indicate that community mental health should be the first line of attack on urban unrest."

In the next months, an incensed Congress, backed by an outraged nation, passed the first of the series of major bills that led to the creation of Operation Inner City, under the joint auspices of the Department of Health, Education, and Welfare and what was then still called the Department of Defense. Despite the heavy drains on the national economy made by American involvement in Ecuador, Eastern Nigeria, and Pakistan, $5 billion were appropriated the first year, with steadily increasing amounts thereafter.

As the concept of urban pathology gained acceptance, police officials referred those detained during urban riots not to jails but to local Community Mental Health Centers. Viewing urban violence as a psychosocial crisis made possible the application of concepts of "crisis therapy" to the violence-ridden inner-city dweller. As predicted, early researchers found very high levels of psychopathology in those referred for treatment, especially in the form of aggravated aggressive-alienation syndrome.

New Statutes Passed in 1971

But it was obviously not enough to treat violence only in its acute phase. Precritical intervention and preventive rehabilitation were also necessary. So city law-enforcement officials and mental health workers began cooperating in efforts to identify those people whose behavior, group-membership patterns, and utterances gave evidence of the pro-drome (early symptoms) of aggressive alienation. New statutes passed by Congress in 1971 empowered mental health teams and local authorities to require therapy of those identified as prodromally violent. In defending this bill in Congress against the congressional group that opposed it on civil-libertarian grounds, Senator Murphy of California noted the widespread acceptance of the principle of compulsory innoculation, mandatory treatment for narcotics addicts, and hospitalization of the psychotic. "Urban violence," he noted, "is no different from any other ill-ness: The welfare of those afflicted requires that the public accept re-sponsibility for their prompt and effective treatment."

Mental health workers, with legal power to institute therapy, and in collaboration with responsible political and law-enforcement authorities, were finally able to implement the Total Saturation Approach in the years from 1972 to the present. Employing local citizens as "pathology detectors," Community Mental Health teams made massive efforts to de-tect all groups and individuals with prodromes of violence, or a predis-position to *advocate* violence. In many communities, the incidence of prepathological conditions was almost perfectly correlated with racial origin; hence, massive resources were funneled into these communities in particular to immediately detect and help those afflicted.

At this point, it became evident that programs attempting to treat inner-city patients still remaining in the same disorganized social envi-ronment that had originally contributed to their pathology were not entirely successful. It was only in 1971, with Rutherford, Cohen, and Robinson's now classic study, "Relapse Rates in Seven Saturation Proj-ects: Multi-Variate Analysis," that it was finally realized that short-term, total-push therapies were not effective in the long run. As the authors pointed out, "The re-entry of the cured patient into the pathogenic dis-acculturating community clearly reverses *all* the therapeutic gains of the inpatient phase."

Remote Treatment Centers Constructed

Armed with the Rutherford study, Congress in 1972 passed a third legislative landmark, the Remote Therapy Center Act. Congress—recognizing that prolonged reacculturative experience in a psychologi-cally healthy community (antidotal therapy) was often necessary for the permanent recompensation of deep-rooted personality disorders—authorized the construction of 247 centers, largely in the Rocky Moun-tain Region, each with a capacity of one thousand patients. The old Department of Defense (now the Department of International Mental Health) cooperated by making available the sites used in World War II for the relocation of Japanese–Americans. On these salubrious sites, the network of Remote Treatment Centers has now been constructed. Although the stringent security arrangements necessary in such centers have been criticized, the retreats now constitute one of our most effective attacks upon the problem of urban mental illness.

The gradual reduction in urban violence, starting in 1973, cannot be attributed to any single factor. But perhaps one idea played the decisive role. During this period mental health workers began to realize that earlier approaches, which attempted to ameliorate the objective, physical, or legal conditions under which inner-city dwellers lived, were not only superficial, but were themselves a reflection of serious psychopathology. Reilly, Bernitsky, and O'Leary's now classic study of ex-patients of the retreats established the correlation between a patient's relapse into violence and his preoccupation with what the investigators termed "objectivist" issues: housing, sanitation, legal rights, jobs, education, medical care, and so on.

Two generations ago Freud taught us that what matters most is not objective reality, but the way it is interpreted by the individual. Freud's insight has finally been perceived in its true light—as an attitude essential for healthy functioning. The fact that previous programs of civil rights, slum clearance, legal reforms, and so on, succeeded only in aggravating violence now became fully understandable. Not only did these programs fail to take account of the importance of basic attitudes and values in determining human behavior—thus treating symptoms rather than underlying psychological problems—but, by encouraging objectivism, they directly *undermined* the mental health of those exposed to these programs. Today's mental health workers recognize objectivism as a prime symptom of individual and community dysfunction, and move swiftly and effectively to institute therapy.

The final step in the development of a community mental health approach to violence came with the development of the Mobile Treatment ("Motreat") Team. In 1972 the Community Mental Health authorities set up a series of forty-five Motreat Teams, organized on a regional basis and consisting of between five hundred and one thousand carefully selected and trained Community Mental Health workers. These heroic groups, wearing their now familiar blue and white garb, were ready on a standby basis to move into areas where violence threatened. Given high mobility by the use of armed helicopters, trained in crisis intervention and emergency treatment, and skilled in the use of modern psychopharmacological sprays and gases, the Motreat Teams have now proved their effectiveness. On numerous occasions during the past years, they

have been able to calm an agitated population, to pinpoint the antiso-
cial-violence leaders and refer them for therapy, and thus to lay the
basis for society's prompt return to healthy functioning. The architects
of the Mobile Treatment Team found that many of their most important
insights were obtained from professionals in the field of law enforcement
and national defense—more evidence of the importance of interdisciplinary cooperation.

As you all know, the past four years have been years of diminishing
urban violence, years when the Community Mental Health movement
has received growing acclaim for its success in dealing with social and
individual pathology, years when the early criticism of the Community
Mental Health movement by the "liberal coalition" in Congress has diminished, largely because of the non-reelection of the members of that
coalition. Today, the Community Mental Health movement has the virtually undivided support of the nation, regardless of political partisan-
ship. The original federal target of 2800 Community Mental Health
Centers has been increased to more than 5000; the principles of Community Mental Health have been extended from the limited "catchment
area" concept to the more relevant concept of "target groups" and beyond; and the Community Mental Health movement faces enormous
new challenges.

But before considering the challenges that lie ahead, let us review
what we have learned theoretically during the past decade.

Doubtless the most important insight was the awareness that *violence and antisocial behavior are deeply rooted in individual and social
pathology*, and must be treated as such. We have at last been able to
apply the insights of writers, historians, sociologists, and psychologists of
the 1950s and 1960s to a new understanding of black character. The
black American—blighted by the deep scars and legacies of his history,
demoralized by what Stanley Elkins described as the concentration-
camp conditions of slavery, devitalized by the primitive, impulse ridden,
and fatherless black families so brilliantly described by Daniel
Moynihan—is the helpless victim of a series of deep deprivations that
almost inevitably lead to intrapsychic and societal pathology. Moreover,
we have begun to understand the communicational networks and
group-pathological processes that spread alienation and violence from
individual to individual, and that make the adolescent especially prone
to succumb to the aggressive-alienation syndrome. To be sure, this view
was contradicted by the report that many of the advocates of violence
—the leaders of the now outlawed black-power group and its precur-
sors, S.N.C.C. and C.O.R.E.—came from relatively nondeprived backgrounds. But later researchers have shown that the virus of aggressive
alienation is communicated even within apparently intact families. As

Rosenbaum and Murphy put it in a recent review paper, "We have learned that social pathology is no less infectious than the black plague."

Another major theoretical contribution has come from our *redefinition of the concept of community*. As the first Community Mental Health Centers were set up, "community" was defined as a geographically limited catchment area, often heterogeneous in social class, ethnicity, and race. But the events of the last decade have made it amply clear that we cannot conceive of the community so narrowly. The artificial boundaries of the catchment area do not prevent the transmission of social pathology across these boundaries; indeed, efforts to prevent personal mobility and communication between catchment areas proved difficult to implement without an anxiety-provoking degree of coercion. It became clear that cutting across catchment areas were certain pathogenic "target groups" in which the bacillus of social pathology was most infectious. Recognition of the target-group concept of community was the theoretical basis for much recent legislation. Rarely have the findings of the behavioral sciences been translated so promptly into enlightened legislation [applause].

This recognition of the too-narrow definition of "community" led to the creation of the Remote Treatment Centers. True, removing the mentally ill from the violence-prone target groups has not solved the problem completely. But the creation of total therapeutic communities in distant parts of the country has had a salubrious and calming effect on the mental health of the groups the patients came from.

It has also become clear that Community Mental Health efforts aimed solely at the disadvantaged are, by their very nature, limited in effectiveness. The suppression of pathology in one group may paradoxically be related to its sudden emergence in others. Stated differently, pathology moves through the entire community, although it tends to be concentrated during any given period in certain target groups. The international events of the past decade, the appearance of comparable psychopathology in Ecuador, Eastern Nigeria, Pakistan, Thailand, and a variety of other countries, raise the question of whether it is possible to have mental health in one country alone.

The Concept of Total Therapy

Another crucial theoretical advance has been the concept of *total therapy*. Patients and groups must be treated *before* symptoms become acute, because the infectiousness of social pathology increases during the acute phase. What has been termed the "pathology multiplier effect" has been widely recognized: This means that it is essential to prevent the formation of pathologically interacting groups, especially when organized around societally disruptive objectivist issues like black power, civil rights, or improvement in living conditions. Furthermore, crisis intervention must be supplemented by *prolonged aftercare*, particularly for those whose involvement in violence has been most intense. Of the many post-rehabilitation follow-up methods attempted, two of the most effective have been the incorporation of rehabilitated patients into mental health teams working in localities other than their own, and the new programs of aftercare involving the continuing rehabilitation of discharged patients in such challenging areas as Ecuador, Eastern Nigeria, and Pakistan. You are all familiar with the many glowing tributes to this aftercare program recently released by International Mental Health Secretary Westmoreland [applause].

The past decade has also demonstrated beyond doubt the importance of *interagency and interdisciplinary collaboration*. The effectiveness of such collaboration has shown how unfounded were the concerns of the First Joint Commission on Mental Health over inadequate manpower. In large measure because of better and better relationships between mental health workers, law-enforcement agencies, local civic authorities, the Department of International Mental Health, the National Guard, the Air Force, and other community agencies, radically new patterns of recruitment into the mental health professions have been established. Indeed, in many communities effective mental health efforts have permitted a major reduction in the size of law-enforcement authorities, and the training of a whole new group of paraprofessionals and subprofessionals who, a decade ago, would have entered law-enforcement agencies.

But lest we become complacent about our accomplishments, let me remind you of the many theoretical problems, difficulties, and challenges that lie before us.

Our program has not been without its critics and detractors, and there is much to be learned from them. To be sure, many of the early criticisms of our work can now be understood either as the result of inadequate understanding of the behavioral sciences, or as symptoms of the objectivist social–pathological process itself. In the years before the liberal coalition became moribund, many so-called civil-libertarian critics persisted in ignoring the humanitarian aspects of our program, focusing instead upon the nineteenth-century concept of civil rights. The political ineffectuality of this group, coupled with the speed with which many of its leaders have recently been reacculturated, suggests the limitations of this viewpoint.

But even within our own midst we have had critics and detractors. We are all familiar with the unhappy story of the American Psychoanalytic Association, which continued its criticisms of our programs until its compulsory incorporation last year into the Community Mental Health Organization. What we must learn from these critics is how easy it is for even the most apparently dedicated mental health workers to lose sight of broader societal goals, neglecting the population and the societal matrix in a misguided attachment to outmoded concepts of individuality, "reality factors," and "insight therapy."

In my remarks so far, I have emphasized our theoretical and practical progress. But those of us who were involved in the Community Mental Health movement from its beginnings in the early 1960s must remind others that almost all of the major concepts that underlie the progress of the past decade were already in existence in 1968. Even a decade ago, the most advanced workers in the field of community health *knew* that crisis intervention was not enough, and were developing plans for preventive intervention and extensive aftercare. Furthermore, many of the most important concepts in this field derived from researches done by Freud, Anna Freud, Moynihan, Caplan, Gruenberg, Keniston, and others. Even the concept of aggressive alienation itself is based on earlier research on alienation done, not in the inner city, but amongst talented college students. Thus, our enthusiasm for the progress of the past decade must be tempered with humility and a sense of indebtedness to those in the pre-Community Mental Health era.

Furthermore, humility is called for because of the many questions whose answers have evaded our search. I will cite but one of the most important: the problem of therapeutic failure.

Extradition of Mentally Ill from Canada

We have much to learn from our failures, perhaps more than from our numerous successes. With some patients, even repeated rehabilitation and maintenance on high doses of long-acting tranquilizers have failed to produce a complete return to prosocial functioning. And the uncooperativeness of the government of Canada has made it extremely difficult to reach those unsuccessfully treated patients who have evaded our detection networks and fled north. Since the Canadian government is unwilling to extradite the large numbers of mentally ill who have flocked to Canadian urban centers, we must support the recent proposal of Secretary Westmoreland that we persuade foreign governments to institute their own programs of Community Mental Health, with the close collaboration and support of American advisors. Indeed, the currently strained relations between Canada and the United States raise a series of far more profound questions, to which I will return in a moment.

Rather than list the many other important research issues that confront us, let me turn to our greatest challenge—the definition of new target groups and the need to broaden still further the concept of community.

New Target Groups

In our focus upon the more visible problems of urban violence, we have neglected other target groups of even greater pathological potential. These new target groups are not always easy to define precisely; but there is a clear consensus that high priority on the list of future targets must be given to college students, to intellectuals with no firm ties to the community, and to disacculturated members of certain ethnico–religious groups who retain close ties with non-American communities.

The passage last year of the College Development Act enables us at last to apply to the college-age group the techniques so successfully used in the inner city. This act will enable the setting up of college mental health centers with a strong community approach. One of the particular strengths of this law should be underlined here: It enables us to treat not only the college student himself, but his professors and mentors, from whom—as recent studies have shown—much of his antisocial acculturation springs.

In our continuing work with new target groups, however, we must not lose sight of certain basic principles. For one, the target-group approach is by its very nature limited. Our practical resources are still so small that we must single out only certain target groups for special interventions. But this should not obscure our long-range goal: nothing less than a society in which all men and women are guaranteed mental health by simple virtue of their citizenship. Thus, the entire community must be our target; we must insist upon *total mental health* from the womb to the grave [applause].

Yet our most serious challenge lies not in America, but outside of our national boundaries. For it has become obvious that the concept of "mental health in one nation" is not tenable. We are surrounded by a world in which the concepts of Community Mental Health have had regrettably little impact. Recent studies conducted by the Department of International Mental Health in Ecuador, Eastern Nigeria, and Thailand have shown an incidence of individual and collective psychopathology even higher than that found in American cities ten years ago. The link between objectivism and violence, first established in America, has been repeatedly shown to exist in other cultures as well. Even young Americans serving abroad with the Overseas Mental Health Corps have been exposed to objectivist influences in their countries that have made their renewed rehabilitation necessary, whether on the battlefield or in the special rehabilitation centers back home.

But it should not be thought that the primary argument against mental health in only one country is mere expediency. Our responsibilities as the most powerful and mentally healthy nation in the world are of a therapeutic nature. Were it simply a matter of expediency, the closing of the Canadian and Mexican borders has shown that it is possible to limit the exodus of non-reacculturated Americans to the merest trickle. Nor would sheer expediency alone justify our involvement, at a heavy price in materials and men, in the mental health struggles of Ecuador, Eastern Nigeria, and Thailand. It is not expediency but our therapeutic commitment to the mental health of our fellow men—regardless of race, color, nationality, and creed—that argues against the concept of mental health in only one nation.

Thus, our greatest challenge is the struggle to create a mentally healthy world. Happy historical accident has given American society a technology and an understanding of human behavior sufficiently advanced to bring about the profound revolution in human behavior that men from Plato's time onward have dreamed of. The lessons of Operation Inner City will continue to be of the utmost importance: the concepts of total saturation, remote therapy, and mandatory treatment; the realization of the close link between objectivism and psychopathology; the need for the closest interdisciplinary cooperation. Already, plans evolved by the Department of International Mental Health and this Community Mental Health Organization call for the international deployment of Mobile Treatment Teams and Overseas Mental Health Corps volunteers, some operating with the assistance of local governments, others courageously risking their lives in communities where pathology has infiltrated even the highest levels of governmental authority. In the years to come, the challenges will be great, the price will be large, and the discouragements will be many. But of one thing there can be no doubt: The Community Mental Health movement will play a leading role in our progress toward a mentally healthy society at the head of a mentally healthy world [applause]. . . .

I stepped back from the podium and tripped. Many hands reached to pull me to my feet. I cried out and awoke to find my wife shaking me. "You've been dreaming and mumbling in your sleep for hours," she said, "and you're feverish." The thermometer revealed a temperature of 103 degrees. I was in bed for several days with a rather severe virus— which, doubtless, explains my dream.

POSTSCRIPT
The Ideologies of Community Intervention

One might get the impression from much of the current community mental health literature, (for example, Adelson & Kalis, 1970), that the concept of community intervention is a discovery of contemporary psychiatry, an impression created by contrasting the contemporary centers with the child guidance clinics of the 1920s. Actually, the settlement houses that flourished at the turn of the century functioned much like today's community centers (Levine & Levine, 1970). And, unlike the staff of the child guidance clinics, the settlement workers were not case-oriented. Although some workers might have felt psychologically more fit than their clients, they never established a formal set of standards comparable to our psychiatric nomenclature. The settlement movement grew out of the reform trend that swept the country before World War I. Settlement workers were responsive to the individual's needs, but, it appears, with the design of winning community support. Once they had this support, the workers proceeded to organize the community around common needs and aspirations. The clients were the "other Americans" of the day, the immigrants, those without power to influence their destiny. It was assumed that community organization would have first an educational and eventually a liberating effect. The people would learn how to transform their lives by transforming the environment. And the settlement workers did not keep a professional distance from their clients or from the community. They identified themselves with the people and fought their political battles. When times changed and the ideology of social reform was no longer acceptable to the American people, the settlement workers either changed their style and became case-oriented social workers, or they gave up in desperation.

There is an important lesson in all this. While forms of community intervention may be justified by scientific theories, in the public mind community intervention is associated with a political ideology. And when public sentiment shifts from an environmentalistic, reform outlook to a point of view that emphasizes individual responsibility, professionals must get in step with the times, or be banished to the sidelines.

Szasz (1970), a psychiatrist who takes a historical perspective, begins his discussion of the political basis for the community mental health movement by comparing a statement by John F. Kennedy, the one political figure most responsible for launching the community movement, with a statement by Prince Karl August Von Hardenburg, who in 1805 urged the building of massive psychiatric institutions. Both leaders seemed to herald a new age for mental health. The comparison, in Szasz's words, is chilling. Furthermore, the similarity goes beyond the fact that both speakers were politicians. It appears as if the liberal Kennedy and the Prussian Von Hardenburg shared a common ideology. Both men were committed to the notion that the state should provide mental health services for the people. They viewed mental health as a disease that eats away at the fabric of society and felt that federal as well as local governments should set up institutional means for wiping out mental illness.

Szasz is unalterably opposed to any form of institutional psychiatry, even if it means that many will never receive psychiatric aid. From his point of view, the state has no responsibility to provide mental health services, and, furthermore, he sees any attempt to set up such services as eventually leading to extralegal means of controlling behavior. Szasz contends that in the name of community mental health, individuals will be harrassed, persecuted, and forced into conforming with community norms. In the end, community mental health may spawn the most effective means for totalitarian behavior and thought control. For Szasz the only safe psychotherapy occurs when one person (the client) freely contracts the services of a professional. The professional can always opt to reject the case, and the client may always fire the therapist when the therapist no longer acts in the client's interest. Szasz, is assuming that people know what is in their own interest and, hence, do not need official agencies to define problems or to impose solutions.

Essentially, Szasz contrasts institutional forms of psychotherapy that are based on the medical or public health models with contractual forms of psychotherapy that are analogous to the legal model. Szasz is convinced that the community mental health practitioners will totally embrace the medical model and treat people like specimens.

Yet there are others who see something entirely different in the community movement. They see hope for the poor, the powerless, the downtrodden, and the oppressed. They are committed to the same ideology of individual freedom expressed by Szasz. But, unlike Szasz, they see the community movement as fostering individual freedom and personal control over one's destiny. They visualize community centers as places where the powerless can pool resources in order to attack social wrongs, bring about social justice, and resist external control. They, too, emphasize the contractual relationship between the professional and the client, but their point of view allows for professionals within the community to work for the people. In fact, community centers can be controlled by local people who then could contract professionals committed to the goals set by the local community. It should be emphasized, though, that the professionals who support this point of view do not seem to expect the people to put a high priority on individual psychotherapy. They expect that professionals will be asked to fight for social reform, especially to combat official agencies, such as the police, the board of education, and the welfare department.

To complete the picture, there are probably those who believe in maximum social control and maximum involvement of the government in the daily lives of the people. Some of these people probably agree with Szasz's contention that community mental health will foster this control and are, therefore, pleased with recent developments.

Community mental health is sufficiently ambiguous to strike fear in the hearts of those committed either to an ideology of social control or to an ideology of individual freedom. And it is probably the case that in centers across the country there are governing bodies with people who represent various positions along this ideological continuum. It is likely that community programs will reflect these ideological conflicts by the way in which they are formulated and carried out.

Prevention and early treatment. One aim of the community center is the prevention of mental illness. Preventive programs develop around essentially two goals: (1) elimination of conditions that cause mental illness and (2) treatment of the diseases in the early stages. It is clear that those who value individual freedom may have serious misgivings about any preventive program that forces people into therapy. Many programs that superficially seem very positive may incur the wrath of those who value individual freedom. No one would oppose a project that emphasized environmental rejuvenation as a means of fostering mental health (for example, cleaning up the city streets), unless this project involved destruction of ethnic neighborhoods and, hence, certain ways of life. Programs that are directed at people, in contrast to environmental structures, will be even more difficult to institute. For example, many parents would object to a procedure by which certain children entering the school system would be selected for special psychotherapy experiences. Some parents might fear that the professionals would use criteria that assure a steady stream of clients for psychotherapy; and there are social scientists who would agree with them (Rubington & Weinberg, 1968).

If preventive programs are ever to get off the ground, then the sponsors must demonstrate a clear awareness of the human costs associated with their programs. They must be prepared to indicate the loss in personal freedom to all members of the community when the attempt is made to change the behavior of a minority. It may turn out that a community is unwilling to accept the negative by-products of a preventive endeavor and would rather tolerate the deviance.

Consultation. The community center is required by law to provide consultation for other agencies, organizations, and institutions in the community, but the government has not provided any guidelines for such activity. How the center relates to the larger community will depend largely on its ideological orientation.

The social-activist consultant who seeks to increase individual freedom will tend to take the point of view of the agency's clients rather than of the agency itself. This is most likely where the consultees are relatively conservative institutions, such as schools, the courts, and the welfare agencies. In these instances the activist may see his mission as one of reforming a backward system. Of course, the community workers run the risk of being exploited by the agency that uses the credentials of their consultant to further legitimize their traditional practices. If the consultant moves too fast or if he is too open about his antiestablishment views, he runs the risk of politically isolating the community center and, hence, making it a convenient target for all other community agencies. On the other hand, the social activist may take the point of view of the agency when the agency is a radical neighborhood group. In fact he may support a group that is clearly not fostering individual mental health but is actually producing social conflict. Although the activist generally values the individual over the group, he also values community power more than individual mental health.

The nonactivist, social-control–minded consultant also runs serious risks consulting with either establishment or radical groups. He may really wish to strengthen established organizations but find that any change tends to disrupt the system and gives the "anarchists" the opportunity to bring the agency to its knees. Or this consultant may set out to co-opt a radical group by supporting its activities while trying to channel its energies in what he feels is the right direction. This strategy is dangerous and may backfire. For example, while it is difficult to document actual cases, it is our impression that many antidrug student groups that are supported by local establishment people, including mental health professionals, are only paying lip service to the notion of reducing drug abuse. These socially conscious student groups are able to use their position in the community to protect dealers and to provide places where drugs can be used safely without interference from the law.

Because consultation may bring about unexpected results, the community mental health center must move cautiously. In almost anything it attempts it is bound to anger both those who want to increase social control and those who want to increase personal freedom. There is one possible solution to this dilemma, although it is not a happy one. The center can align itself with particular forces in the community, that is, embrace an ideology. This may be a workable solution if the center does not appear to be too powerful and if the community-at-large feels that the center is open about its objectives. Reasonable men may be able to support an agency that fights for the underprivileged as long as it does not try to hide behind mental health double-talk.

The alternative to facing ideological conflict is ignoring it. Professionals have been doing this for years, but it is a deadly game. Essentially, it means assuming the posture of the technician who just carries out orders. To our mind this is a morally bankrupt position, for those in power can then merely exploit the knowledge and abilities of others. The community mental health practitioner can act as if he were morally neutral, but meantime be manipulated by the politicians and businessmen who have an interest in mental health. It may very well be that heretofore science had to suppress moral concerns in order to foster technological progress, but it has gotten to the point at which we can no longer tolerate a blind technology run by morally insensitive professionals. The reintegration of science and morality, of values and facts, of theoretical and ideological perspectives, cannot be anything but a painful task. Science and technology have traditionally acted as if questions of value should be banished from disciplined minds. To a great extent this educational effort was successful. What now?

We now appreciate that psychological intervention has an impact on the moral and ethical life of the people and of the community. But our knowledge in this area is scanty and incomplete. We have justified programs on the basis of intrapsychic theories that are suspect even in their own realm. To be candid, we really do not know what happens to a community when a program is launched. So it may be time to begin finding out. Studies in planned social change that examine the relationship between social–political factors and the experience of the people undergoing the change are desperately needed. Only now, thirty years after instituting the welfare system, are we beginning to study the impact of welfare on personal lives (May, 1965). If we had known thirty years ago what we know now, we could have avoided years of human misery.

In planning for social change we cannot introduce the notion of ethnic, cultural, and social differences as an afterthought. The current model for the community mental health center was formulated on the federal level by a body of mental health professionals who claimed to know the diseases of the mind and at least some cures. The local community is required to follow the general guidelines and provide certain basic services. Beyond that it is up to the local mental health professionals to elaborate specific strategies of intervention. This works well when the people serviced by the Mental Health Center share the same ethnic and cultural background as the professionals who drew up the original guidelines. Difficulties arise in those areas of the country where, because of a variety of social factors, local people do not share the values of the educated, professional class. Yet it was the unmet needs of these people that were used to justify launching an expensive and elaborate mental health program. Has the middle class in this country exploited the agony of the working class? Did middle-class researchers stimulate interest in mental health by documenting the high rates of mental illness in the deteriorated communities only to obtain federal funds to better the lot of the middle class? Without anyone wanting it to turn out this way, the current community mental health program may benefit only the middle-class client because the model upon which this program is based introduces ethnic and cultural differences as an afterthought. Alternative models for community intervention that would be acceptable to different peoples need to be explored. Various hypothetical models come to mind:

Community Mental Health Center No. 1. The concepts and programs of the center are traditional. Deviance is interpreted in mentalistic and intrapsychic terms. Most individuals seen in the clinic come voluntarily because they are unhappy about their personal adjustment. The exceptions to this general rule are children (who are brought by their parents), acute psychotics, and criminals whose mental state is in question. The center offers diagnostic, therapeutic, and some consulting services (for example, to the schools and the courts). Policy is set by the professional staff, although there is a citizens' advisory board. Upper-middle-class and some working-class ethnic clients with a conservative, individualistic orientation may find this model the most acceptable.

Community Mental Health Center No. 2. The concepts and programs of the center are not based upon the traditional psychiatric conception of mental illness. The orientation is rather environmentalistic. Individuals come to the center voluntarily because they have personal problems. But the clinicians "treat" the clients by helping them alter their environment. Diagnosis is ignored, and therapy tends to be brief and crisis-oriented. Consultation may go on with a variety of other agencies, including agencies that send involuntary patients, but the center is likely to take the point of view of the client rather than the agency. Policy is set by the professionals in the center, although they may feel accountable to a citizens' advisory board. Americans with a strong liberal tradition could support this model, especially if it operated in a working-class neighborhood. Reform-minded people who are not prepared to reject totally the mental health establishment may be most at home with this center.

Community Mental Health Center No. 3. This center is, in fact, a base for social action. All forms of diagnostic and therapeutic activity are kept at a minimum. In fact, workers here may view mental illness as a form of "copping out" or refusal to work with "the people" to effect revolutionary change. The center's programs deal with certain basic social problems, such as drug addiction, crime, poverty, substandard housing, and racism. In dealing with these problems, the center is likely to come into open conflict with established agencies, institutions, and governmental bodies. Policy is set by local social activists who might hire some professionals or purchase the time of some professionals when it becomes necessary. Militant people, black and white, who embrace the radical and populist view would probably find this model most acceptable.

Community Mental Health Center No. 4. Professionals and nonprofessionals associated with this center avoid the term "illness" and instead talk about growth experiences. Some cases may be handled individually, but the emphasis is upon group experiences. Some efforts clearly derive from an educational orientation, for example, the evening classes on child development and on handling the emotional aspects of divorce. Other programs have an existential bent. Integral to this center are weekend marathons, T-Groups, sensitivity training, and black–white, union–management, and teacher–student encounter groups. Because the stigma of mental illness is not associated with the services offered by this center, the clients talk openly about their experiences. Hence, the community can easily keep an eye on the center without resorting to formal advisory or regulatory boards. This model would appeal most to the educated or to those people who place a high value on moral, ethical, self-improvement along intellectual, secular lines. This model might also appeal to agencies, businesses, institutions, and varieties of social groups that have members who do not share the above values but whose administrators embrace the value of self-improvement.

The above models are not really mutually exclusive. It is conceivable that one community could support two or more centers with different missions. Also, it might be argued that at different times in the history of a community one type of center is more appropriate than another. Unfortunately, institutions are often perpetuated by an established bureaucracy long after their services have become meaningless or even harmful. Perhaps communities thinking of establishing a mental health center should not think in terms of a permanent institution but in terms of time-limited programs to cope with specific problems. It follows that an institution that is based upon the value system of a community and the people's way of life should be open for change as time alters the values and way of life.

REFERENCES

Adelson, D., and Kalis, B. (Eds.) *Community psychology and mental health*. Scranton: Chandler, 1970.

Levine, M., and Levine, A. *A social history of helping services: Clinic, court, school and community*. New York: Appleton-Century-Crofts, 1970.

May, E. *The wasted Americans*. New York: Signet Books, 1965.

Rubington, E., and Weinberg, M. *Deviance: The interactionist perspective*. New York: Macmillan, 1968.

Szasz, T. *Ideology and Insanity*. Garden City, New York: Doubleday & Co., 1970.

INDEX

A

Aberle, David F., 286, 294
Accountability, 196, 290, 292–294
Adelson, D., 352, 359
Adoption, 206–207
Agoglia, Vincent T., 161
Aides, career ladders, 122
  class shift, 123–124
  as community, 290–291
  community caretakers, 86
  education, 123, 275
  indigenous nonprofessionals, 42–44
  new, 113, 115
  non-professionals, 99
  pay checks, 273
  personal account, 127–135
  police as, 115, 150, 160
  professionals (non-mental health), 102–107
  revolt, potential, 10
  rivalries, 121–122, 129, 134, 273–274
  role, 117–118
  training method, 118–121, 123, 128–129
  status quo, 205–206
  success of, 121
  working method, 129–134
Alcoholics Anonymous, 42
Alcoholism, 8, 314–315, 317
Alinsky, Saul, 70, 260
Anderson, Franklyn, 70
Anti-poverty program (*see* Model Cities program; Office of Economic Opportunity; Poverty program)
Apartheid, 210–211
Ardrey, R., 246, 259
Arensberg, C. M., 245, 258
ARRIBA, 320–325
Assassination, 4
Association for Mentally Retarded Children (ASMIC), dissension, internal, 327–328, 331–332
  founded, 328–329
  "United Agency," 329–330

"Urban Action," 330–331
Autism, 327–332

B

Back-of-the-Yards movement, 260
Baker, B., 313, 325
Banfield, Edward G., 306, 311, 324, 325
Bard, Morton, 146, 149–150, 152, 160
Bell, Winifred, 211
Berkowitz, Bernard, 146, 152
Bernstein, Bernice, 262–263, 267, 269
Biestek, Felix J., 204
Billingsely, Andrew, 205
Bindman, A. J., 286, 295
Bittner, E., 136, 145–146
Black Panthers, 9, 279, 282–283
"Black Students," alcoholism program, 314–315, 317
  development of, 299–300
  meetings, 300–305
  subcontract, 313
  theory, 307
"Blaming the Victim," 17, 25
Bloom, B., 286, 294
Bloom, B. S., 173, 180
Bodkin, John E., 151–152, 155–156
Bourgeois, Black, 210–211
Brager, George A., 218n, 228n
Branch, J. D., 288, 295
Breggin, P. R., 166, 180
Briar, Scott, 195n, 208, 218n, 224n
Brower, M., 71, 73
Brown, DeForest, 70
Brown, M., 181n, 192
Bryant, Ernest, 159

C

Calvinism, 25
Caplan, G., 6, 15, 37, 86, 97, 349
Captor-captive settings (*see* Prisons)

Please remember that this is a library book,
and that it belongs only temporarily to each
person who uses it. Be considerate. Do
not write in this, or any, library book.